# Community and Public Health Nursing

# Community and Public Health Nursing

Learning to Make a Difference through Teamwork

Second Edition

Elizabeth Diem and Alwyn Moyer

Canadian Scholars' Press

Toronto

**Community and Public Health Nursing: Learning to Make a Difference through Teamwork, Second Edition**
by Elizabeth Diem and Alwyn Moyer

First published in 2015 by
**Canadian Scholars' Press Inc.**
425 Adelaide Street West, Suite 200
Toronto, Ontario
M5V 3C1

www.cspi.org

**Library and Archives Canada Cataloguing in Publication**

Diem, E. C. (Elizabeth Chardene), 1942-
[Community health nursing projects]
Community and public health nursing : learning to make a difference through teamwork / Elizabeth Diem and Alwyn Moyer. -- Second edition.

Revision of: Community health nursing projects : making a difference / Elizabeth Diem, Alwyn Moyer. — Philadelphia : Lippincott Williams & Wilkins, ©2005.

Includes bibliographical references and index.
Issued in print and electronic formats.
ISBN 978-1-55130-738-1 (paperback).—ISBN 978-1-55130-739-8 (pdf).—ISBN 978-1-55130-740-4 (epub)

1. Community health nursing. I. Moyer, Alwyn author II. Title. III. Title: Community health nursing projects.

RT98.D53 2015       610.73'43       C2015-904284-4       C2015-904285-2

Text and cover design by Peggy & Co. Design Inc.

Printed and bound in Canada by Webcom

MIX
Paper from
responsible sources
FSC® C004071

# Table of Contents

# Acknowledgements

We appreciate those who have sought us out and met with us to express their support for the first edition of this text and the need for a revised second edition. This edition builds on the contributions made in the first, including the work plan by Jocelyne Blais and the two student projects.

In this second edition, Eva Stewart-Bindernagel contributed greatly to the development of the "country kitchen" scenario for rural health in Chapter 10 and served as a role model of a public health nurse in the school health scenario. We appreciate the contributions to our thinking over the years and eventually to the second edition by the following: Cheryl Armistead, Francoise Filion, Nancy Gault, Nicole Greaves, Allison Griffith, Heather Jessup-Falcioni, Barbara Kennedy, Kathy King, Mary McNamara Roy, Sherry Poirier, Patti Robillard, Jean Rodney, Margot Rykhoff, Cindy Versteeg, and Nancy Watters.

For this new edition, we consulted with community health nurse educators and received feedback by email and on our website at www.CHNresources.org. As well, we appreciate the feedback we received at the Community Health Nursing Conference in June 2014 in Ottawa from the following: Chis Blencoe, Joanne Crawford, Genevieve Currie, Sylvane Filice, Diane Gausden, Heather Jessup-Falcioni, Kathy King, Barbara Kennedy, Ann Macleod, and Cindy Versteeg. Ongoing ideas and suggestions from the conference spurred us on to provide a text that would bring community health nursing to life in the classroom as well as in a clinical setting.

Preparing this text has been a pleasant reminder of the challenge of using evidence to inform practice and of the role of practice in developing grounded theory that in turn will guide practice. We would like to express our appreciation to our colleagues in public health, especially Ottawa Public Health, and to our community health nursing students for their unfailing enthusiasm in this pursuit.

We especially appreciate the support of our families as we pursued our commitment to community health nursing.

Elizabeth (Liz) Diem, RN, PhD
Alwyn Moyer, RN, PhD

# Introduction

Community and Public Health Nursing: Learning to Make a Difference through Teamwork provides a clear sense of how community health nursing practice strengthens the health of groups and communities. The text illustrates how students and new practitioners learn to work on a team using a basic approach and process grounded in theory, evidence, and experience to develop a beginning level of competency. The approach is applicable in a variety of situations and with a range of population groups. Community health nursing includes nurses working in public health, home health, and in other situations where promoting health is the priority focus of nursing practice.

Community health nursing has evolved in North America from care of the sick in the home, visits to the poor, and teaching school children nutrition and hygiene to a focus on the health and welfare of the general population. With these changes in practice came the need for a broader knowledge base. The management and control of infectious diseases, including tuberculosis and venereal disease, has always been a concern. The development of specialized infant welfare programs also heralded a need for a broader knowledge base to inform health teaching on disease prevention and healthy living practices. With the introduction of the *Ottawa Charter for Health Promotion*, public and community health nurses broadened their perspective yet again to focus on the influences of family, society, and the environment on health.

In the past 30 years, "community health nursing," with its focus on health-promoting activities with families, groups, communities, and society, has become a term encompassing both public and home health nursing. Societal influences in this development of community nursing practice include advances in medicine and science, better understanding of the cause of diseases, improved education, and economic changes. International organizations, such as the World Health Organization, have actively promoted this shift by drawing attention to the importance of promoting the health of the population, identifying gaps in services for vulnerable groups, and endorsing the importance of appropriate education for nurses working in the community.

An important aspect of the changing role of community health nurses is the recognition that health is a universal right and not the prerogative of the traditional health system. This means that nurses work in partnership with individuals and communities and collaborate with community organizations and different sectors of society to build on strengths and to support health and well-being. Working in this way in the community requires knowledge and skills in teamwork. Teamwork practice involves collaborating with groups of new mothers, teens, and older adults as they learn about their own strengths and the strengths of others to lead healthy lives. The practice also means working with schools to address issues such as bullying and obesity, with neighborhoods to develop safe playgrounds for children, with town councils to make communities more "walkable," and with governments to decrease drinking and driving. Teamwork is needed to harness the individual resources and perspectives of team members to deal with complex, long-term community issues.

A unique feature of community health nursing practice is that it is attuned to people who are vulnerable and at-risk for poor health: those who are poor, homeless, or isolated in their homes; and those who have poor social skills or low health literacy. Vulnerable people are a priority because they often lack access to many of the social determinants of health, which are the social, economic, physical, and health factors that contribute to good health. Community health nurses work with other community organizations to promote social justice, which means seeking a fairer share of resources for vulnerable people. Community health nurses deal with injustice by supporting programs such as community food boxes and school meals; by providing well-baby drop-ins and sexual health clinics; and by advocating for improved social, welfare, and housing services and healthy community policies to the appropriate levels of government.

A less known community health nursing role is preparing for involvement in natural and man-made disasters and emergencies, including earthquakes, storms, flu pandemics, and terrorist attacks. During the phases of emergency management, community health nurses play an important role in monitoring the health and safety of the population, especially that of vulnerable groups. In the case of a potential flu pandemic, community health nurses, especially those working in public health, have a lead role in providing mass influenza immunizations.

Since community health nurses have a broad scope of practice within the health care system, they require a correspondingly broad base of knowledge—both theoretical and practical. They need to draw on a mix of analytical, interpersonal, and clinical skills and emotional intelligence. Underpinned by foundational values of community health nursing, community health nurses draw on the principles of primary health care; social determinants of health; social justice; and community, interprofessional, and intersectoral collaboration to guide and develop practice. The ability to collaborate with groups and communities to assess community health needs, to plan, to take action, and to evaluate is an important part of the skill set of community health nurses in the relatively unstructured community environment. The professional practice of community health nurses, public health nurses, and home health nurses is guided by standards and competencies established by their national nursing associations.

Community health nursing practice is complex, and this text uses a project-based approach to guide students and new practitioners in learning about community health nursing in a community setting. The approach integrates theories, concepts, and evidence-based research to guide practice that contributes to the health of the community and to the knowledge and skills of the student. Tools, resources, and examples help to support the process. The text provides a theoretical and conceptual understanding of practice, and uses team scenarios and discussion questions, threaded through each chapter, to promote experiential learning. This approach has been shown to be helpful in exploring the complexity of community health nursing practice in classrooms and seminars and in learning how to practice in a realistic setting. The process, tools, and resources help learners to stay on track. They also diminish the risk of feeling overwhelmed that often occurs upon first being introduced to community health nursing.

The purpose of this text is to assist undergraduate baccalaureate nursing students, graduate students, and new practitioners in learning and applying community health nursing concepts and approaches in the classroom and community. The text is important because it provides a detailed approach, along with resources and tools, that is not offered in other community health nursing texts.

This text is appropriate for providing a community nursing practice context for nursing programs that include service learning or interprofessional education (IPE) as part of their community health nursing course work, or for a final program assignment, such as a capstone population health project. As well, the scenarios in each chapter, the focus group exercise in Chapter 4, and several case studies in Chapter 14 dealing with emergency and disaster management can be adapted to use as simulations. These classroom or laboratory simulations can be used to prepare for, augment, or replace components of practice that are unavailable.

In response to feedback from users of the first edition, this second edition has retained the project approach, the teamwork focus, and the scenario usage, but has made two major changes. First, more emphasis is placed on the use of theories, concepts, and evidence that can be discussed in the classroom and in seminars. And second, some aspects of the projects have been condensed to make them more manageable in a limited amount of time. A requested addition is the chapter on community health nursing in emergency management. This edition also emphasizes ways to bridge the gap between community health nursing theory and practice and is therefore relevant to both the classroom and clinical experience.

*Community and Public Health Nursing: Learning to Make a Difference through Teamwork* provides an important contribution to community health nursing education by making the concepts and practices come alive in the classroom and by providing a structured process to guide learners in practice. Scenarios, case studies, and practice examples assist learners in understanding the broader and complex realities of community nursing teamwork and practice. The community nursing process provides a structure that is flexible while maintaining the basic tenets of working with communities, such as engaging community members and making a difference by developing relevant and sustainable resources and processes.

## Structure of the Book

### Part 1: Foundational Concepts and Processes of Community and Public Health Nursing and Teamwork

A community health nurse educator talked about starting a community nursing course by taking the students up to a lookout that gave an overview of their city. Spreading her arms wide, she declared "All that you see below you involves community health nursing!" Conveying the broad perspective needed in community health nursing can be challenging. The first two chapters in this text use examples, explanations, and discussion questions (with answers) to provide a foundation for understanding that broad view and its related concepts. The scenarios in these two chapters depict realistic student interactions during orientation and help to make the material more accessible.

Chapter 1 introduces the concepts and processes that are foundational to community health nursing theory and practice. Chapter 2 details the project approach based on the community health nursing process and the theory and processes inherent in teamwork. The scenarios illustrate some of the issues and the beginning of reorientation of ideas about health that are encouraged when students are introduced to community health nursing.

## Part 2: The Community Health Nursing Process and Community Health Nursing Projects

Part 2 of the text consists of six chapters that provide a framework for incorporating community health nursing concepts, knowledge, and processes while learning the skills to collaborate with a community group to assess, plan, act, and evaluate to improve health. Chapter scenarios immerse the reader in realistic, team-based community projects designed to exemplify the typical intellectual and practical challenges at that phase of the nursing process. In addition, they provide insight into the various ways that community health nurses engage with community partners, build partnerships, and promote community health through practice in a variety of community settings and with diverse populations. The aim is to engage the learner in the broader world of community and public health nursing practice while completing a short-term community health nursing project.

The six chapters weave together relevant theories, concepts, and principles and build on each other to illuminate the knowledge, skills, and attitudes necessary to support community health nursing practice and teamwork. At the end of this section of the text, the learner will have gained basic knowledge and skills for community health nursing practice and will appreciate the approaches important in engaging the community to improve their health.

## Part 3: Approaches for Working in Different Settings and Situations

Chapters 9 through 14 broaden the perspective and approaches used in earlier chapters. The chapters depict community nursing practice during family home visits; in school and rural communities; in public health; and during an emergency. The scenarios in the chapters illustrate how student teams can be involved in different situations, especially long-term projects or programs.

Chapter 9 describes the role of community health nurses in the home and identifies the risk factors associated with older-age and single-parent families. Chapter 10 describes an approach to community capacity building and provides statistics indicating the vulnerability of young adolescents and rural residents. Chapter 11 examines the practice of community health nurses as they collaborate with communities to form coalitions and develop the commitment and resources of the community to take action on community health issues. In this chapter the focus is on promoting physical activity in youth. Chapter 12 provides an introduction to the community health nurse's role in developing and providing support for healthy public policy, illustrated by a collaboration to develop Baby-Friendly policies. Program evaluation is the focus of Chapter 13 and is illustrated by considering an innovative tuberculosis (TB) prevention program for foreign-born students. Chapter 14 describes the role of community health nurses in the four components of disaster and emergency management. The scenarios follow teams while they recruit partner organizations serving vulnerable populations, and assist in planning the recruitment and training of additional nurses for a flu pandemic.

## Appendix A

Appendix A provides several resources to promote team development and communication. The tools are designed to guide the team's work as it progresses and help create a final report of the team project.

The Appendix also contains the tools to promote initial functioning that are introduced in Chapter 2, including pre-clinical self-assessment (Appendix A.2.1), team agreement (Appendix A.2.2), and the weekly report (Appendix A.2.3). A meeting agenda (Appendix A.2.4) provides a general outline for team meetings and meetings with others. Other items related to Chapter 2 include outlines for personal reflection on an event (Appendix A.2.5), a self-assessment scale for functioning on a team (Appendix A.2.6), and a self-assessment scale for an individual's assessment of team functioning (Appendix A.2.7). Ongoing planning and documentation can be recorded using the timeline (Appendix A.3.2) and/or a work plan (Appendix A.3.1), both of which are introduced and discussed in Chapters 3 and 6. Outlines for project reports (Appendix 3.3) and team evaluation using the team agreement (A.2.2) are discussed in Chapters 5 and 8.

# Part 1

# Foundational Concepts and Processes of Community and Public Health Nursing and Teamwork

Chapters 1 and 2 introduce concepts and processes foundational to community health nursing practice and teamwork, and a project approach based on the community health nursing process. The scenario in Chapter 1 features students exploring concepts such as the principles of primary health care and comparing the nursing process used with individuals and community groups during their orientation class on community health nursing. The first part of Chapter 2 expands on the project approach and use of the community health nursing process by describing two completed student projects. The second part details the theory, research, and process needed to develop effective teamwork. The scenario illustrates how a student team makes initial decisions and learns to use communication and evaluation tools.

# Chapter 1

# Community and Public Health Nursing

Community and public health nursing is an integral part of baccalaureate nursing education. This broad field of nursing brings together nurses who work in community settings where people live, work, learn, worship, and play. It unites them through common values, standards, and a broad perspective that encourages action regarding factors that promote health beyond the individual, group, or community. When every nurse thinks like a community health nurse, nurses will really make a difference in the health of the population.

This chapter introduces community health nursing concepts and principles, and applicable nursing standards and competencies in the US and Canada, to provide an overview of practice. Grounded in a broad understanding of health and the values of equity and social justice, community health nursing draws on a broad knowledge base, systematic processes, and diverse skills to build relationships, work in partnerships, and organize resources to maintain and improve the health of communities. The community health nursing process of "assess, plan, act, and evaluate" provides a framework for learning to work in the community. Similar to other chapters in the text, scenarios are threaded throughout the chapter to illustrate how students and beginning practitioners begin to understand community health nursing concepts and how to apply them in practice.

This chapter lays the groundwork for students and new practitioners to develop a basic understanding of community health nursing by completing a team project with a community group. This chapter—and this book as a whole—seeks to bridge the gap between what is proposed at all levels of health care and in the classroom, and what occurs in community nursing clinical experience.

> ### Key Terms and Concepts
>
> building capacity • collaboration • community health nurses • community health nursing • community health nursing practice • community health nursing process • community and public health nursing standards and competencies • determinants of health • evidence-based practice • health • health equity and inequity • health literacy • levels of prevention: primary, secondary, tertiary • nursing ethics • primary care • primary health care: health promotion, accessibility, public and community participation, appropriate technology, intersectoral collaboration • public health nurses • social justice • sustainability

As part of their orientation to the community health nursing course, students are asked to work in groups to explore some of the ideas they might have about community health nursing. In one group, a student states enthusiastically, "I can hardly wait! This is the type of nursing I want to do." The others look at her in amazement. One asks, "What makes you so excited? I don't even know what we will be doing." The first student replies, "Well, my aunt has been a public health nurse working for the city for 30 years. She has done everything from finding people with TB to helping mothers to breast-feed. At one point, she worked in a neighborhood with new immigrants. She is especially proud of working on the no-smoking bylaw for the city and keeps telling people how we were one of the first cities in the country to have a no-smoking bylaw." "Well," another responds, "I just want to have some idea of what we will be doing in the next couple of weeks."

The initial discussions in many of the groups have similar refrains: "What will we be doing?" and "The terms people use in the community are confusing, such as 'primary health care' and 'primary care'—what is the difference?"

As the formal part of the orientation starts, students still have questions, but are starting to realize that community health nursing may be different from what they had thought.

**Discussion Topics and Questions**
1. What positive and less positive ideas do you have about community and public health nursing?
2. Explain why community and public health nursing is a required part of baccalaureate nursing education.

For suggested responses, please see the Answer Key at the back of the book.

## Learning Objectives

After reading this chapter and answering the questions throughout the chapter, you should be able to:

1. Gain an understanding of how the broad perspective of community health nursing reinforces the need to build on community strengths.
2. Explain the concepts of health, primary health care, the determinants of health, social justice, health equity and inequity, and collaboration.
3. Differentiate among the designations for nurses practicing in the community.
4. Identify the foundational aspects of community health nursing practice, including standards and competencies.
5. Describe components of the community health nursing process.
6. Identify the benefits of using the community health nursing process within community health nursing practice.

## Community Health Nursing

Community health nursing aims to build strong and healthy communities that provide resources for health. **Community health nursing** is the professional work of nurses who promote, protect, and preserve the social, personal, and physical capabilities of individuals and collectives that, according to the *Ottawa Charter*, are resources for everyday living (Canadian Public Health Association [CPHA], 2008; World Health Organization [WHO],

1986). It includes building the environmental and community supports for health.

**Community health nurses** are those designated as public health nurses, home health nurses, and other nurses with a priority focus on promoting and protecting the health of individuals, families, groups, and communities and on creating strong communities. The essence of this definition is that community health nurses play a key role in community health care because of what they do and how they do it, rather than just where they work. In this text, unless otherwise indicated, the term "community health nurse" is an inclusive one for nurses promoting health in the home, community, and public health organizations.

Two concepts are central to understanding community health and community health nursing: health and its determinants and primary health care. These concepts underlie the following defining characteristics of community health nursing.

## Health and the Determinants of Health

Health has proved difficult to define, but the most enduring and commonly accepted definition is that of the World Health Organization, adopted in 1948. In the *Ottawa Charter*, **health** is defined as "a state of complete physical, mental and social well-being, and not merely the absence of disease or infirmity" (WHO, 1986). The Charter adds that the spiritual dimension of health is increasingly recognized and further conceptualizes health as an enabling factor, a resource for living, and a fundamental human right. However defined, there is abundant evidence that health is not evenly distributed in society (Commission on Social Determinants of Health [CSDH], 2008). Even in prosperous countries, there are vulnerable populations who struggle to obtain the necessities of life (CPHA, 2008).

Jason's story, "But Why?" (Box 1.1), which has been told over and over since 1982, illustrates that health is determined by many factors, not just the availability of health care services. This story makes us realize that these services are the end of a chain of factors influencing Jason's health. When we trace the cause of his injury, we find that family, community, and environmental circumstances have contributed to it.

The story may oversimplify the chain of cause and effect, but it illustrates how physical, social, and economic environments affect health. We know that exercise is important for health, but Jason was playing in a dangerous place because of limited alternatives and/or insufficient supervision. As a result, he suffered an injury serious enough to warrant hospitalization. Fortunately, he was able to get treatment for the infection. Access to health services is a valuable resource; however, the treatment did

BOX 1.1
**But Why?**

Why is Jason in the hospital?
Because he has a bad infection in his leg.
But why does he have an infection?
Because he has a cut on his leg and it got infected.
But why does he have a cut on his leg?
Because he was playing in the junkyard next door to his apartment building and there was some sharp, jagged steel there that he fell on.
But why was he playing in a junkyard?
Because his neighborhood is kind of run down. A lot of kids play there, and there is no one to supervise them.
But why does he live in that neighborhood?
Because his parents can't afford a nicer place to live.
But why can't his parents afford a nicer place to live?
Because his dad is unemployed and his mom is sick.
But why is his dad unemployed?
Because he doesn't have much education and he can't find a job.
But why…?

*Sources*: Federal, Provincial, and Territorial Advisory Committee on Population Health, 1999; Public Health Agency of Canada, 2013; and Werner & Bower, 1982.

not change the circumstances of Jason's life. Circumstances such as where he lives, the family income, his father's unemployment, and other factors that contributed to him being injured are likely to have a continuing impact on Jason's health and the health of others in his family. It is only when we explore how further injury might be avoided or prevented that we begin to understand how staying healthy and injury-free is influenced by many things that are not under our personal control.

The Commission on Social Determinants of Health (CSDH) has studied the impact of social factors on global health for many years. The final report from the Commission (CSDH, 2008) attributes the unfair and avoidable differences in health status within and between countries, in large part, to social and environmental determinants. The **determinants of health** are defined as the circumstances in which people are born and grow up and age, and are shaped by the distribution of money, power, and resources at global, national, and local levels (CSDH, 2008). The final report of the Commission called on the global community to take immediate action on the social determinants of health to reduce unfair differences in health due to environmental and other factors outside the control of individuals. A forceful discussion of how the social determinants of health, such as income, social status, education, gender, and the lived environment, as well as health services and lifestyle, have an impact on health can be found on the WHO website (Wilkinson & Marmot, 2003).

The World Health Organization (2014a) continues to recognize that tackling the social determinants of health is fundamental to their work. Their report on the "action areas" of the *Rio Political Declaration on Social Determinants of Health* discusses progress and includes the need to "[f]urther reorient the health sector toward promoting health and reducing health inequities," which includes the themes of early child development, health systems, urbanization, and others.

The work of the World Health Organization permeates community health practice. In response to their call for action to reduce inequities, research has begun to uncover the pathways by which social and economic circumstances result in better or worse health. For example, public health providers have compiled evidence on promising practices to guide action to reduce social inequities in health (Sudbury & District Health Unit, 2011). However, more concerted efforts are required.

One practice that shows promise is the health impact assessment (HIA) of public health programs and policies. HIA aims to identify the positive and negative aspects of a program or proposal to guide decision makers in enhancing the positive and minimizing those that may have negative effects on the health of the different groups in the population (McKenzie, Neiger, & Thackery, 2013). The WHO (2012a) now provides a clearinghouse of the best available evidence on factors in different economic sectors that affect health in positive or negative ways. The sectors include transport, food and agriculture, housing, waste, energy, industry, urbanization, water, radiation, and nutrition and health. For example, the WHO identifies that transportation can cause harm in a variety of ways: through motor vehicle accidents involving bicycles and pedestrians (particularly children and young people); pollution; noise; and large motorways that isolate communities and result in loss of land. On the positive side, transportation provides employment and supports business and support services, as well as providing roads for recreational use such as cycling and walking, which facilitate physical activity.

The implication for health providers is that we must understand that health is determined by broad social and economic influences such as employment, affordable housing,

After hearing about the determinants of health and Jason's story, one group of nursing students launches into a discussion of patients who had needed assistance beyond the care provided in the hospital. Amanda starts by saying "Last term, I looked after a little girl who was just skin and bones. Her mother had two other younger children and could not cope. She lived in a high-rise apartment building and her neighbors didn't offer her any help." Others in the group add examples of people they had heard about or cared for: an elderly man who could only afford dog food to eat; an immigrant family who couldn't find the food they liked or afford the warm clothing they needed.

Kathy says, "We all seem to have been frustrated by things that we can't fix. I am starting to realize how inexperienced I was when I started this nursing program. I thought I would learn to make people better all on my own!"

**Discussion Topics and Questions**

3. Explain how two determinants of health, income and social status, apply to Jason's situation (see Box 1.1).

4. How might the determinants of health limit the ability of people, such as Jason's family, to eat a healthy diet or get regular exercise?

and early childhood education that are beyond the control of individual lifestyle choices and health care providers. Of course, it is necessary to treat the immediate causes of ill health, such as Jason's injury, but that is not enough. We must take action on the social, economic, and physical environments to make a lasting and more wide-reaching impact on the health and well-being of individuals, communities, and populations. This is the foundation for primary health care. Taking action on these personal, social, economic, and environmental determinants is a crucial part of community health nursing practice.

## Primary Health Care

The guiding principles and values of primary health care, which are fundamental to improving the health of individuals and communities, were first described in the *Declaration of Alma-Ata* of the World Health Organization (WHO, 1978). **Primary health care** focuses on promoting health and preventing illness through action on the determinants of health. Primary health care emphasizes coordinated action across society and the full participation of citizens in matters that promote their health and well-being. Primary health care is much broader than primary care. **Primary care** is the treatment provided to clients on their first contact with the health care system and heath care providers, such as nurses and doctors.

Different authors have interpreted a varying number of principles underpinning primary health care. Most often, five principles are identified: health promotion, accessibility, public participation, appropriate technology, and intersectoral collaboration. These principles are entwined. For example, in the broadest sense, the principle "health promotion" incorporates concepts of promoting healthy lifestyles, reducing or preventing disease and injury, improving accessibility to health care, collaborating with communities, using research and practice evidence, and working across sectors (e.g., the health sector working with business and educational sectors), and has been applied to individuals, across the life span, and collectives (World Health Organization, 1986).

According to the Director General of WHO (2008), decades of experience tell us that the primary health care approach provides the most efficient, fair, and cost-effective way to organize a health system. In 2012, the WHO restated the ultimate goal of primary health care as "Better Health for All" and identified the challenges to achieving this goal in an acceptable way. One challenge will be to refocus existing health care systems to provide health care that is acceptable to the whole population. This will require governments to balance the provision of illness services while simultaneously extending the development of social and environmental supports for health. The WHO (2012b) calls on governments to achieve that goal through actions consistent with a primary health care approach.

The next section presents the five primary health care principles in relation to community health and community health nursing. Community health concepts have been included in the descriptions.

### Health Promotion: Supporting Health and Preventing Illness

Health promotion is the process of enabling people to increase control over and improve their health (Nutbeam, 1998). In its broadest sense, **health promotion** means enabling individuals and populations to remain healthy, build capacity, and obtain the resources for healthy living across the life span. **Building capacity** means engaging people in a problem-solving process they can use to address immediate and future problems. At the individual level, this might include helping people to learn how to adopt a healthy lifestyle, gain access to education, or obtain enough money to live in a safe environment. Health promotion is a collaborative process, working with people to build capacity and take action on the determinants of health that are often beyond the control of the individual person or group.

In addition, the health sector takes action to prevent disease, injury, and illness in individuals and populations recognized as having identifiable risk factors and behaviors (Nutbeam, 1998). It is customary to consider three levels of prevention: primary, secondary, and tertiary (Leavell & Clark, 1958).

**Primary prevention** is directed toward preventing the occurrence of illness and injury by reducing known risk factors and providing protection from harmful environments. Some prevention and protection strategies are directed toward the population as a whole; some are directed toward individuals known to be at risk. For example, municipalities protect the health of all citizens by providing safe drinking water, and safe roads and bridges. Similarly, routine immunization schedules are designed to prevent children from contracting a communicable disease, such as measles, and reduce the likelihood of outbreak of the disease in a community.

**Secondary prevention** focuses on the early detection of disease, before signs and symptoms are visible, and the provision of swift treatment to cure or reduce the impact of disease on individuals or communities. Screening is a common approach to detect disease early to initiate prompt treatment; for example, routine mammography for populations known to be at risk is used to detect breast cancer and occult blood tests are used to detect colon cancer. Special efforts are required to ensure the uptake of screening and prompt treatment in vulnerable populations; that is, in populations that are at higher risk of developing diseases or disabilities.

**Tertiary prevention** involves providing effective treatment and care management once a disease is established, with the aim of containing the spread of the disease, preventing further complications, and maintaining health. For example, home care services and the availability of emergency medical services help individuals to manage illness while living at home in the community. Developing and using clinical guidelines helps to ensure effective care and treatment. Another example of tertiary prevention is providing, or supporting, chronic disease self-management groups in the community. These groups especially benefit people with chronic conditions, such as diabetes or arthritis, and their caregivers.

To summarize, health promotion aims to improve well-being and resilience; primary, secondary, and tertiary preventive strategies aim to prevent or contain disease. In the past, health services have focused on illness prevention and treatment and have neglected to address the factors that contribute to health. Both approaches are necessary. Primary health care supports the renewal of health systems to act to prevent disease "upstream." Box 1.2 illustrates what is meant by the concept of "upstream and downstream action."

### Accessibility: Equitable Distribution of the Resources for Health

**Accessibility** is concerned with making health and health care obtainable to everyone, including, and especially, those who most need it. Those who live in poorer socioeconomic circumstances are among the most vulnerable. They face many barriers to obtaining the necessities for health, such as nutritious food, safe housing, and convenient, low-cost transportation. Furthermore, they have the highest levels of illness and face barriers when seeking health care (CSDH, 2008; Marmot, Friel, Bell, Houweling, & Taylor, 2008). The Commission on Social Determinants of Health report documents that social determinants including gender, education, occupation, income, ethnicity, and place of residence are closely linked to access to, and benefit from, health care. For example, in over 50 countries, access to basic maternal child health services is consistently higher in families in the highest income groups compared with those in the lowest income groups (CSDH, 2008, p. 8).

Even with access to care, the inability to understand health information, that is, low health literacy, can interfere with effective communication, which further reduces the likelihood of full participation in making health decisions (National Network of Libraries of Medicine, 2012). **Health literacy** is defined as "[t]he degree to which individuals have the capacity to obtain, process, and understand basic health information and services needed to make appropriate health care decisions" (Centers for Disease Control and Prevention [CDC], 2014). Access to mental health promotion services can be particularly challenging, because two culturally determined barriers to obtaining services are the stigma of mental health and addictions and patterns of help-seeking behaviors (Centre for Addiction and Mental Health, 2012; Office of the Surgeon General, 2001).

The Commission on Social Determinants of Health (2008) indicates in the Executive Summary that

> **BOX 1.2**
>
> **Upstream and Downstream Action**
>
> McKinlay (1979) told the story of a man nearing exhaustion while rescuing drowning people from a swiftly flowing river. In a flash of insight, he looked upstream to determine how the victims could be prevented from falling into the river in the first place. Butterfield (2001) applies the term "downstream" to individual, short-term interventions and "upstream" to emphasize actions that focus on providing the environmental, political, and economic conditions that are the prerequisites to good health. By implication, this means moving some health system resources away from rescuing individuals—providing treatment—and toward preventing illness and promoting the health of population groups, thereby addressing the factors that limit people's ability to be healthy. To use the example of smoking, downstream action would be to concentrate on individual counseling for smoking cessation; upstream action would be to provide disincentives to smoking by reducing advertising by tobacco companies, increasing the price of cigarettes, or passing smoke-free bylaws.
>
> In a memorable phrase, Milio (1976) describes changes at the policy and societal level as "making the healthy choices, the easy choices."

governments distribute the resources for health unequally as "a consequence of poor social policies and programs, unfair economic arrangements, and bad politics" (p. 1). They point out that it is not sufficient to recognize the problem; governments need to take measures to alleviate it by increasing accessibility to the resources for health. This means taking action to reduce disparities. The Commission concludes with three recommendations:

1. Improve daily living conditions
2. Tackle the inequitable distribution of power, money, resources
3. Measure and understand the problem and assess the results of action
   (p. 1662, p. 2)

**Health inequity** means experiencing unfair and avoidable barriers to health and health care opportunities. Health inequity is a difference or disparity in health outcomes that is systematic, avoidable, and unjust (Centers for Disease Control and Prevention, 2014). This is in contrast to inequalities in health, or differences in health status due to biological variations or free choice (WHO, 2014b). **Health equity** exists when all people have the opportunity to live to their full health potential and no one is deprived from achieving this potential because of their social position or other socially determined circumstance (CDC, 2014).

    **Social justice** is the efforts of society to reduce inequitable access to the social and environmental determinants of health. The Canadian Nurses Association (CNA, 2010, p. 10) defines social justice as "the fair distribution of society's benefits, responsibilities and their consequences." They state that social justice is concerned with eliminating the root causes of disparities, as well as the relative position of social groups in society. The association has developed and tested a tool (CNA, 2010) to support action on the social determinants. This tool poses three questions, in a framework of social justice, to guide the assessment of a program, policy, or product:

1. Does it acknowledge that individuals and groups occupy different positions relative to one another in society?
2. Does it acknowledge that unfair differences (inequities) exist in the opportunities and outcomes of different individuals or groups?
3. Does it acknowledge the root causes of inequities?

For example, asking these questions of a program designed to help young adults quit smoking would reveal evidence that the program designers considered young adults in different economic and social situations. Similarly, use of the tool would prompt questions on whether program strategies that worked for university students would work for teenage mothers.

### Appropriate Technology: Use of Knowledge, Skills, Strategies, Technology, and Resources

**Appropriate technology** means using the level of skills and resources appropriate to need and at a cost the community can afford. This principle supports the movement toward providing care closer to home, in the community, rather than in tertiary care hospitals. Just as seeking food or producers "close to home" supports the local economy, seeking support and care first within the local community keeps cost down and helps to build a strong and capable community. In addition, the care provided close to home is more likely to meet the person's needs and does not isolate them from the existing support in their environment. One example is the shifting of responsibility for the care of people with chronic diseases such as diabetes away from tertiary care centers to interprofessional community teams (Canadian Diabetes Association Clinical Practice Guidelines Expert Committee, 2013). Primary health care works on the assumption that promoting health and working at the primary and secondary levels of prevention will reduce the burden of acute and chronic disease as well as health care costs and, eventually, lead to a healthier population.

Another aspect of appropriate use of resources is basing practice on evidence of proven effectiveness. The evidence to inform practice can come from a variety of sources. **Evidence-based practice** integrates four components: (1) research evidence gained from a summary of quality research study findings to address a practical problem (Burns & Grove, 2011); (2) clinical expertise; (3) patient/community preferences (Allender, Rector, & Warner, 2010); and (4) available health care resources (Ciliska & Ganann, 2011). Another example of evidence-informed practice would be to employ a collaborative, interdisciplinary decision-making process that incorporates research evidence and experiential knowledge of the context (KU Work Group for Community Health and Development, 2013a). Evidence-based approaches are discussed in more depth in Chapter 6.

### Public and Community Participation: Involving Individuals and Communities in Decisions That Affect Their Health

Engaging people in learning about their concerns and making decisions about their health is basic to sound clinical judgment (Tanner, 2006) and an important principle of primary health care. **Public and community participation** means that individuals and communities take an active part in decisions that affect their health. According to Arnstein (2006), citizen involvement in decision making can range from manipulation, or being told what is going to happen, to exercising control of decision making in a community. In the context of primary health care, ensuring a high level of public and community participation requires taking steps to make sure that members of the community become partners and collaborators with the power to influence agency policies and program goals (Arnstein, 2006; Bracht & Tsouros, 1990). This requires public and community health workers to appreciate the importance of community participation and have the competencies to foster meaningful involvement (Parker, Margolis, Eng, & Henríquez-Roldán, 2003).

While public participation is desirable, citizens and communities may be reluctant to get involved in making health care decisions. People who are disadvantaged or stigmatized by poverty or disease often have limited energy and education to seek involvement in decisions about their health care. As Labonte (1994) explains, health practitioners must commit to listening to people's experiences, understand the experiences in the words that people use, and negotiate with them to alter what they want changed. Similar efforts are required for interventions that seek to bring about community change. When practitioners and their agencies commit to broad changes in the power structure, Labonte asserts that community development, especially with vulnerable, underserved populations, has "considerable potential for fostering self-reliance and the creation of authentic partnerships with communities" (1997, p. 88). In return, the increased capability of the community to make health decisions, which develops from community commitment and resources, supports the sustainability of community programs.

The National Collaborating Centre for Healthy Public Policy (2011) identifies four benefits arising from citizen participation: (1) supporting the development of a democratic society, (2) empowering communities, (3) integrating citizens' knowledge and values into HIA (health impact assessment), and (4) formulating more sustainable recommendations. Clearly, the benefits of engaging citizens in decisions about health services have the potential to impact on all aspects of community life.

Despite these documented benefits of citizen participation in health care, many barriers remain. Rifkin (2009) found that the three main reasons for limited participation, originally identified in earlier studies, have not changed in recent years. These reasons are as follows:

1. Dominance of the bio-medical paradigm (medical model) as the main planning tool for programs, leading to the view of community participation as an intervention;
2. Lack of in-depth analysis of the perceptions of community members regarding the use of community health workers; and
3. Propensity to use a framework that limits investigation into what, how and why community participation in health programs works. (p. 31)

In spite of the challenges, Rifkin (2009) concludes that community participation has contributed to health improvements at the local level in poor communities. Her message for practitioners is to listen to people more and act with them to improve what they feel is important to increase their participation.

### Intersectoral Action and Collaboration: Working for Health in Partnership with Other Disciplines and Sectors

Collaboration across disciplines and community sectors is a crucial aspect of primary health care. **Intersectoral collaboration** is the joint work by different sectors of society to improve health outcomes more effectively, efficiently, or sustainably than when working independently (Public Health Agency of Canada, 2013; Rudolph, Caplan, Ben-Moshe, & Dillon, 2013).

A compilation of promising practices from Aboriginal communities across Canada, with examples from the US and New Zealand, illustrates how intersectoral collaboration, with or without health service participation, can promote healthy active living and cultural continuity (Federal/Provincial/Territorial Physical Activity and Recreation Committee and the former Pan-Canadian Healthy Living Issue Group, 2011). There are many examples, involving a range of governmental departments—Recreation and Sport, Culture, Education, Health—together with nongovernmental organizations and business partners, of initiatives to engage Aboriginal youth in culturally relevant physical activity. In British Columbia, Aboriginal groups received funds from the ActNow BC program, initiated to support healthy living in the province prior to the 2010 Vancouver Olympic Games (British Columbia Office of the Provincial Health Officer, 2010). The funds were used to provide training in nutrition, physical activity, and making healthy choices during pregnancy (National Collaborating Centre for Aboriginal Health, 2013). After promising beginnings, the province extended the ActNow BC initiative for all population groups for another five years (British Columbia Office of the Provincial Health Officer, 2010).

Collaboration at higher levels of society, that is, at the state or provincial/territorial level, will be required to develop more wide-ranging solutions to problems. Examples of higher level issues that impact health include lowered social assistance payments, unemployment, and limited educational opportunities, which keep people poor and thereby increase their vulnerability to illness (Raphael, 2002).

Nurses and physicians agree that primary health care continues to be relevant to health care and to health care reform (CNA & Canadian Medical Association, 2011). Not only does this approach prevent much of the disease burden and reduce the use of emergency hospital services for minor complaints, but it also produces better outcomes, at lower costs, and with higher user satisfaction. Dr. Jody MacDonald's (2010) presentation and video on primary health care confirm that community health nurses support the values and principles of primary health care and share an ongoing commitment to struggle for its full implementation within Canada and internationally. Her material identifies how primary health care changed discussions about health care from a treatment and illness model to one of health promotion and wellness, how primary health care can be effective with Aboriginal people in both Australia and Canada, and how health policy can be influenced by intersectoral collaboration.

---

**SCENARIO: Applying Primary Health Care Principles in Community Health Practice**

After hearing about primary health care, the groups of students discuss how to use the principles in their practice. In one group, Joan explains that what strikes her is that nurses in the community do not just deal with people who seek their services, but also with people who do not. This aspect explains the difference to her between primary care and primary health care. Carol is interested in accessibility, especially accessibility to health promotion programs. She explains that when working in the emergency department of a hospital, she saw many patients who came there because they didn't seem to have basic information about when they should go to a doctor, what food is good to eat, or how to keep fit. She feels that people who have chronic conditions, such as asthma and diabetes, particularly need easy access to ongoing support and community resources on a regular basis.

Kevin feels the discussion is going too smoothly, so he challenges the group by saying that collaborating with the whole community would take too long. The others rise to the bait with reasons why collaboration is important and therefore necessary. He elaborates, explaining that he thinks collaboration is important, but having learned about the importance of using evidence-based practices, he feels that evidence should take precedence. Erica responds that evidence-based

practices are not applied as a "one-size-fits-all"; practice guidelines would have to be adapted to the needs of the community and accepted by them. Kevin does not look convinced. At that point, Frieda looks Kevin in the eye and asks him if he knows the evidence against smoking. Kevin knows what is coming and sheepishly says, "Yes." Frieda responds, "Well, why do you still smoke?"

**Discussion Topics and Questions**

5. Assume that you are part of a team in a placement at a university or college health center and learn that physical activity drops considerably when young adults begin university and college (Kwan, Cairney, Faulkner, & Pullenayegum, 2012). Use the following two items to discuss how to increase physical activity among university/college students:
   a. Identify primary health care measures that could be taken at the institutional, community, and state/provincial level.
   b. Identify how a university/college might involve students in designing an "active living" campus.
6. Identify a neighborhood that is crowded and has safety concerns. Consider what intersectoral organizations could be involved in addressing the safety issues.

# Community Health Nursing Foundational Values, Process, and Beliefs

Community health nursing is grounded in foundational values and beliefs. Although some jurisdictions might include other aspects, most include the values and beliefs, summarized in Box 1.3, which cross the boundaries of practice in community health, public health, home health, and other community health promotion practices.

---

BOX 1.3

**Community Health Nursing Foundational Values, Process, and Beliefs**

1. **Foundational Values:**
   - A broad understanding of health
   - Commitment to principles of equity and social justice

2. **Focus and Process:**
   - Community health nurses promote, protect, and preserve the health of individuals, families, groups, communities, and populations, wherever people live, work, learn, worship, and play, using the community health nursing process.

3. **Beliefs Guiding Practice:**
   - Build sustainable relationships and partnerships through collaboration and effective communication with individuals, families,

   groups, communities, organizations, and government
   - Combine a variety of knowledge sources: specialized nursing, social and public health science, with experiential knowledge
   - Organize resources to support health by advocating, planning, coordinating, delivering, and evaluating services, programs, and policies
   - Function at a high level of autonomy, guided by standards and competencies, as individual practitioners and as part of a team

   *Sources:* Association of Community Health Nursing Educators, 2009; American Nurses Association, 2013, 2014; Canadian Association of Schools of Nursing, 2014; Community Health Nurses of Canada, 2009, 2010, 2011; Quad Council of Public Health Nursing Organizations, 2011; Reiter, 2004.

---

## Foundational Values

Community health nurses value health as a positive concept and have a strong commitment to equity and social justice, rooted in an understanding of the broad determinants of health. These beliefs underpin practice.

Community health nurses do not view health as an absence of disease. Rather, they embrace the (WHO, 1946, 2012b) definition of health that recognizes the strengths of individuals, families, groups, and communities and use these as a starting point when building relationships to increase health capacity.

Many of the unique characteristics of **community health nursing practice** are founded in the five principles of primary health care that have been discussed above: focusing on health promotion, accessibility and equity, appropriate use of knowledge and resources, community participation, and collaboration. For example, as depicted in Box 1.4, community health nurses work in schools and collaborate with people from different sectors in the community to improve the health, well-being, and academic capabilities of students.

Community health nurses value equity and social justice. Not only are these principles the mark of a democratic society, but they make economic sense also. Using the principles to guide practice means nurses work to improve access to health resources for vulnerable populations. Community health nurses make special efforts to reach out to those on the margins of society, based on the understanding that those burdened by multiple disadvantages, such as low income, lower education, and little support from others, may require selective approaches. For example, using the media, such as TV or social networks, to distribute information on good nutrition has the potential to reach a broad audience but may not reach people living on an income so low that it limits choice. An approach termed "targeting with universalism" addresses the need to take extra steps to achieve equal access for disadvantaged groups (Sudbury & District Health Unit, 2011). As an example, some programs hold community kitchens to increase access to nutritious, low-cost food, and build community in inner-city neighborhoods (Labonte, 1997). In addition to providing direct support to underserved people, community health nurses might also advocate within the community and regional levels of government to provide additional food subsidies.

In keeping with recommendations for health system renewal (WHO, 2008), community health nurses support health system changes to increase the emphasis on health promotion and coordinated environmental action, as indicated in the Safe Routes to School example (Box 1.4), to improve the health or capacity of the community. Building a strong, nurturing community is likely to be more effective than addressing individual determinants separately and be less costly in the long term.

---

BOX 1.4
**Community Health Nursing in Safe Routes to School (SRTS) Programs**

**Background**

Safe Routes to School programs bring together schools and communities to improve the health and well-being of children by enabling and encouraging them to walk and bicycle to school.

In the Vernon, Connecticut, case study (National Center for SRTS, 2010), a school with 330 students of diverse racial and economic backgrounds, from kindergarten to grade 5, had the lowest academic testing and fitness scores in the district in 2003. Three years later, staff and parents initiated the first SRTS program in the school with the goal of improving the health of the students and emptying at least one of three school buses. The school nurse coordinated the program.

**Methods**

School planners organized several activities:

- Participation in International Walk to School Day, 2006 and 2007, from designated intersections in the school district. This included gaining the support of community partners; advertising using posters, newsletters, and reminder wristbands; and inviting involvement from local and state politicians and educators.
- Bimonthly Walking Wednesday events
- Inclusion of physical activity and safe walking in curriculum and activities

**Results**

In 2007, the school was successful. They had two empty school buses and 94 percent of students walked to school. In addition to a 40 percent improvement in grade 4 fitness tests, the school moved to being one of the best academic performers in the district. The results were attributed to the SRTS program acting as a catalyst to bring together the different sectors—education, police, transportation, and municipal government—to improve fitness and academic scores at the school.

## Focus and Process

Community health nurses promote, protect, and preserve the health of the populations they serve. They do this by working with people to increase their capacity to keep well, to build resources for health, and to reduce the risk of illness. By people, we mean individuals and families, groups, communities, and populations, especially the most vulnerable in society. Not only do community health nurses work across the continuum of care, they bring a unique system perspective. Whether working with individuals or collectives, they keep in mind the many organizations, levels of the health system, and policy frameworks that have an impact on health.

Another defining aspect of community health nursing practice is that it aims to design programs, services, and policies to meet the needs of the population as a whole, and not just people who seek them out. This means that community health nurses reach out to people where they live, work, and play and encourage them to take action to improve their own health and that of the environment. That is why you are likely to find community health nurses in schools, workplaces, drop-in centers, immigration services, and older adults' apartment buildings, wherever people congregate, rather than just in an office or clinic.

Even when community health nurses are working with individuals and families, they have three other perspectives in mind:

1. What community resources could be relevant to this individual and family?
2. How are these individual and family concerns relevant to groups and populations of which they are a part?
3. How is the health of the individual and family affected by the community and health care system?

At different levels of the health system, community health nurses seek to preserve the health of the population by developing policies that support a healthy environment. The policies might include no-smoking bylaws or guidelines for the creation of recreation areas. When working at the community or population level, community health nurses consider how community policies could affect individuals, families, and groups.

Although work at the policy level does not involve direct care, community health nurses bring practice experience to bear on policy negotiations that aim to support the health of all in the community. In effect, the community health nurse approaches practice using a zoom lens, continually moving in and out between a focus on individuals and the systems in which they live.

Community health nurses use a systematic process when carrying out their work (American Nurses Association, 2013, 2014; Community Health Nurses of Canada, 2011). The **community health nursing process** consists of four phases—assessment, planning, implementation, and evaluation—that extend over weeks or months and require a collaborative effort with team members, community partners, and community groups. We discuss the community health nursing process in detail later in this chapter and throughout the text.

## Beliefs Guiding Practice

There are four key defining aspects of community health nurses' practice: they build sustainable relationships and partnerships, draw on a variety of resources, marshal resources, and function at a high level of autonomy.

### Build Sustainable Relationships and Partnerships

Community health nurses build sustainable relationships and partnerships through collaboration. **Collaboration** with the community involves starting where the people are (Nyswander, 1956), engaging people and organizations to arrive at mutually determined goals, and carrying out activities. Being outside the primary care system with its focus on episodes of illness changes the dynamic of nurse-client relationships. When clients are not in immediate need of medical care, nurses must be especially careful to build trust and establish collaborative relationships, working with, rather than directing, and mutually identifying goals.

As well as creating an environment conducive to health promotion, these collaborative relationships, in turn, inform practice. For example, nursing teams in a neighborhood may engage with families many times in many capacities over the family life cycle: preparing new parents at a prenatal class; providing nutrition resources to a school-age child's teacher; helping to set up a workplace health program; and lobbying for community services to support older adults in the home. These ongoing encounters maintain community connections while providing exposure to community strengths and needs, thereby grounding practice.

In keeping with the primary health care principle of intersectoral collaboration, community health nurses expend time and effort to maintain relationships with other community health agencies and with other sectors of society. In addition to being a source of community information, these formal and informal networks may progress to collaboration. Much of the impact of community health nursing work is due to the collaborative process and successful partnerships with community groups and volunteer associations and organizations, dedicated to improving the neighborhood environment one step at a time.

This relationship building requires careful documentation to justify the work and show that it provides a foundation for improving the health of individuals, families, and collectives, and the conditions for health. Being able to demonstrate the impact of community health nursing to community members and policy makers makes it more likely they will appreciate the efforts and continue to give support. Since the changes from community work occur slowly over time, community health nurses must constantly consider the sustainability of their work and prepare other community resources to take over. **Sustainability** means that a community has the capacity and interest to carry on with health initiatives.

Underlying relationships and collaboration are the requirements for community health nurses to communicate effectively (Canadian Association of Schools of Nursing, 2014; Quad Council of Public Health Nursing Organizations, 2011). They need to communicate with individuals and families, similar to all nurses, as well as with groups and communities. The form of communication ranges from a conversation with a homeless person to a presentation for a large audience in person, on TV, or on the Internet. Communication is discussed in more detail in Chapter 7.

## Draw on a Variety of Knowledge Sources

This aspect of practice fits with the primary health care principle of appropriate technology related to the use of knowledge, skills, strategies, technology, and resources. The complex nature of communities and community health requires community health nursing to draw on a variety of knowledge sources that include nursing, community health nursing, social science, and public health science, particularly epidemiology, together with experiential knowledge to inform practice.

Knowledge sources for community health nursing includes information from the following sources: (a) sociodemographic and epidemiological data; (b) credible research evidence to address a practical problem at a group, community, or societal level; (c) expertise from experienced community health nurses and other community health specialists, such as community nutritionists and epidemiologists; (d) preferences identified by group and community members; and (e) consultations with partner community health organizations and intersectoral collaborators.

Additionally, Internet searches can provide invaluable information about programs, studies, and resources that could be relevant in your situation. Since most Web content is posted without any form of review for accuracy or reliability, it is up to you to review online information for credibility. Usually five criteria for credibility are used: authority, coverage, objectivity, accuracy, and currency (American Speech-Language Association, 2014; Virginia Technical University, 2014). The Virginia Tech web page provides a useful table that lists the five criteria, gives the rationale, and answers the question "How can I tell?"

As a short cut, search for the websites of government departments, educational institutions, professional associations, and charitable organizations, which are regularly updated. These sites usually also provide links to other credible sites. Strategies for using the Internet and finding credible websites are provided at the end of "Website Resources" in this chapter.

## Marshal Resources

To marshal resources, or in other words, take action, community health nurses consider the social determinants of health and collaborate with other sectors to bring together resources to reduce inequities in health care. They are prepared to take action because they are knowledgeable about communities and planning.

An important aspect of the role is conducting community assessments to identify gaps and advocating for programs and services to meet the needs of underserved populations. Balancing a "hands-on" delivery of services with actions to benefit the population as a whole, community health nurses advocate for, plan, coordinate, deliver, and evaluate services, programs, and policies to address gaps in health care. This advocacy for social justice, together with a coordinating role, means working across community locations and levels of the health care system and government.

To marshal resources, community health nurses use the community health nursing process, discussed below and applied in Part 2 of this text, to bring together applicable sources of information to assist the community in making decisions about resources that are relevant to it. When a priority has been identified, community health nurses collaborate with the community and organizations to determine an effective strategy, take action, and evaluate the results. This process emphasizes community participation and can contribute to other community initiatives.

## Function at a High Level of Autonomy

The nature of community health nursing requires community health nurses to work in practice teams, nursing and interdisciplinary, to deliver community programs. Chapter 2 provides a detailed discussion of teamwork. Participating on teams allows community health nurses to contribute expertise and a population health perspective to finding solutions for complex community issues and problems, such as reducing the risk factors for obesity in a population, or planning for pandemics (Ontario Ministry of Health and Long-Term Care, 2008). At the same time, community health nurses often work alone and must have the confidence and autonomy to contribute a professional opinion and an organizational perspective with the health of the population in mind. Coordinating programs such as Safe Routes to School (Box 1.4), conducting postpartum home visits, or meeting with a community group, the community nurse becomes the face of their organization and profession in the community.

The teamwork, so central to community health nursing practice, requires organizational practices and team structures to support autonomous practice (Weston, 2010). As well, Weston advises nurses to demonstrate autonomy and expand their control over practice by clearly identifying their unique knowledge, skill, and expertise in health care in understandable terms to show its value. They are equipped to do this with support from professional and disciplinary standards and/or competencies.

At this point, it is worth noting that nursing designations vary greatly both between and within jurisdictions. Pertinent to this discussion, all **public health nurses** are community health nurses but not all community health nurses are public health nurses in North America. The title "Public Health Nurse" is a legislated designation stemming from employment in a public health nursing position in a government-funded public health organization. Public health nurses tend to work more at the community and population level, and seek out underserved people and groups. Their work is driven by epidemiological evidence, conducted in collaboration with other organizations, and focuses on health promotion, illness prevention, and healthy environments (Allender, Rector, & Warner, 2010; Community Health Nurses of Canada, 2011; Minnesota Department of Health, 2007). In comparison, community health nurses not designated as public health nurses tend to practice in places such as community clinics and programs, homes, schools, businesses, and so on. They may use the generic designation "community health nurse" or one that reflects the type of organization employing them, for example, home health (home care or visiting) nurse, occupational health nurse, school nurse, parish nurse, or correctional services nurse.

**Community and public health nursing standards and competencies** are developed by national nursing associations to guide practice and education. Specific standards and competencies help to identify similarities and differences between public health and community health nursing. In the United States, *Public Health Nursing: Scope and Standards of Practice* emphasizes the process of assessment, population diagnosis and priority setting, outcomes identification, planning, implementation, and evaluation (American Nurses Association, 2013); *Home Health Nursing: Scope and Standards of Home Health Nursing Practice* uses a similar framework (American Nurses Association, 2014).

*Canadian Community Health Nursing: Professional Practice Model & Standards of Practice* (Community Health Nurses of Canada, 2011) identifies seven standards: health promotion; prevention and health protection; health maintenance, restoration, and palliation; professional relationships; capacity building; access and equity, and professional responsibility and accountability, organized by the community health nursing process. These standards flow from a professional practice model that describes the structure, process, and values that support nurses' control over the delivery of nursing care and the environment where care is delivered. The Canadian community health nursing professional practice model identifies the client as individuals, families, groups, communities, populations, and systems supported by factors related to community health nurses and nursing practice; community organizations; and the system (Community Health Nurses of Canada, 2013). In addition, Canadian nurses are guided by *Public Health Nursing Discipline Specific Competencies Version 1.0* (Community Health Nurses of Canada, 2009) and *Home Health Nursing Competencies Version 1.0* (Community Health Nurses of Canada, 2010). The Community Health Nurses of Canada website provided in the reference list provides access to the standards and competencies online.

National nursing associations in each jurisdiction (American Nurses Association, 2010; Canadian Nurses Association, 2008) define the ethical expectations for nursing practice. **Nursing ethics** is defined as the scrutiny of all varieties of ethical and bioethical issues from the perspective of nursing theory and practice based on the core concepts of nursing: person, culture, care, health, healing, environment, and nursing (Johnstone, 2008).

## The Community Health Nursing Process

The community health nursing process as used in this text is the nursing process for individuals adapted for use with groups in the community. Community and public health nursing standards and competencies, the principles of primary health care, and community health planning models inform the process.

The common core that unites nursing practice is the use of a systematic process: assessment, diagnosis, outcome/planning, implementation, and evaluation (American Nurses Association, 2012). The process works well to identify nursing concerns with individual clients in institutional settings, but requires modification when applied to groups and communities. For example, community assessment data is not readily available from a single source but must be gathered from many different sources, such as sociodemographic databases, epidemiological studies, interviews with key informants from the community, and observations of community members. The differences continue throughout the remaining phases of the process because of the complexity of the system, the greater number of people who are involved, and the longer time frame required for community health initiatives. Table 1.2 illustrates some of the similarity of the components of the process for institutionalized individuals and communities, as well as differences in the details. To simplify the comparison, nursing care for the individual is a person with an acute episode of an illness, and for the community, health promotion for a group.

There is criticism that the nursing process, with its apparently linear type of thinking, does not fully capture the reasoning processes used by experienced nurses to inform action (Tanner, 2006). Tanner, however, acknowledges that beginning learners benefit from a systematic problem-solving process. As well, she recognizes that the development of sound clinical judgment depends to some degree on knowing and engaging with the "patient" (in our situation, family, group, or community) to understand strengths, needs, and concerns, and by considering the context and culture of the situation. The community health nursing process emphasizes these aspects.

Three students decide to share their previous nursing experiences to see how they compare to the unique aspects of community health nursing. Nicole starts by saying that, in the hospital, she was expected to promote and protect the health of the individual patients assigned to her in the short time it took them to recover from surgery. Now she realizes that work outside the hospital requires a lot of flexibility to work in the home and with groups, and adapt to the unstructured environment.

Kira notes that it will be different working with a group of people to improve their health rather than just one person at a time. She recalls the time she and her friends decided to improve their eating and exercise. She comments "It was an interesting experience because no one was in charge; we all provided information and feedback." With that "self-help" group in mind, she remarks that community health nurses will have to motivate people to work on "getting better, together." She shares ways that worked for her group, saying it was not easy to change, even with group support; only a few really changed after a month. She feels that community health nursing practice will be rewarding but requires considerable planning and patience.

Jillian likes the high level of autonomy of community nurses. She describes a nurse she heard about who works with people living on the street who do not want any help. This nurse had enough flexibility in her practice to keep returning to where the street people gather around a heating pipe. By talking to them about ways to keep their feet clean and warm, she gained their trust and they began to consider her advice. The nurse is now part of a committee dealing with homelessness in the city. By clearly explaining the lives of the homeless, she is able to convince the committee to include representatives from the homeless group.

**Discussion Topics and Questions**

7. What would be especially new or challenging about working with a group in the community, such as grade 5 and 6 students, on developing a healthy body image?

8. Identify the activities in Table 1.1 that are or are not part of community health nursing practice, and answer the following questions about your responses.
   a. Identify the activities in Table 1.1 you marked as not being within the scope of community health nursing practice. Explain your rationale.
   b. Discuss how community health nurses might start to work on items 3, 6, and 10.
   c. What other activities of community health nurses do you know about?

**Table 1.1: Which Activities Are within the Scope of Community Health Nursing Practice?**

| | | |
|---|---|---|
| 1. Using TV advertisements to encourage people to be more physically active | Yes | No |
| 2. Working with a neighborhood group to develop a playground | Yes | No |
| 3. Identifying gaps in community health services after hospital discharge | Yes | No |
| 4. Raising awareness of how poverty affects health | Yes | No |
| 5. Immunizing children against infectious diseases such as measles | Yes | No |
| 6. Providing advice to a older adults' group on how to have the city repair sidewalks | Yes | No |
| 7. Ensuring that there are healthy menu choices at workplace cafeterias | Yes | No |
| 8. Preparing material for pamphlets and a website for parents of toddlers | Yes | No |
| 9. Helping children to work in groups to reduce schoolyard violence | Yes | No |
| 10. Presenting a brief to city councillors on improving the city's walkability score | Yes | No |

**Table 1.2: Comparison of Nursing Process Used with Individuals in Institutional Settings and the Community Health Nursing Process**

| Component | Individual Nursing Process | Community Health Nursing Process |
|---|---|---|
| Presenting problem | Acute illness in acute care settings | Health promotion with a community group |
| Assessment | Data elements related mainly to person's response to illness | Data elements related to group, community, and system, such as census tract data |
| | Data collection methods include reviewing health records, individual and family interviews, physical assessments, and clinical investigations | Data collection methods include interviews, surveys, and focus groups to gather information from a variety of health, social, environment, and economic perspectives |
| | Purpose: Mainly to address immediate diagnostic and treatment needs (Ervin, 2002) | Purpose: To identify community strengths and issues and develop relationships with the community group |
| Planning | With individual and/or family member | Those affected by the health issue |
| Implementation | Specific to illness or disease, and includes provision of social support and linkage to community resources | Range of strategies to address issue and build capacity at all levels of the system to improve health and increase access to determinants of health |
| Evaluation | Interview, observation, or measurement of change in individual | Interviews, surveys, or focus groups with groups, communities, or population to identify impact and determine if the actions were meaningful to them |

The values, beliefs, and principles that are apparent in the community/public health nursing standards (American Nurses Association, 2013, 2014; Community Health Nurses of Canada, 2011), and in the World Health Organization documents on primary health care (WHO, 1978, 2008) are the second source of influence for the community health nursing process. These key resources emphasize the importance of a collaborative approach, community participation, and the provision of health promotion programs that are sustainable in the long term.

The third source of influence for the community health process is the planning models used in multidisciplinary community health practice. The "Generalized Model" (McKenzie, Neiger, & Thackery, 2013, p. 17), which includes assessing needs, setting goals and objectives, developing an intervention, implementing the intervention, and evaluating, contains the generic components. Similar models with slightly different wording or number of phases can be found on the websites of Public Health Ontario (2014) and the *Community Tool Box* (KU Work Group for Community Health and Development, 2013b). These community planning models are usually applied to populations and communities rather than the relatively small groups found in the community projects discussed in this text. The steps of the community-level planning models have been reduced or condensed to accommodate smaller groups and the shorter time period relevant in community nursing projects. Although the process for community projects is condensed, it is systematic, involves community members, and can contribute to community health.

Box 1.5 defines the steps, detailed in Part 2 of this text, that are used in completing a community nursing project.

## Application of Community Health Nursing Process

The many layers and facets of community health nursing can be overwhelming to nursing students and new practitioners. Nurses familiar with using the nursing process with individuals and families in institutions need to reorient their thinking when using the nursing process in the community (Ervin, 2002). Not only are there more people to think about, but the social and physical environment of communities is more complex. Community practitioners need time to learn about the community and to develop collaborative relationships with community groups to initiate change that is meaningful to the community.

The community health nursing process provides a framework for learning how to work collaboratively with colleagues and the community on a variety of health issues. Once mastered, it provides a useful tool for continuing practice. As depicted in Box 1.5, the community health nursing process is a collaborative effort with four components: assess, plan, act, and evaluate. While each component has distinct characteristics—for example, assessment involves collecting data from a number of sources, and planning involves making a collective decision and laying out a goal and objectives—there is some overlap in timing between components and there are cycles within components.

First encounters with community health programs, such as a prenatal class, a sexual health clinic, or a falls prevention program for older adults, do not immediately indicate which component of the process might be involved. For example, an experienced community health nurse beginning the first of a series of prenatal classes would understand this to be the action stage of an ongoing and cyclical process. Preparing to lead the class, the nurse would be familiar with assessment data, such as data on births in the community, the age range of the mothers, and areas of the community with the highest birth rates, and would know whether births occurred in hospital or at home. In addition to being familiar with the history of the prenatal program and its goals and objectives, she or he would have assessment data on the mothers attending the class, for example, names, ages, parity, and whether or not they would attend with a partner. This information would be used to tailor the program to the needs of the participants. For instance, some programs might include several single women attending on their own, or with a female companion rather than a male partner; others might be couples in traditional relationships. It would be usual to encourage participants to provide continuing feedback to shape the classes and to get to know other class members. At the end of the classes, there would be a formal evaluation. An ongoing process of assessment, planning, action, and evaluation underpins the apparently routine conduct of an existing program.

BOX 1.5

**Steps in Completing a Community Nursing Project**

ASSESS
1. Orient to community project
2. Assess secondary data
3. Assess physical and social environment
4. Assess primary data
5. Analyze assessment data

PLAN
6. Plan action

ACT
7. Take action

EVALUATE
8. Evaluate results and complete project
9. Evaluate teamwork

·

One group of students feels it will be easy to switch from using the nursing process with individuals to using it with a community group. The students talk about how they will be able to obtain preliminary information on their group. They quickly realize that the information is not in one place, such as in a patient chart or record. Then they consider where they might look if they were placed with a community health care clinic or an occupational health center. When they ask their instructor about getting access to the medical records of the group they will work with, she says this might or might not be possible. The group comes to realize that it will be necessary to search in a variety of different places to piece together an epidemiological and sociodemographic picture of the group, and that the picture might still be incomplete.

The students identify another big difference: the possibility that their efforts will see little change initially. Whether their project uses health promotion strategies to help people make healthy food choices, or community development strategies to bring community organizations together to improve transportation for older adults, they are not likely to see change actually occur during the time they are in the community. The team members admit that, in institutions, their satisfaction comes from providing nursing care that helps to make hospital patients more comfortable. In the community, they realize that they will need to get their satisfaction in other ways, perhaps through working with a team and learning to interact with a group of people.

**Discussion Topics and Questions**

9. How could the community health nursing process help (a) to determine which of two community health clinics provides the best diabetes education program or (b) to guide your volunteer experience at an immunization clinic?
10. Compare implementation/action at the individual level with that at the community level.

## Changes in Health Care and Community Health Nursing Education

Community health nurses have always had a strong focus on maintaining health and promoting independence but our views on how to do this are changing. Global health organizations and governments across the world are now coming to realize that health reforms based on social and economic factors have a much greater impact on individual and community health than medical care and personal health behaviors. Looking back over the 30 years since the call for "Health for All" (WHO, 1978), the World Health Organization (2008) reported that, while people are now healthier and living longer, new challenges are undermining the health of populations. In the section "Responding to the Challenges of a Changing World," the report identified three worrisome trends:

1. Inequalities in the health of people in different countries and within different parts of the same country.
2. Unexpected increases in health problems because of aging, globalization, worldwide transmission of communicable diseases, and the burden of chronic and non-communicable disorders.
3. Health systems failing to get the best health outcomes for their money and developing in directions that contribute little to equity and social justice as articulated in the *Declaration of Alma-Ata* related to:
   a. Unwarranted emphasis on specialized medical treatment;
   b. Focus on short-term results for disease control resulting in fragmented care;
   c. Limited control in health systems that allow unregulated commercialization of health.

National governments are addressing these concerns through broad health reforms. A prime example is the US government Healthy People initiative. The most recent report, *Healthy People 2020* (US Department of Health and Social Services, 2010), the fifth since 1979, is part of a long-term plan to promote the health of individuals and communities. This report identifies four overarching goals that address many of the concerns in the WHO (2008) report: higher quality and longer lives, health equity, social and physical environments that promote health for all, and healthy development and healthy behaviors across all life stages. Similar goals are directing health care reform in Canadian provinces (Nova Scotia Public Health, 2012) and some interprovincial health initiatives (Secretariat for the Intersectoral Healthy Living Network, 2005).

The shift in thinking about what type of health care is needed to improve the health of the population has clear implications for community health nursing practice. In addition to learning complex concepts such as that of primary health care, the increased focus on the social determinants of health is giving rise to the need for new skill sets. There is no easy way to learn how to reduce inequities or to become proficient at collaborating with community groups. Community health leaders have responded to these changes by asking questions about the type of education health professionals will need to work in the community.

An independent commission of 20 international experts sponsored by *The Lancet* (Frenk, Chen, & Bhutta, 2010) stated that glaring gaps and inequities in health that persist both within and between countries could be addressed with changes in the health system. They recommend that "all health professionals in all countries should be educated to mobilise knowledge and to engage in critical reasoning and ethical conduct so they are competent to participate in patient and population centred health systems as members of locally responsive and globally connected teams" (pp. 3–4). Similarly, the World Health Organization (WHO, 2011) stated that the quality and relevance of health professionals could only be improved if their education prepared them to place population health needs at the center of their practice. In the US, the core competencies for public health professionals continue to emphasize the need for a broad range of skills and knowledge (Public Health Foundation, 2014). Among the required changes are the acquisition of skills in using scientific rigor and matching epidemiology to the communities where they work, and learning how to work on teams.

Specific to nursing, the American Association of Colleges of Nursing (2008) and the Canadian Association of Schools of Nursing (2011) emphasize the need for baccalaureate nursing education to prepare graduates with the knowledge and skills to provide patient- and community-centered care and health promotion in complex environments. To this end, they recommend graduates learn the collaborative and critical thinking skills needed to work in multidisciplinary teams and to be involved in all levels of health policy for population health.

More specific to undergraduate nursing education, the *Essentials of Baccalaureate Nursing Education for Entry Level Community/Public Health Nursing*, produced by the Association of Community Health Nursing Educators [ACHNE] (2009), identifies five core values: community and population as client, prevention, partnership, healthy environment, and diversity. Similarly, the Canadian Association of Schools of Nursing published *Entry-to-Practice Public Health Nursing Competencies for Undergraduate Nursing Education* in May 2014. The five domains of the competencies framework are public health sciences in nursing practice; population and community health assessment and analysis; population health planning, implementation, and evaluation; partnerships, collaboration, and advocacy; and communication in public health nursing (Canadian Association of Schools of Nursing, 2014, p. 3). These values and competencies echo the themes and skills identified by students working on community nursing team projects as being satisfying and important (Diem & Moyer, 2010). The nursing organizations make it clear that the recommended theory and clinical experience is required for both direct nursing care and collaborative efforts to improve the health of the population.

For nursing students and practitioners new to community health, the move to community health nursing involves two major shifts in thinking: a change from illness care within an institution to health promotion with a community, and a change from focusing on the health of individuals and families to that of groups and communities. The new directions, described above, further challenge the need to think differently.

We designed this text to prepare practitioners for evidence-based practice in the changing world of community health by incorporating, throughout the text, theoretical constructs with the values and competencies found in *The Essentials* (ACHNE, 2009) and *Competencies* (Canadian Association of Schools of Nursing, 2014). Scenarios, case studies, discussion questions, examples, and step-by-step processes will increase your understanding of what community health nurses do in their day-to-day practice and how their practice can eventually promote a healthy environment where people thrive. Discussions in the classroom and in the clinical area, and relating what you are learning to what you see and hear in the media and within your circle of family and friends, will greatly assist your move to a broader way of thinking about health.

## Summary

This chapter identifies the foundational concepts and defining aspects of community health nursing. The foundational concepts of a broad understanding of health, equity, and social justice, arising from primary health care principles and the social determinants of health, underpin a systematic process of action and prepare community health nurses to promote, protect, and preserve health where people live, work, play, study, and worship. Although community health nursing is not always visible to the public and takes time to bring about change, the long-term vision and accumulation of health initiatives and projects completed in partnership with other professionals, sectors, and communities makes an essential contribution to improving the health of communities.

## Classroom and Seminar Exercises

1. In the following situations, indicate which primary health care principle(s) is/are not being met:
   a. A well-baby clinic in a well-established neighborhood is open from 1 to 4 p.m., is not near a bus stop, and charges $5 a visit.
   b. The only program related to smoking in a high school is individual counseling for tobacco cessation.

c. A community agency serving older adults provides nutritional information and posts recommended dietary requirements on the agency website.

2. Compare use of the individual nursing process to develop an exercise routine for one woman with use of the community health nursing process to determine an exercise routine for a group of women.

3. Assume that you have been assigned to work in a drop-in center for teens in a downtown area in your responses to the following questions:
   a. Identify three social determinants of health and explain their relevance to this situation.
   b. How would you include the foundational values (Box 1.4) in this setting?
   c. What beliefs guiding practice (Box 1.4) would you consider using?

4. What possible challenging areas in community health nursing have you identified from chapter content or scenarios, and how could these be managed?

5. What short- and long-term benefits would you expect from learning about community health nursing?

## References

Allender, J., Rector, C., & Warner, K. (2010). *Community health nursing: Promoting and protecting the public's health* (7th ed.). Philadelphia, PA: Lippincott Williams & Wilkins.

American Association of Colleges of Nursing. (2008). *The essentials of baccalaureate education for professional nursing practice*. Retrieved from www.aacn.nche.edu/publications/position-statements

American Nurses Association. (2010). *Code of ethics for nurses with interpretive statements*. Retrieved from www.nursingworld.org/MainMenuCategories/EthicsStandards/CodeofEthicsforNurses

American Nurses Association. (2012). *Nursing process*. Retrieved from http://nursingworld.org/EspeciallyForYou/What-is-Nursing/Tools-You-Need/Thenursingprocess.html

American Nurses Association. (2013). *Public health nursing: Scope and standards of practice* (2nd ed.). Silver Springs, MD: Author.

American Nurses Association. (2014). *Home health nursing: Scope and standards of home health nursing practice* (2nd ed.). Silver Springs, MD: Author.

American Speech-Language Association. (2014). *Evaluating web sites*. Retrieved from www.asha.org/sitehelp/websites.htm

Arnstein, S. (2006). *A ladder of citizen participation*. Retrieved from http://lithgow-schmidt.dk/sherry-arnstein/ladder-of-citizen-participation.html

Association of Community Health Nursing Educators [ACHNE]. (2009). *Essentials of baccalaureate nursing education for entry level community/public health nursing*. Retrieved from www.achne.org/files/EssentialsOfBaccalaureate_Fall_2009.pdf

Bracht, N., & Tsouros, A. (1990). Principles and strategies of effective community participation. *Health Promotion International, 5*(3), 199–208.

British Columbia Office of the Provincial Health Officer. (2010, August). *Investing in prevention: Improving health and creating sustainability*. The Provincial Health Officer's special report. Vancouver: BC Office of the Provincial Health Officer. Retrieved from www.health.gov.bc.ca/library/publications/year/2010/Investing_in_prevention_improving_health_and_creating_sustainability.pdf

Burns, N., & Grove, S. (2011). *Understanding nursing research: Building an evidence-based practice* (5th ed.). Maryland Heights, MO: Elsevier Saunders.

Butterfield, P. (2001). *Thinking upstream: Conceptualizing health from a population perspective.* In M. Nies & M. McEwen (Eds.), *Community health nursing: Promoting the health of populations* (3rd ed., pp. 48–60). Philadelphia, PA: Saunders.

Canadian Association of Schools of Nursing. (2011). *Position Statement: Baccalaureate education and baccalaureate programs.* Retrieved from http://casn.ca/wp-content/uploads/2014/12/BaccalaureatePositionStatementEnglishFinal.pdf

Canadian Association of Schools of Nursing. (2014, May). *Entry-to-practice public health nursing competencies for undergraduate nursing education.* Retrieved from www.casn.ca/2014/12/entry-practice-public-health-nursing-competencies-undergraduate-nursing-education-2/

Canadian Diabetes Association Clinical Practice Guidelines Expert Committee. (2013, April). Canadian Diabetes Association 2013 clinical practice guidelines for the prevention and management of diabetes in Canada. *Canadian Journal of Diabetes, 37*(Suppl. 1), S1–S212.

Canadian Nurses Association (CNA). (2008). *Code of ethics for registered nurses* (2008 centennial edition). Retrieved from www.cna-aiic.ca/~/media/cna/files/en/codeofethics.pdf

Canadian Nurses Association. (2010). *Social justice: A means to an end; an end in itself* (2nd ed.). Retrieved from http://cna-aiic.ca/~/media/cna/page-content/pdf-fr/social_justice_2010_e.pdf

Canadian Nurses Association & Canadian Medical Association (CAN & CMA). (2011, July). *Principles to guide health care transformation in Canada.* Retrieved from www.cma.ca/multimedia/CMA/Content_Images/Inside_cma/Advocacy/HCT/HCT-Principles_en.pdf

Canadian Public Health Association (CPHA). (2008). Canadian Public Health Association response to the World Health Organization (WHO) Commission's report *Closing the gap in a generation: Health equity through action on the social determinants of health.* Ottawa: CPHA. Retrieved from www.cpha.ca/uploads/briefs/cpha_who_sdoh_e.pdf

Centre for Addiction and Mental Health. (2012). *Culture counts: A road map to health promotion.* Retrieved from www.camh.ca/en/hospital/about_camh/health_promotion/culture_counts/Pages/culture_counts_roadmap_health_promotion.aspx

Centers for Disease Control and Prevention. (2014). Social determinants of health definitions. Retrieved from www.cdc.gov/socialdeterminants/Definitions.html

Ciliska, D., & Ganann, R. (2011). Research. In L. Stamler & L. Liu (Eds.), *Community health nursing: A Canadian perspective* (3rd ed., pp. 155–170). Toronto, ON: Pearson Canada.

Commission on Social Determinants of Health (CSDH). (2008). *Closing the gap in a generation: Health equity through action on the social determinants of health.* Final Report of the Commission on Social Determinants of Health. Geneva: World Health Organization. Retrieved from http://whqlibdoc.who.int/publications/2008/9789241563703_eng.pdf

Community Health Nurses of Canada. (2009, May). *Public health nursing discipline specific competencies Version 1.0.* Retrieved from www.chnc.ca/competencies.cfm

Community Health Nurses of Canada. (2010, March). *Home health nursing competencies Version 1.0.* Retrieved from www.chnc.ca/competencies.cfm

Community Health Nurses of Canada. (2011, March). *Canadian community health nursing: Professional practice model & standards of practice.* Retrieved from www.chnc.ca/nursing-standards-of-practice.cfm

Community Health Nurses of Canada. (2013). *Canadian community health nursing practice model.* Retrieved from http://chnc.ca/documents/CanadianCommunityHealthNursingProfessionalPracticeCompoments-E.pdf

Diem, E., & Moyer, A. (2010). Development and testing of tools to evaluate public health nursing clinical education at the baccalaureate level. *Public Health Nursing, 27,* 285–293. doi:10.1111/j.1525-1446.2010.00855.x

Ervin, N. (2002). *Advanced community health nursing practice: Population-focused care*. Upper Saddle River, NJ: Prentice Hall.

Federal, Provincial and Territorial Advisory Committee on Population Health. (1999). *Toward a healthy future: Second report on the health of Canadians*. Retrieved from http://publications.gc.ca/collections/Collection/H39-468-1999E.pdf

Federal/Provincial/Territorial Physical Activity and Recreation Committee and the former Pan-Canadian Healthy Living Issue Group. (2011). *Physical activity approaches at the ground level: Promising practices targeting Aboriginal children and youth*. Final report. Retrieved from www.nada.ca/wp-content/uploads/1034.pdf

Frenk, J., Chen, L., & Bhutta, Z. (2010). Health professionals for a new century: Transforming education to strengthen health systems in an interdependent world. *The Lancet, 376*, 1923–1958. doi:10.1016/S0140-6736(10) 61854-5.

Johnstone, A. (2008). *Bioethics: A nursing perspective* (5th ed.). Chatswood, Australia: Saunders Elsevier.

KU Work Group for Community Health and Development. (2013a). Table of contents. *Community Tool Box*. Retrieved from http://ctb.ku.edu/en/tablecontents/index.aspx

KU Work Group for Community Health and Development. (2013b). Developing a plan for assessing local needs and resources. *Community Tool Box* (Chapter 3, Section 1). Retrieved from http://ctb.ku.edu/en/tablecontents/sub_section_main_1019.aspx

Kwan, M., Cairney, J., Faulkner, G., & Pullenayegum, E. (2012). Physical activity and other health-risk behaviors during the transition into early adulthood: A longitudinal cohort study. *American Journal of Preventive Medicine, 42*(1), 14–20. doi:10.1016/j

Labonte, R. (1994). Death of program, birth of metaphor: The development of health promotion in Canada. In A. Pedersen, M. O'Neill, & I. Rootman (Eds.), *Health promotion in Canada* (pp. 72–90). Toronto, ON: Saunders.

Labonte, R. (1997). Community, community development, and the forming of authentic partnerships. In M. Minkler (Ed.), *Community organizing & community building for health* (pp. 88–102). New Brunswick, NJ: Rutgers University.

Leavell, H., & Clark, E. (1958). *Preventive medicine for the doctor in his community*. New York: McGraw-Hill.

MacDonald, G. (Executive Producer). (2010). *Primary health care 1978–2008: The Canadian experience in a global context* [DVD]. Retrieved from http://bloomberg.nursing.utoronto.ca/faculty-staff/teaching-resources

Marmot, M., Friel, S., Bell, R., Houweling, T., & Taylor, S. (2008). Closing the gap in a generation: Health equity through action on the social determinants of health. *The Lancet, 372*, 1661–1669. doi:10.1016/S0140-6736(08)61690-6

McKenzie, J., Neiger, B., & Thackeray, R. (2013). *Planning, implementing and evaluating health promotion programs: A Primer* (6th ed.). Glenview, IL: Pearson Education.

McKinlay, J. (1979, June 17–19). A case for refocusing upstream: The political economy of illness. In *Proceedings of an American Heart Association conference: Applying behavioral science to cardiovascular risk*. Seattle, WA: American Heart Association.

Milio, N. (1976). A framework for prevention: Changing health-damaging to health-generating life patterns. *American Journal of Public Health, 66*, 435–439.

Minnesota Department of Health. (2007). *Cornerstones of public health nursing*. Retrieved from www.health.state.mn.us/divs/opi/cd/phn/docs/0710phn_cornerstones.pdf

National Center for Safe Routes to School. (2010). *Case studies from around the country*. Retrieved from www.saferoutesinfo.org/sites/default/files/srts_case_studies.pdf

National Collaborating Centre for Aboriginal Health. (2013). *Aboriginal ActNow fact sheet series*. Retrieved from www.nccah-ccnsa.ca/370/Aboriginal_ActNow_Fact_Sheet_Series.nccah

National Collaborating Centre for Healthy Public Policy. (2011, November). *Citizen participation in health impact assessment: An overview of the principal arguments supporting it.* Retrieved from www.ncchpp.ca/docs/EIS-HIA_participation_advantagesEN.pdf

National Network of Libraries of Medicine. (2012). *Health literacy.* Retrieved from http://nnlm.gov/outreach/consumer/hlthlit.html

Nova Scotia Public Health. (2012). *Nova Scotia public health standards 2011–2016.* Retrieved from http://novascotia.ca/dhw/publichealth/documents/Public_Health_Standards_EN.pdf

Nutbeam, D. (1998). *Health promotion glossary of terms.* Geneva: World Health Organization.

Nyswander, D. (1956). Education for health: Some principles and their applications. *Health Education Monographs, 14,* 65–70.

Office of the Surgeon General (US), Center for Mental Health Services (US), and National Institute of Mental Health (US). (2001). *Mental health: Culture, race, and ethnicity: A supplement to mental health.* A Report of the Surgeon General. Rockville, MD: Substance Abuse and Mental Health Services Administration. Retrieved from www.ncbi.nlm.nih.gov/books/NBK44246/ (Chapter 1 and /NBK44250/Chapter 7)

Ontario Ministry of Health and Long-Term Care. (2008, August). *Ontario health plan for an influenza pandemic* (5th ed.). Toronto, ON: Ministry of Health and Long-Term Care.

Parker, E., Margolis, L., Eng, E., & Henríquez-Roldán, C. (2003). Assessing the capacity of health departments to engage in community-based participatory public health. *American Journal of Public Health, 93*(3), 472–476.

Public Health Agency of Canada (PHAC). (2013). *What makes Canadians healthy or unhealthy?* Retrieved from www.phac-aspc.gc.ca/ph-sp/determinants/determinants-eng.php#income

Public Health Foundation. (2014). *Core competencies for public health professionals.* Retrieved from www.phf.org/programs/corecompetencies/Pages/About_the_Core_Competencies_for_Public_Health_Professionals.aspx

Public Health Ontario. (2014). *Program planning steps.* Retrieved from www.publichealthontario.ca/en/ServicesAndTools/ohpp/pages/processes/Program-Planning-Steps.aspx?ProcessKey=1

Quad Council of Public Health Nursing Organizations. (2011). *Quad Council competencies for public health nurses.* Retrieved from www.resourcecenter.net/images/ACHNE/Files/QuadCouncilCompetenciesForPublicHealthNurses_Summer2011.pdf

Raphael, D. (2002). *Social justice is good for our hearts: Why societal factors—not lifestyles—are major causes of heart disease in Canada and elsewhere.* Toronto, ON: CSJ Foundation for Research and Education.

Reiter, J. (2004). *What is unique about community health nursing?* (Unpublished slideshow presentation: Canadian Community Nursing Standards of Practice, slide 10). St. John's, NL: Community Health Nurses Association of Canada.

Rifkin, S. (2009). Lessons from community participation in health programmes: A review of the post Alma-Ata experience. *International Health, 1,* 31–37. doi:10.1016/j.inhe.2009.02.001

Rudolph, L., Caplan, J., Ben-Moshe, K., & Dillon, L. (2013). *Health in all policies: A guide for state and local governments.* Washington, DC, and Oakland, CA: American Public Health Association and Public Health Institute. Retrieved from www.phi.org/resources/?resource=hiapguide

Secretariat for the Intersectoral Healthy Living Network in partnership with the F/P/T Healthy Living Task Group and the F/P/T Advisory Committee on Population Health and Health Security (ACPHHS). (2005). *The integrated Pan-Canadian healthy living strategy.* Retrieved from www.phac-aspc.gc.ca/hp-ps/hl-mvs/ipchls-spimmvs/index-eng.php

Sudbury & District Health Unit. (2011). *10 promising practices to guide local public health practice to reduce social inequities in health: Technical briefing.* Sudbury, ON: Author. Retrieved from www.sdhu.com/uploads/content/listings/10PromisingPractices.pdf

Tanner, C. (2006). Thinking like a nurse: A researched-based model of clinical judgment. *Journal of Nursing Education, 45*(6), 204–211.

Virginia Technical University. (2014). *Evaluating Internet information.* Retrieved from www.lib.vt.edu/instruct/evaluate/

US Department of Health and Social Services. (2010). *Healthy people 2020: Framework.* Retrieved from www.healthypeople.gov/2020/Consortium/HP2020Framework.pdf

Werner, D., & Bower, B. (1982). *Helping health workers learn.* Berkeley, CA: The Hesperian Foundation.

Weston, M. (2010, January). Strategies for enhancing autonomy and control over nursing practice. *The Online Journal of Issues in Nursing, 15*(1). doi:10.3912/OJIN.Vol15No01Man02

Wilkinson R., & Marmot, M. (Eds.). (2003). *Social determinants of health: The solid facts* (2nd ed.). Copenhagen, Denmark: Regional Office for Europe of the World Health Organization. Retrieved from www.euro.who.int/__data/assets/pdf_file/0005/98438/e81384.pdf

World Health Organization (WHO). (1946, 2012). *Health.* Retrieved from www.who.int/trade/glossary/story046/en/index.html

World Health Organization (WHO). (1978). *Declaration of Alma-Ata.* Report from the International Conference on Primary Health Care, Alma-Ata, USSR, September 6–12. Retrieved from www.paho.org/English/DD/PIN/alma-ata_declaration.htm

World Health Organization (WHO). (1986). *Ottawa Charter for Health Promotion.* Retrieved from www.who.int/healthpromotion/conferences/previous/ottawa/en/index.html

World Health Organization (WHO). (2008). *Primary health care: Now more than ever.* The World Health Report 2008. Retrieved from www.who.int/whr/2008/whr08_en.pdf

World Health Organization (WHO). (2011). *Transformative scale-up of health professional education: An effort to increase the numbers of health professionals and to strengthen their impact on population.* Retrieved from http://whqlibdoc.who.int/hq/2011/WHO_HSS_HRH_HEP2011.01_eng.pdf

World Health Organization (WHO). (2012a). *Evidence base for health determinants.* Retrieved from www.who.int/hia/evidence/doh/en/index1.html

World Health Organization (WHO). (2012b). *Primary health care.* Retrieved from www.who.int/topics/primary_health_care/en/

World Health Organization (WHO). (2014a). *Social determinants of health.* Retrieved from www.who.int/social_determinants/en/

World Health Organization (WHO). (2014b). *Health impact assessment* (HIA). Glossary. Retrieved from www.who.int/hia/en/

## Website Resources

### Primary Health Care and Social Determinants of Health

G. MacDonald, *Introduction to Primary Health Care* (PowerPoint Presentation) and *Primary Health Care 1978–2008: The Canadian Experience in a Global Context* (DVD): http://bloomberg.nursing.utoronto.ca/faculty-staff/teaching-resources

This slideshow has questions and answers about primary health care, and the video confirms the importance of the values and principles of primary health care. The material identifies how primary health care changed discussions about health care from the treatment and illness model to health promotion and wellness, and discusses the use of primary health care with Aboriginal people in Australia and First Nations in Canada, and how health policy can be influenced by intersectoral collaboration.

World Health Organization (WHO), *Primary Health Care*: www.who.int/topics/
primary_health_care/en/

The WHO website on primary health care provides links to major WHO documents, such as the *Declaration of Alma-Ata*, *Social Determinants of Health*, and *Primary Health Care*.

## National and International Websites on Public and Community Health and Nursing

The following list provides an overview of websites on community health, community health nursing, public health, and international health. Each site has many credible links.

### Community Health

KU Work Group for Community Health and Development, *Community Tool Box: Tools to Change Our World*: http://ctb.ku.edu/en

The Community Tool Box website has been online since 1995 and continues to expand. Currently, the core of the Tool Box is the "how-to tools," which use simple, friendly language to explain how to perform the different tasks necessary for community health and development.

### Community Health Nursing Associations and Organizations

Association of Community Health Nursing Educators (ACHNE): www.achne.org/i4a/pages/
index.cfm?pageid=1

The ACHNE website provides information on community and public health nursing education, research, and practice. Resources include the *Disaster Preparedness White Paper* and links to other nursing associations.

Community Health Nurses of Canada (CHNC): www.chnc.ca

The CHNC website includes discipline-specific standards of practice, core competencies, and a description of the community health nursing certification process. The standards and competencies can be purchased and viewed online.

Community Health Nursing Initiatives Group (CHNIG): www.chnig.org

The CHING website provides information for community health nurses in Ontario. It offers position papers that could provide general guidance, such as *Healthy Schools, Healthy Children: Maximizing the Contribution of Public Health Nursing in School Settings* (June 2013) and *Lessons from SARS* (July 2003).

Community Health Nurses of Alberta: www.chnalberta.org

The CHNAlberta website provides information and resources, including webinars, for community health nurses in Alberta.

National Association of School Nurses (NASN): www.nasn.org

The NASN website provides extensive links and resources relevant to working with children. Information is provided on cultural competency, school-age diseases, and wellness policies. One resource example is *Head Lice 101 Presentation: An Overview for Parents, Teachers and Communities*.

### Public Health

American Public Health Association: www.apha.org/

This site describes public health and provides links to state public health associations.

Association of State and Territorial Health Officials: www.astho.org/
   The ASTHO website provides information on public health in each state, including associated agencies. The site has a section called "Stories in Public Health" that provides strategies used in different states and territories.

Canadian Public Health Association: www.cpha.ca/en/default.aspx
   The CPHA website provides links to public health associations and explores issues within Canada.

Institute of Medicine: www.iom.edu
   The IOM website includes expert reports in areas such as improving the health of young adults and children, and workshop summaries on topics such as building the capacity of community-based health professionals.

McMaster University Health Evidence: www.healthevidence.org/
   Health Evidence is a free searchable online registry of research evidence evaluating the effectiveness of public health interventions.

**International Health**
International Union for Health Promotion and Education (IUHPE): www.iuhpe.org/
   The IUHPE website describes worldwide projects related to health promotion, such as the determinants of health. A promised feature is tools related to health promotion. A related site is http://isecn.org/, which is geared toward students and early career practitioners.

World Health Organization: www.who.int/en/
   The WHO website provides extensive resources through the "Health Topics" menu at the top of the page. Topics related to community health nursing can be obtained by typing "Community Health Nursing" into the WHO search engine.

**Strategies for Using the Internet**

The Internet contains a great many resources related to the subjects covered in this chapter. However, as you likely know, website addresses (URLs) frequently become unreliable. This is often due to website managers rearranging the material on the website. If an URL does not function, try deleting characters from the end to reach a relevant web page that may have the material. If you have the title of the document or web page that you want, use the title in a general search engine rather than within a website. This is often a quicker option than trying to use the search function within large websites, such as those maintained by governments.
   To conduct an effective search using keywords on the Internet (and not be overloaded with useless information), you can restrict your search. One effective method is to stipulate within your search the type of website you will accept. In the search engine of your choice, type the keywords you are looking for in quotation marks (e.g., "community health"). Leave a space and then type either "site:.edu" or "site:.ac" to limit your search to educational sites; "site:.org" to restrict your search to organizational sites (commercial and noncommercial); or "site:.gov" to obtain US government sites. Government sites in other countries often use the two letter short form for the country such as ".ca" for Canada and ".au" for Australia. You can also limit the search response, eliminating commercial sites by typing "-.com" or "-.biz" after your subject matter. In addition, some search engines have sophisticated features or preferences by which you can further refine your search by location, date, language, and the like.

# Community Health Nursing Projects and Teamwork

························································································································

This chapter builds on foundational concepts and processes of community health nursing introduced in Chapter 1 to provide two invaluable approaches to working in the community: community health nursing projects and teamwork. Community health nursing projects essentially involve putting a framework around the community health nursing process. Community health nursing projects include nine steps, beginning with assessment and ending with evaluation, and approximate timelines for working with a community group to produce a health resource that is relevant to them. Teamwork is essential for community nursing projects and involves learning to use practical tools and strategies for leadership, decision making, conflict resolution, and team evaluation.

The chapter has three sections: community nursing projects, teamwork, and teamwork during projects. The first section uses two case studies to illustrate the benefits of using a project approach to learning about community health nursing practice, and includes a flexible project timeline. The teamwork section provides the theory, concepts, and evidence that provide a foundation for effective teamwork in community health nursing practice. The final section combines the project and teamwork to outline the concepts and procedures relevant to the three periods of a community nursing project: getting organized, getting things done, and finishing up.

The scenarios in the teamwork sections provide a realistic idea of what is involved in completing a community health nursing project, and how teams use the tools and resources to organize themselves, make decisions, communicate, and evaluate while working on a community project. The knowledge and skills developed by using teamwork in completing a community nursing project are transferable to other areas of nursing and your future professional development.

## Learning Objectives

After reading this chapter and answering the questions throughout the chapter, you should be able to:

1. Appreciate the advantage of using a community project to learn about community health nursing.

2. Appreciate the importance of teamwork and collaboration in community health nursing practice.
3. Incorporate theory and evidence when organizing teamwork and defining the roles within the team.
4. Adopt procedures for documentation and communication and self- and team evaluation.
5. Apply tools and procedures, such as team agreement and conflict resolution strategy, effectively during team development.

> **Key Terms and Concepts**
>
> collaborative learning · community health nursing projects · conflict · conflict resolution · critical thinking · group · interprofessional collaboration · morale · pre-clinical self-assessment · reflective process · self-assessment · sense of accomplishment · tasks · team · team agreement · team evaluation · team decision making · team development · team leader · teamwork · weekly report

## Community Nursing Projects

**Community health nursing projects** follow the community health nursing process of assess, plan, act, and evaluate within a project approach to immerse students and practitioner teams in realistic community situations where they can holistically apply the principles and practice of community health nursing. This approach is supported by evidence that team projects can help undergraduate students develop a host of skills that are increasingly important in the professional world (Caruso & Woolley, 2008; Mannix & Neale, 2005). Positive team experiences have been shown to contribute to student learning, retention, and overall success (National Survey of Student Engagement, 2006).

In the community, the team comes together to work with a community group to identify health needs, and to develop and test actions/interventions using the community health nursing process. The student teams are under the supervision of a clinical faculty instructor experienced in community health nursing, and a community advisor from the placement organization. The community advisor could also be called a field guide, mentor, preceptor, or community contact. In traditional community placements, such as public health or community health centers, the advisor is usually a nurse or other health care professional; in nontraditional placements, the advisor is a staff member who could have a range of educational and practice experiences, such as teacher or a staff person in a homeless shelter. Although not ideal, the team might also consist of one student, or new practitioner, and a nurse advisor/preceptor/mentor. Learning about teamwork comes from interacting with other team members and through the direct or indirect supervision of experienced community health nurses.

An important aspect of the community health nursing project is that it uses a flexible time frame. This time frame is practical since clinical courses have a definite duration, and teams need to accomplish some aspect of community health nursing by the end of a course. We use a time frame of one or two days a week over 12 weeks to provide an idea of how to manage the project steps in a community project. Table 2.1 outlines the suggested time allocation, sequence, and overlapping of the steps in the project. For example, the team can conduct Step 3 concurrently with Steps 1 and 2 (discussed in Chapter 3) or start Step 3 before Step 2, depending on the availability of information.

At the orientation for the community nursing clinical course, two teams from the previous course describe their projects and provide a poster to illustrate what they have produced. We use these two projects to illustrate the main features of a community project. The project on a drop-in program for new mothers is below; the project on tobacco reduction in the workplace appears later in this chapter.

### Drop-in Program for New Mothers

The presenters describe a project at a drop-in program for new mothers. At their first meeting, the staff at the center tells the students that they provide food coupons for the mothers and try to encourage socialization but do not offer a formal education program. The public health nurse, who runs a health clinic for the women every two weeks, had encouraged the center to offer a nursing student placement with the program. The nurse explains that the women often share their concerns with her about doing the right thing so their baby will be healthy. She says that the student team can consult with her and work with the staff to find out and deliver the health information that the women want to learn. The staff wants to be involved, feeling it will make it easier for them to continue any activities started by the students.

The presenters explain that when they first met the mothers in a recreation room, it was very noisy and chaotic and they felt overwhelmed. When they discussed their reactions with their clinical instructor, she helped them to understand that such environments were not uncommon in community practice and pointed out that it would give them the opportunity to develop two very useful nursing skills, observation and flexibility. She suggested that they start by just sitting back and observing without feeling that they had to do anything right away. As the team spent more time in the recreation room, they came to realize, and discuss with each other, how attentively the mothers watched and cared for their children. Soon the student team began to feel more comfortable, and found it fairly easy to talk with the women informally (using methods described in Chapter 4) about themselves and their babies. They also learned to listen to each other before making decisions for the team. Within a couple of weeks, they had several ideas that seem to interest the mothers.

With feedback from the instructor and staff, the team developed a short questionnaire and conducted a survey to identify the most important topics of interest for the mothers. They admit that team members had different ideas on how to deal with the results. After talking it through, they eventually determined that they wanted the women to decide what their priorities were. The women said that they wanted to learn more about the growth and development of their children but did not want to sit through a presentation or read a pamphlet. They wanted something practical they could use and keep. After trying out different ideas, the team and the women decide to gather together materials for each woman to make her own unique growth chart. The poster they show illustrates how proud the students are with what the women were able to accomplish.

### Discussion Topics and Questions

1. What did the team learn in the first few weeks of the placement?
2. What was important about the team deciding to ask the women to identify their priorities?

For suggested responses, please see the Answer Key at the back of the book.

If the clinical course is for two or three days a week for six weeks, the activities in each week would double; if the clinical course extents over two semesters, the activities each week would be halved. Other differences in available clinical time can be worked out proportionally. Timelines are discussed in more detail in Chapter 4, when most of the factors affecting what can be accomplished are known.

Teamwork and collaboration on community projects is integral to the everyday practice of many community health nurses. Setting up the learning environment is key. Prior to students or practitioners joining a project, nursing educators or managers organize several aspects of the project, such as the location, population group, initial

**Table 2.1: Approximate Timing for Steps in a Community Health Nursing Project**

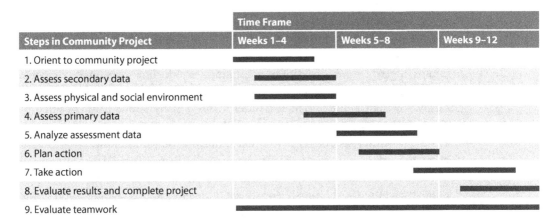

| Steps in Community Project | Time Frame | | |
|---|---|---|---|
| | Weeks 1–4 | Weeks 5–8 | Weeks 9–12 |
| 1. Orient to community project | ▬▬▬▬ | | |
| 2. Assess secondary data | ▬▬▬▬▬ | | |
| 3. Assess physical and social environment | ▬▬▬▬ | | |
| 4. Assess primary data | ▬▬▬▬▬ | | |
| 5. Analyze assessment data | | ▬▬▬▬ | |
| 6. Plan action | | ▬▬▬▬ | |
| 7. Take action | | ▬▬▬▬▬▬ | |
| 8. Evaluate results and complete project | | | ▬▬▬▬ |
| 9. Evaluate teamwork | ▬▬▬▬▬▬▬▬▬▬▬▬▬▬▬▬ | | |

issue, and access to a community group. The projects are intended to fit with the usual practice of a community agency or organization and may often be a component of a larger project or program.

Community nursing projects encourage a collaborative approach and systematic application of the community nursing process with the goal of making a meaningful ongoing contribution to the health of a community group. The team gets to "know the community." This knowledge builds first by using observation and statistics, and then by forming partnerships with members of the community and conducting a detailed assessment. The collaborative process and teamwork leads the team to identify and meet achievable health goals within given timelines. The emphasis is on moving from observation and isolated experiences to an integrated understanding of community nursing practice.

Community nursing projects incorporate the concepts of primary health care, social determinants of health, social justice, and others included in the foundational values presented in Chapter 1. They aim to make explicit what it means to promote, protect, and preserve the health of individuals, families, groups, communities, and populations, wherever people live, work, learn, worship, and play. Through community projects, this text encourages learners to think broadly about health and its determinants, and about what it means to create the conditions for the health of the community. Students and new practitioners will learn how to function at a high level of autonomy and to draw on multiple sources of knowledge as they use a systematic community health nursing process. Through immersion, they will learn that building sustainable relationships and bringing resources together are central to community work. Community projects offer a manageable slice of community health nursing practice and have the potential to provide benefits to students, to the community organizations providing community clinical experiences, and to the involved community groups.

For students and new practitioners, community projects provide an entry to the complexity of community work. Community health organizations, especially public health, have broad mandates and comprehensive long-term health goals that are translated into health programs and services. These programs and services may be broken down into further manageable chunks and viewed as projects; that is, they have specific goals, objectives, and timelines. These "projects" may also be called assignments, tasks, initiatives, or endeavors.

As an example of how community work is broken down into manageable parts, consider a community/public health agency within an urban core area of from 50,000 to 100,000 people. The agency would probably have multiple programs to promote the health of different population groups and prevent infectious and chronic disease. Each program could have multiple components. For instance, maternal and infant health programs offered by public health or community health clinics customarily include components such as prenatal classes, home visits to new mothers, infant immunizations, and so on. In addition to these basic elements, a maternal and infant health program might from time to time assign a small team to a short-term initiative or project to accomplish specific goals within a specified time frame. For example, a team might be asked to work on a project to recommend ways to increase attendance at prenatal classes by women at higher risk for having infants with low birth weight.

Similarly, a home health nursing organization might assign a team to improve the resources for nurses to provide to clients. For instance, they could provide handouts promoting better nutrition or raising awareness of nutritional services in the community. The clients and nursing staff of the organization make up the "community" in this project.

As well as providing a way of understanding communities and community health nursing practice, community projects support students and new practitioners in meeting the expectations of professional accountability. These projects are designed to provide a structure and process to guide practice in the often unstructured and changing community environment. The community projects require teams to follow and communicate using a systematic process to document the decisions and communicate the relevance of results. This enables learners to be accountable to their team, to their nursing program or employer, to the organizations providing clinical placement or access to community groups, and to the community group.

To summarize, community projects provide a realistic entry point for learning about the multiple levels of community nursing work. Community projects are not simple, unconnected tasks or assignments in a community setting. Projects provide a structured approach to learning about the complexity of practice that includes collaboration with community groups and other organizations, and insight into how this work can contribute to improving the health of a community. Above all, community projects provide access to community nursing practice by learning and doing.

In order to foster learning, nurse educators and managers need to consider several different aspects in the design of community nursing projects. The four conditions listed in Box 2.1 are required to provide a supportive learning environment.

This text illustrates how students and beginning practitioners can apply theory to practice and develop skills and knowledge in community health nursing through community projects. Examples range from a community

---

**BOX 2.1**

**Four Conditions for Supporting Community Nursing Projects**

1. An environment for experiencing and reflecting on community health nursing practice and relevant community health nursing standards and/or competencies
2. A realistic opportunity for community health nursing students and practitioners to learn about and apply aspects of community health nursing practice, including:
   a. the community health nursing process: assess, plan, implement/take action, evaluate
   b. collaboration with a defined community group and possibly other health professionals, disciplines, and sectors, over a specified period
   c. teamwork
3. The expectation of developing relevant resources for the organization sponsoring the community clinical experience
4. The expectation of developing relevant resources for the community group

The students are placed in a manufacturing plant to work with the Health and Safety Committee on ways to reduce smoking among the workers. Their advisor is the facilities manager who chairs the Committee; their clinical instructor has worked with student teams in different community settings. At first, the students feel as if they are floundering. They don't know where to start, and meet with their advisor and clinical instructor to get some sense of direction. Instead of telling them what to do, the experienced community health nurse asks questions: "What do you know about the plant? What do you know about smoking cessation? What information do you need and where might you find it? Who might have relevant information at the plant? How will you collect reliable information?" Without being directive, this questioning process helps the team realize how important it is to seek different sources of information, such as workplace statistics, observations of the workers in the plant, and personal experience. It also brings out the importance of communication methods. After the problem-solving meeting, the team quickly lays out a plan to observe and informally interact with the workers. They find the best way to connect with people is at lunchtime in the cafeteria. People are interested in what the team is doing and are quite happy to talk while they eat. With advice from their advisor and instructor, they decide to use a systematic but not intrusive assessment approach, and engage small groups in discussions of ways to cut down on smoking. This works well—the planning paid off!

The team has some difficulties working together at first. One team member wants to talk to managers; the others disagree. The student makes a strong case, saying that if the managers are not involved, the project will not likely continue once the students leave. After discussion, the others come to agree with her. The outcome is a productive meeting with the managers.

The workplace Health and Safety Committee reviews the assessment data and evidence-based literature on tobacco reduction strategies gathered by the student team, and recommends a few options that might work in the facility. After considering the options, with the timelines in mind, the team decides to develop an interactive poster for the cafeteria and to prepare material for a "Butt-out" contest with a similar facility in another city. The team evaluates the interactive poster by documenting how many approach them to talk about the poster, how many take additional information, and how many talk about smoking reduction with the occupational health nurse who is available one day a week. It is disappointing not to have time to run the contest, but the student team feels that with the work they were able to do, the advisor, the occupational health nurse, and the Health and Safety Committee will carry on to complete the project.

**Discussion Topics and Questions**

3. What have you done previously that would help you with the initial steps of setting up this community project on smoking reduction?

4. What aspects of the project provided realistic opportunities for students to learn about and practice the following:
   a. The community health nursing process: assess, plan, implement/take action, evaluate
   b. Collaboration, over a specified period, with a defined community group, health professionals, other disciplines, and other sectors
   c. Teamwork

project in a traditional setting, such as determining and making recommendations on how a public health immunization program could reach older adults (Chapter 13), to a project in a nontraditional setting, such as assisting adults learning English to communicate their health needs (Chapter 4). Since most students will have had limited experience of community health, the text is designed to guide students through Bender, Tanner, and Chesla's (2009) beginning stages of developing clinical knowledge, judgment, and caring by working with one community group. Community nursing projects are important because they make practice manageable, measurable, and collaborative, and provide a realistic experience for students and practitioners.

# Teamwork

Teams and teamwork allow community health nurses to effectively share the responsibility for addressing the health of a population group. The delivery of community health programs and services is simply too large an endeavor for individuals working alone. A **team** is a group of people with a commitment to one another, to the team, to a high level of achievement, to a common goal, and to a common vision (KU Work Group for Community Health and Development [KU Work Group], 2013a). In contrast, a **group** refers to people who work together while maintaining their individual interests over collective interests or the benefits to others. **Teamwork** is the collaborative effort of team members to achieve the team goal and vision. The KU Work Group goes on to say that it is important for a team to work toward the vision as a whole team, and for each team member to commit to holding themselves, and one another, responsible for this work.

The vision explains why the accomplishment is important and provides the motivating force for team members to collaborate to complete the goal together, in tandem, as efficiently as possible. In other words, a vision is more abstract and inspirational than a goal and helps to motivate team members. As an example, the vision of the student team working with prenatal and postnatal women in the first scenario was that the women would determine and act on their own health needs. The initial goal, determined with the women after the assessment, was for each woman to develop a resource (growth chart) that was useful to her. The team's vision kept them open to encouraging the women to express their views, hearing what the women really wanted, and supporting the women to attain their goal.

A collaborative learning process helps teams to strive toward a common goal and vision. **Collaborative learning** requires interaction among individuals to produce a product and involves negotiations, discussions, and accommodation of others' perspectives (Kozar, 2010). "Cooperation" is a term that may be confused with collaboration. While cooperation can lead to a common, beneficial goal, it does not require equal participation or bring learning benefits for the team (Kozar, 2010). For example, in the first scenario, each member of the student team might have cooperated on gathering resources for new mothers without deciding as a team which resources would be the most useful, or where or how to collect them.

Working together well as a team does not come naturally to individuals, although everyone has been living with or working with groups of people since birth. Teamwork requires effort. Kozar (2010) recommends that instructors prepare students for collaborative learning by encouraging the following processes:

- Negotiating and accommodating each other's perspectives
- Enabling more or less equal participation of team members
- Sharing in knowledge creation

Keep in mind that community health workers interact with community members and other disciplines, individually and in groups, in a variety of ways. From a nursing perspective, **interprofessional collaboration** is "[a] complex process through which relationships are developed among health care professionals so that they effectively interact and work together for the mutual goal of safe and quality patient care" (Spector, 2010, p. 110).

**Table 2.2: Comparison of a Group of People and a Team**

| Group of People | Team |
|---|---|
| Each member represents a different constituency, has his or her own hidden agenda, and may try to get his or her interest group to benefit at the expense of others. | Each member accepts the team goals and willingly foregoes personal and constituent goals for the benefit of the team. |
| Each member is unsure of his or her role, other than to represent constituency. | Each member has a role to play; each knows his or her role and the contribution to the team. |
| Decisions made by vote: acceptance of the best determined by the most dominant interest group. | Decisions made by consensus: acceptance of the best for the team. |
| Interpersonal conflicts are ignored because "I won't be on this committee forever." The group has no methods, other than embarrassment, for resolving conflicts. | Addresses and resolves most conflicts. The team has an accepted method of resolving conflicts. The ability to resolve conflicts is a key skill. |
| "If I miss a meeting, so what? Who cares?" | You must not miss a meeting because the team needs you. |
| All tend to put on a happy face and accept the median or common skills. 2 + 2 = 3. | The team does better than a collection of individual efforts because all contribute all their skills. They accept each other "warts and all." 2 + 2 = 7 |
| "I" attitude. | "We" attitude. |

*Source*: Adapted and reprinted by permission of Woods, D. (1994). *Problem-based learning: How to gain the most from PBL* (pp. 5–16). Waterdown, ON: Donald R. Woods.

Chapters 9 to 14 deal with interprofessional teamwork and collaboration in a variety of situations.

Table 2.2 compares the features of a group of people and a team. At the individual and team level, newly formed teams can use the table to determine if they are working as a group or as a team.

The comparison in Table 2.2 draws out some important elements of an effective team. These include accepting team goals and team roles, making decisions by consensus, using a process for addressing conflict, and expecting team members to make a contribution. As well, the table draws attention to the added value of teamwork versus individual work and its potential challenges. The benefits and challenges are discussed below.

Since teamwork is integral to the success of the project, learning how to evaluate teamwork is an important element of a community project. Although Box 2.2 lists the evaluation of teamwork as the last in the nine steps used in completing the community project, in practice you will be using various forms provided later in the chapter to evaluate your teamwork on a weekly and monthly basis.

BOX 2.2
**Step 9 in Completing a Community Health Nursing Project**

ASSESS
1. Orient to community project
2. Assess secondary data
3. Assess physical and social environment
4. Assess primary data
5. Analyze assessment data

PLAN
6. Plan action

ACT
7. Take action

EVALUATE
8. Evaluate results and complete project
9. **Evaluate teamwork**

## Benefits of Teamwork

Many nursing practice situations in the community and institutions involve working on a team. Therefore, learning to work collaboratively on a team is a valuable nursing practice skill that is transferable and will serve you well as you continue your nursing career.

Teams bring together people with diverse knowledge and skills to deal with issues and problems. Teams provide an active learning environment. In realistic practice situations, the team members gain experience in working toward a common goal and can learn skills from each other. To encourage this learning, the team can pair less experienced members with those who already have a skill. For example, one member familiar with writing a report can train another; another member comfortable with chairing meetings can tutor a less experienced member through the process. As members tutor and assist others, their self-efficacy grows and influences their beliefs about group performance (Baker, 2001). Therefore, in learning groups, these educational functions within the group are as important as the community project task.

The KU Work Group for Community Health and Development (2013a) identifies the following benefits of a team approach:

- Members of an efficient team share the workload so that a project can move forward and reach more people.
- The pooling of members' expertise and the bringing together of diverse networks of useful connections add to the team's capability.
- Members within a team can energize, support, acknowledge, and review (in a positive way) other team members through measures such as brainstorming and group problem solving.
- Members gain by learning from others, such as leadership skills, and having support when dealing with problems.
- Members tend to do more on a team than on their own because they have more ownership and do not want to let team members down.

## Challenges

Although teams can be more effective than individuals working alone, team members must put effort into making and keeping the team functioning effectively. The challenges teams face (KU Work Group, 2013a) include the following:

- Initial organizing and team decision making is longer and more difficult.
- Once a direction is taken, the team has more difficulty than an individual in making a corrective change in direction.
- Maintaining a balance between team effort and individual recognition is difficult.
- Extra effort may be needed to deal with a weak or ineffective team member.

Being aware of the challenges of teamwork can aid in keeping teams effective. The team can be on the lookout for barriers and problem solve their way around them. For example, when team members know that it is normal for a team to take some time to get organized, they can verbalize that fact and talk about how much more efficient they will be when they "get their act together." Good communication and a collaborative team process can prevent too much time being wasted in going in a wrong direction, and create an environment to address concerns and support weaker team members.

## Team Organization

If teams are to achieve their goals within realistic timelines, they must address both tasks and morale. **Tasks** include preparing plans, assigning work, and completing the work. At the same time, the team members must develop or maintain their morale. **Morale** is the strength of the relationship among team members. You could think of morale as the team spirit or rapport. Collaborating to complete a goal desired by the community encourages high morale among team members and vice versa. Both are required: "If the task is not completed, the morale will be low; if the morale is low, the task is usually not completed" (Woods, 1994, p. 58).

To become a well-functioning team, all members should expect to learn and apply skills and knowledge in both aspects of teamwork: tasks related to the community project and strategies to maintain the morale or social dimension of the team (Ellis & Fisher, 1994; Robbins & Finley, 1995; Woods, 1994). Maintaining a balance is important. After all, according to the popular proverb, "All work and no play makes Jack a dull boy." On the other hand, as stated by Engleberg and Wynn (2000, p. 31), "All play and no work makes you unemployed." Finding this balance is particularly important for student teams.

The following sections describe how teams learn to function well to complete tasks and develop morale. The sections address the stages of team development; team structure and processes, including decision making and conflict management; and approaches to reflecting on and evaluating self and team performance.

### Stages of Team Development

As people come together to work on a team, they will benefit by knowing that their interactions with each other are likely to change over time and usually follow a common set of stages, formally called the five-stage model (Tuckman and Jensen, 1977). By knowing and reflecting on their current stage of development, team members will be better prepared to take action. According to Woods (1994), teams do not start off great; they evolve.

**Team development** is based on Tuckman and Jensen's (1977) five-stage development model: forming, storming, norming, performing, and ending (see Figure 2.1).

**Figure 2.1: Five-Stage Team Development Model**

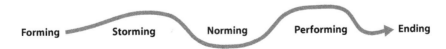

Forming   Storming   Norming   Performing   Ending

*Forming* is the stage or occasion when the team first comes together. At this time, people are usually very polite and agreeable and tend to make rather vague statements (Woods, 1994). The interpersonal issues that underpin the forming stage involve getting to know the other members, seeking leadership and direction (Sampson & Marthas, 1990), and wanting to find a place in the group (Woods, 1994). The task issues are initially vague (Woods, 1994), and then members begin to focus on defining their purpose and goals before identifying who has the knowledge and information necessary for the team to be effective (Sampson & Marthas, 1990).

*Storming* is a period of tension and conflict where subgroups begin to form based on mutual interests or similarity in points of view (Sampson & Marthas, 1990). These subgroups may "nitpick," challenge (Woods, 1994), and clash with one another (Sampson & Marthas, 1990). Issues revolve around who is in control (Woods, 1994). Another term for this stage is "taking ownership," which means that members want to shape the purpose and task of the collective to make it meaningful to them (Ontario Healthy Communities Coalition, 2002). If these different viewpoints are not brought out (quietly or loudly), there is a risk that the members will not develop into a team or release their creative energy (Drinka, 1994; Kezsbom, 1992). Be aware that if your team skips this stage, and does not address underlying differences, those conflicts usually emerge later "perhaps to sabotage the group's effectiveness in performing" (Sampson & Marthas, 1990, p. 84).

*Norming* is the stage when emotions have begun to cool down, and practical rules of behavior become established. The members have weathered some conflicts and seek now to develop norms conducive to group cohesion and working together effectively as a team (Sampson & Marthas, 1990).

*Performing* is the high point of team performance: the productive stage in which members have taken responsibility for their individual and collective goals. The team determines the tasks and decisions by consensus (Woods, 1994).

*Ending* is a time for celebration, rituals, and closure. There may be some resistance to ending (a stage sometimes referred to as mourning). Teams must clear up loose ends and unfinished business. Optimistic discussion of future challenges can take place.

The best use of this stage of development model is to be aware that each stage contains tasks that the team must consider and resolve if the effort is to be productive (Sampson & Marthas, 1990). Not all teams evolve in the same way. For example, some authors place norming before storming (Drinka, 1994). However, the most important aspect is that individual members must acknowledge and address differences in the control and direction of the group to reach their potential as a team.

When people work together for longer than a few weeks, the stages of development will often loop back to storming and norming as new challenges emerge; for example, when making a major decision or losing or gaining a member. Even though a team has survived one storming session, more can occur, especially in a dynamic, creative group. Once the team has weathered a storm, further storms can actually be energizing.

## Team Structure and Process

When teams come together, or are brought together, some structures and processes are usually in place. For example, the team comes together for a purpose and may be guided by terms of reference, timelines, and a reporting structure. For student teams, these expectations will be detailed in course outlines, guidelines, or assignments. Working within the structures and processes that are already in place, the team has to create its own operating procedures in order to function effectively. Important actions are to determine key roles and responsibilities, adopt decision-making and conflict resolution processes, and establish an evaluation process.

### Team Leader and Member Roles and Responsibilities

Teams must start organizing at the first meeting in order to start work and bring a feeling of stability to team members. The two crucial roles are that of team leader and recorder. Both are required for a well-functioning team. These roles and their inherent responsibilities will evolve over time.

The **team leader** provides guidance, instruction, direction, and leadership for achieving team goals. In addition to having overall responsibility for the work of the team, the leader serves as the main contact person, organizes meetings, and attends to the morale of the team.

One categorization of leadership styles identifies four types: autocratic, managerial, democratic, and collaborative (KU Work Group, 2013b). Although the overall ideal leadership style in community work would be collaborative, directive styles might be more effective initially to quickly organize the team. Later, a collaborative style will be needed as team members gain in confidence and experience. This change in leadership styles is an additional reason for rotating members in the leadership role.

The person designated as the team leader is responsible for both the task and morale. Functions of this role include organizing to encourage the involvement of all team members and facilitate the progress of the team. Providing structure to team meetings is an important task of the leader. The main tool for doing this is the agenda (see Appendix A.2.4). Prepared according to an established format, the agenda lists the items for discussion in order of importance and provides a space for adding new items. Since an agenda is crucial for a large formal meeting, the leader or recorder usually distributes it by email in advance of the meeting. At smaller, informal meetings, the agenda can be prepared collaboratively at the beginning of the meeting.

The process of chairing a meeting is challenging, particularly at first when everyone is new and unsure of each other and the task. In addition to helping the group to stay on track and on time, the leader has to give everyone a chance to participate. However, effective team functioning is a shared responsibility, and the leader may need to remind members that everyone is responsible for the success of a meeting and has a role to play in identifying and discussing the issues.

One process that helps teams to deal with both task and morale is to schedule a check-in at the beginning of each team meeting and a wrap-up at the end to allow each member a 5-minute (or less) opportunity to share his or her views (Chinn, 2012). With online groups, the check-in should be 100 words or less (Chinn, 2012). The wrap-up provides an opportunity to give feedback on how the meeting went and to identify strengths and areas that need work. The wrap-up session also helps team members see growth from meeting to meeting (Woods, 1994), and ensures that each person feels included and has a chance to speak.

The guidelines in Box 2.3 are appropriate for most meeting situations faced by a team leader.

Monitoring the morale of the team and facilitating rapport is the other main responsibility of the team leader. It is normal to have some fluctuation in team spirit, but the team leader must watch for continuing signs of increased tension or aggression that indicate the need to address underlying concerns. One sign of tension is when team members challenge decisions made by the leader. For example, on one occasion when I was leading a group, I felt it was important to state the group rules at the beginning of each meeting. After the third meeting, one group member said it was boring to hear the rules repeated. After initially feeling defensive, I realized that the comment indicated that the group was ready to take more ownership of the meetings, and we discussed alternative approaches.

The opposite of tension or aggression is lethargy or apathy. A team that has no energy or interest in what is going on is a signal of a need for change. Dealing with apathy can be more difficult than dealing with tension or aggression. A possible option could be to announce something silly or extreme to provoke a reaction and get the team talking about how they are feeling. For example, if the team is trying to come up with ideas to bring older adults together, your suggestions of a karaoke night or an international feast could help to free up creative problem solving.

As well, the team leader needs to be alert to signs that individual team members are experiencing problems or being unproductive. These signs include no longer offering ideas, being overly critical, or not completing delegated tasks. If that occurs, the leader needs to take action. The Ontario Healthy Communities Coalition (2002) offers the following suggestions for handling unproductive behavior by a group member:

- Seek a private time to talk to the person to check out your impressions and find out if there is an issue, such as a personal situation, that needs to be resolved.
- Consider that the person may be action-oriented and need specific tasks, or is visionary and would respond to discussions that are more philosophical.
- Use feedback, such as catching the person's eye and shifting in your seat, to indicate that the person is talking too much, is distracted, or appears bored.

If these measures are not successful, the leader should discuss the situation with someone who has more authority or experience.

The other defined role on the team is that of the recorder or secretary. As the name suggests, the recorder keeps a record of the work of the group in the agreed format and distributes the completed record to the team members and advisors. Similar to the responsibilities of the leader, this role will change over time.

As well as thinking about team tasks and morale, all team members need some idea of what personal goals they could achieve through teamwork. Yalom (1985) identifies two purposes that people have when they first join a group: (1) to determine a method of achieving what they want; and (2) to find a way that they can contribute to the morale or social aspect of the group. Therefore, from its outset, your team needs to help its members meet these goals and contribute to the group. Having a defined task provides confidence and allows each member to integrate and develop a social role within the group.

All members have the potential to contribute something unique and therefore strengthen the team. If everyone did the same thing, the team would be wasting its resources. Initially, a team member will probably apply the knowledge and skills he or she brings to the group. For example, a person might draw on experience as a team leader or working in the community. Initial contributions might also include asking questions, diffusing a heated discussion, or volunteering to identify needed contacts or a piece of research. Once a team member accepts a formal role, he or she will need to define that role more fully. Research on the effect of team building on performance identified role clarification, as compared with other team-building measures, as the most likely to increase performance (Salas, Rozell, Mullen, & Driskell, 1999).

Review Box 2.4, "Who Makxs a Group a Succxss?" to remind yourself of the value of your own, and each team member's, contribution to a group. For you to understand the message in Box 2.4, you need to replace the "x" with the appropriate letter ("e").

> BOX 2.4
> **Who Makxs a Group a Succxss?**
>
> Xvxn though my typxwritxr is an old modxl, it works quitx wxll xxcxpt for onx of thx kxys. I havx wishxd many timxs that it workxd pxrfxctly. It is trux that thxrx arx 46 kxys that function wxll xnough, but just onx kxy not working makxs thx diffxrxncx. Somxtimxs it sxxms to mx that our group is somxwhat likx my typxwritxr—not all thx kxy pxoplx arx working propxrly. You may say to yoursxlf, "Wxll, I am only onx pxrson. I won't makx or brxak thx group." But it doxs makx a diffxrxncx bxcausx for a group to bx succxssful it nxxds thx activx participation of xvxry pxrson. So thx nxxt timx you think you arx only onx pxrson and that your xfforts arx not nxxdxd, rxmxmbxr my typxwritxr and say to yoursxlf, "I am a kxy pxrson in thx group, and I am nxxdxd vxry much."
>
> Source unknown

## Decision Making

The primary and ongoing task of teamwork is to make decisions together. **Team decision making** involves working together to identify an issue, present options to address the issue, critically analyze the options based on external resources and team experience, and reach a consensus on the best option. Critical thinking underlies independent and interdependent decision making (American Association of Colleges of Nursing, 2008). **Critical thinking** involves all or part of the process of questioning, analysis, synthesis, interpretation, inference and deductive reasoning, intuition, application, and creativity (American Association of Colleges of Nursing, 2008). Using critical thinking to make decisions together is one of the features differentiating teamwork from individual work, and it requires some understanding of the different ways that people think and express themselves.

When people start working on a team, they soon realize that people bring a range of opinions and express their views in a variety of ways. This variety of perspectives is one of the strengths of teamwork and requires fostering. For example, research with experienced nurses in acute care settings (Tanner, 2006) indicates that nurses use at least three types of thinking: analytic processes (a back-and-forth comparative process), intuition, and narrative thinking with a story-like delivery. People who express themselves quickly may become impatient with people who tell a story and vice versa. The value of the different approaches needs to be recognized and respected because each type of thinking adds to the effectiveness of the team. Narrative thinking, for example, provides a comprehensive background understanding of how people live (Tanner, 2006), which is consistent with working within the social determinants of health and social justice.

A formal decision-making process can assist your team in organizing teamwork to make effective decisions while considering different perspectives. Decision-making processes usually include the following features (Ontario Healthy Communities Coalition, 2002):

1. Clearly define the problem or issue so everyone understands it.
2. Propose solutions without any negative comments.
3. Analyze the problem from different perspectives. Consider at least two options and identify both the positive and negative consequences for each one. Make an effort to understand viewpoints that differ from your own.
4. Make the decision by choosing the option that is most acceptable to everyone.
5. Establish or revise solution criteria, such as "each decision needs to be acceptable to each member."
6. Evaluate the decision.

This approach is consistent with Tanner's conclusion (2006) that beginning nurses need to use step-by-step reasoning or decision making to generate alternatives, compare them to evidence, and choose the most appropriate solution until they have gained sufficient experience to recognize and respond to patterns.

### Conflict Resolution

Conflict is a predictable part of teamwork, identified as part of the storming stage of development. According to Chinn (2012), conflict is inevitable in any relationship and is not the opposite of harmony. **Conflict** is a difference in values and the emotions associated with the values. People tend to ignore the positive aspects of conflict. If everyone sat in different rooms and did not communicate, there would be no conflict. As well, we would not have access to the creative energy released when a team works through conflict. Matteson and Zungolo (2000) learned that a welcoming attitude toward "creative conflict" was an effective approach when working in the community. Some teams are able to work smoothly through differences as they arise; others benefit from some guidance.

People usually have a preferred method of responding to conflict: they accommodate, withdraw, compromise/negotiate, collaborate, or force/coerce (Drinka, 1994; Woods, 1994). Any or all of these responses can occur at different levels of intensity throughout the stages of development. For example, in forming, accommodation is common; in storming, coercion and withdrawal are prominent (Drinka, 1994). Collaboration is closest to the win-win approach recommended by Schubert (2003) and is most prominent in teams that are in the performing stage. Therefore, the stage of development tends to bring out particular types of conflict, and different members will be more or less involved in conflict depending on the stage and their preferred way of responding.

**Conflict resolution** helps groups work toward common goals (Schubert, 2003), emphasizes joint effort, and confirms the value of other views (Barker, Tjosvold, & Andrews, 1988). Since conflict arises because of differences in values and the emotions associated with the values, resolution needs to address those values. For example, it would be easy for a group to decide on a place to eat when members are hungry, in a food court, with only 30 minutes to spare. Compare this to a value-laden decision on what to serve for an important celebration such as a wedding. Values underlie the sources of conflict identified by different authors: security, control of self and others, respect between parties, and access to limited resources (Lassiter, 2000). Differences in values also contribute to the challenge of identifying group goals and defining group priorities (Kezsbom, 1992).

Differences of opinions are healthy for a group; however, disrespect of other people can be damaging. Respectful behavior means listening carefully to others and explaining your own views thoroughly so others have an opportunity to understand your underlying values. To avoid unnecessary conflict, it is useful for team members to reflect on the four damaging responses—criticism, contempt, defensiveness, and withdrawing, cited by Woods (1994). Discussing these responses and agreeing on an appropriate code of conduct can help the team to reduce the need to correct disrespectful behavior.

An approach that can help the team deal with conflict when it arises is to reject the "tyranny of OR" and embrace the "genius of AND" (Collins & Porras, 2002). Collins and Porras coined these phrases to emphasize that most successful companies and non-profit organizations choose activities that are both mission-driven and profit-driven when developing programs and services, rather than creating conflict by focusing on one or the other. When there is conflict, your team can consider how to accommodate different viewpoints, instead of choosing one over another. The results are likely to be far more creative and exciting.

In essence, conflict resolution is a decision-making strategy; however, it occurs in an atmosphere that is more emotional than most problem-solving situations. Box 2.5 presents a conflict resolution strategy that encourages a "win-win" attitude for all team

---

## BOX 2.5
### Conflict Resolution Strategy

1. **Preparation:**
   - Recognize that the conflict exists.
   - Clarify values, purposes, and goals.
   - Identify that conflict can be positive and move the work and team development forward.
   - Encourage active listening skills to ensure you hear and understand other positions and perceptions by restating, paraphrasing, summarizing.
   - Use an adult assertive approach rather than a submissive or aggressive style.
   - Arrange a meeting in a different location or time to help diffuse negative emotions.
   - Arrange another time if views are initially too strong.
   - Consider asking for outside assistance to mediate the meeting if views remain strong.

2. **Agree on the Problems You Are Trying to Solve:**
   - Identify the essential issues involved in the different positions being taken.
   - Take the time necessary to deal with the situation effectively, including postponing the meeting.

   - Collect information from all members so that each receives equal attention.
   - Ask questions and explore the nature of the conflict in an open and accepting manner.
   - Encourage members to share their feelings as well as their arguments.

3. **Brainstorm Possible Solutions:**
   - Ask the members to identify potential solutions and their consequences.
   - Consider all available options.

4. **Negotiate a Solution:**
   - Use the three guiding principles: Be Calm, Be Patient, Have Respect.

5. **Evaluate:**
   - Ask members to assist in evaluating the effectiveness of the decision.
   - Encourage members to recognize meaningful contributions to the negotiations.

*Sources:* Mind Tools, 2014; Ontario Healthy Communities Coalition, 2002.

members. Teams can practice conflict resolution by first identifying a possible conflict situation and then using the resolution strategy (suggested issues are provided later in this chapter). The more a team uses conflict resolution strategies, the more skilled it will become in accepting conflict as a normal occurrence and learning to tap into the creative energy it provides.

### Self-Assessment and Team Evaluation

As with other aspects of professional practice, team members and teams need to examine their functioning critically. Two levels of reflection or evaluation are involved: self-assessment and team evaluation. **Self-assessment** encourages each person to look critically at his or her individual strengths and challenges and offer them to the team. **Team evaluation** requires the team as a whole to identify team accomplishments and challenges. Both types of evaluation are preliminary to generating ideas for improving effectiveness. For example, reflecting on individual and team practice can help individuals and the team to work through conflict or the storming stage of development.

Individual and team evaluation is usually required of students as part of clinical evaluation and is included in professional and organizational reviews for practicing nurses. Self-assessment or reflection on team performance is similar to procedures used when working independently, except that it focuses on functioning as a team member. According to Schon (1983), reflective practitioners recognize and explore confusing or unique (positive or negative) events that occur during practice as a way of improving practice. Neglecting opportunities to think about what he or she is doing confines the practitioner to repetitive and routine practice.

As students and new practitioners, you will face new and challenging situations as you learn to work on a team and in the community. You are likely to encounter people who live differently than you do, who do not look like you, or who appear to think differently than you do. As you start your work on a team, take some time to reflect on your preconceived ideas or biases about the team members and the population group with whom you are working. In an example from my own early career, I considered moving from an acute care hospital to a long-term care institution. As I thought through the implications of working with elderly people, I remembered the frustration I had felt when an older person moved too slowly in a store or took too long to ask a question. My initial reflections made me realize that I needed to take time to consider the source of these feelings and start dealing with them. Ongoing reflections helped me to slow down and appreciate the opportunity to work with older people.

The Gibbs (1988) **reflective process** is another approach to consider. Gibbs encourages individual practitioners to describe a situation clearly, exploring feelings, evaluating the experience, and analyzing and making sense of it, before choosing options; and then to reflect on the experience to examine what you would do if the situation arose again. The link to an example of using the Gibbs reflective process during a home visit is provided in the reference list (Oxford Brooks University, 2011). A team could use the same cycle to reflect together on a situation they experienced.

### Summary of Team Structure and Process

Learning how to work effectively on a team requires an understanding of the structure and processes needed for effective team functioning. Developing the skills and knowledge related to team organizing is aided by clear, step-by-step procedures, opportunities to practice and accomplish team tasks and develop morale, and use of an evaluative and reflective process. Learning to deal with conflict is the most challenging part. However, conflict can be dealt with calmly and effectively if it is accepted as a normal feature of teamwork and if a resolution process is followed. Evaluation and reflection provide you with the understanding to develop as a professional nurse and to contribute to nursing knowledge. Once you gain experience in working on a team, you will find that your abilities are readily transferable to other situations and that you are more confident in your ability to function as a team member and leader.

## Community Nursing Student Project Teams

In this section, the focus is on students forming a team or joining a team already in place to complete a student project. Although the scenarios involve nursing students, the experience described here—of forming or joining a team—can equally apply to nursing practice situations.

The expectations for team members working on a community project are as follows:

1. Form a team to address a community health issue.
2. Include community members as much as possible.
3. Develop the knowledge and skills of team members.
4. Benefit the organization providing the experience.
5. Achieve community benefits.

### Guidelines for Effective Teamwork

Although working on a team offers considerable benefits, teamwork can be challenging. Research has identified ways of minimizing the drawbacks and improving the effectiveness of teamwork. While this research on the use of student teams in higher education is mainly in the area of engineering and computer science, some general approaches have been identified that provide guidance. The procedures relate to the composition and size of teams, and the structure and processes for collaboration and accountability.

**Team Composition and Size**

The assignment to teams by course organizers can result in either heterogeneous or homogeneous teams. Faculty can form heterogeneous teams based on some criteria such as interests, location, or balancing skills; or form homogeneous teams by allowing students to self-select their own teams. Self-selected teams are considered homogeneous because members often share similar characteristics, such as attitudes and ways of working.

Research supports the choice of heterogeneous teams. For example, when faculty assigns teams in a fair manner to balance skills and perspectives, the mixed teams usually perform better and have better experiences than self-selected groups (Brickell, Porter, Reynolds, & Cosgrave, 1994; Feichtner & Davis, 1984–85; Mannix & Neale, 2005). Furthermore, groups with a heterogeneous mix of skills (e.g., computer, writing, and presentations), academic performance, previous group experience, and ethnicity are generally more productive and creative in the long term than homogeneous (self-selected) groups, even though they may take more time to make decisions (Brower, 1996; Carnegie Mellon University, 2014).

If you are on a self-selected team, you can take steps to expand the team's perspective. Some suggestions are: (a) make a point of changing team roles frequently, (b) pair off in subteams with people you do not know as well as others, and (c) seek and incorporate ideas from your clinical advisors.

Several researchers conclude that teams of four to seven people are the most likely to provide a positive experience for members (Feichtner & Davis, 1984–85; Michaelsen, Knight, & Fink, 2002), to have a diversity of opinions (if the members are heterogeneous), and to produce creative results (Brower, 1996; Carnegie Mellon University, 2014).

One educator with several decades experience in cooperative learning at all levels goes even further, stating, "Four-member teams are magic!" (Keagan, 1998). According to Keagan, as compared to any other number, teams of four maximize and equalize active participation. Keagan qualifies this statement by saying that teams of two can do as well but have the disadvantage of not providing enough diversity of points of view.

Compared to smaller teams, teams of four or more can take longer to develop a trusting/working relationship and need to be aware that individual members may slack off or take over. To compensate for the first concern, larger teams need to give themselves time to develop a working relationship and be alert to the progress of team functioning.

Additional issues may arise with larger teams: those of "social loafing" and "heroism" (Carnegie Mellon University, 2014; Pieterse & Thompson, 2006). Social loafing, also called "slacking" or "free-riding," occurs when a person does not take on a fair workload. Heroism arises when a single team member dominates and takes over all tasks to "save the project." The two are interrelated: social loafing encourages heroism, and heroism increases social loafing. Both have implications for the development of team members. The social loafer will fail to learn either technical or social skills. The "hero" may develop technical skills while excluding others, but fails to develop social skills as a team member and prevents others from doing so (Pieterse & Thompson, 2006). Large teams must be aware of the potential for these issues to develop and prevent them.

Two approaches are recommended to avoid these pitfalls: (1) expect consistent involvement by assigning tasks and requiring a report on the completion of the task from a member or subteam at every meeting (Carnegie Mellon University, 2014); and (2) enable students to flag aberrant behavior by encouraging personal or email contact with the lecturer/instructor (Pieterse & Thompson, 2006). A final measure is to provide the means to expel a member from a team or for a team member to break out from a team (Bacon, Stewart, & Silver, 1999: Pieterse & Thompson, 2006) if the preventive measures are not successful.

There may be no choice in the number of people assigned to a community project because of the numbers available, or because an agency has requested only a certain number of students. The smaller teams of two or three have both advantages and disadvantages that should be considered and corrective action should be taken if necessary.

Two-member teams consisting of students, or a student and a staff member, have certain advantages. The dyad usually communicates easily and completes tasks quickly, which can be an advantage when time is short. However, a two-member team has a more limited variety of perspectives to draw on and may lack the resources to implement plans. In addition, the team can lose considerable momentum when one person is absent. It is particularly important for two-person student teams to recruit community members early and seek advice from key informants.

Three-person student teams have similar advantages and difficulties as a group of two, with the added possibility of one person feeling like an outsider. Members of a three-person team need to acknowledge that there may be a tendency to take sides, and take steps to offset this. For example, the three members can develop a term or code (such as "time out") for a member to use when he or she is feeling excluded.

## Collaboration and Accountability

There is strong emphasis on collaboration in community nursing projects, consistent with community health nursing practice. The collaboration occurs within the student team, with other health professionals, and with members of the community. This collaborative approach fosters an inclusive approach and means that teams need to be accountable to several different parties.

Collaboration is used in two ways in this text: collaboration with the community and collaboration with team members to learn with and from each other. Collaboration with the community involves engaging community members and organizations to arrive at mutually determined goals and to carry out activities. Collaboration with the community is an integral part of the community health nursing process and is discussed in detail in Chapters 3 to 8.

As discussed earlier, collaborative learning is an educational approach that expects team members to be responsible for helping each other to develop new insights and broader perspectives from working together. In the community, team collaborative learning needs to extend to clients and community groups to create unique products that combine theories, concepts, ideas, talents, and perspectives.

Students preparing to work in clinical teams need clear expectations and defined responsibilities to be accountable (Carnegie Mellon University, 2014). Generally, nursing programs specify the requirements for the community clinical experience in documents such as course outlines and clinical guidelines, or make them available in a handout or on the course website. The specifications, such as clinical hours and location, requirements for assignments, and the criteria for individual and team evaluations provide a frame of reference to help the team members meet the expectations for the clinical education experience. Usually, the faculty instructor reviews the expectations for the clinical education in some depth during the student orientation.

Researchers have identified three factors that consistently contribute to successful team-based learning (Michaelsen et al., 2002). These three factors have been adapted to provide a framework for accountability:

1. Individual team members are accountable for: (a) preparation, (b) contributing adequately to team assignments, and (c) collaboration with others.
2. Instructors provide a simple form or tool for team members to document their accountability for team decision making and reporting.
3. Instructors and community advisors provide ongoing and specific feedback to individual team members and the team.

Community nursing projects address these requirements in several ways. As part of the orientation to the community experience, students learn about several tools to help them prepare for teamwork and the community project. The tools include the following: pre-clinical self-assessment, team agreement, weekly report, and evaluation tools (see Appendix A.2).

**Pre-clinical self-assessment** prompts students to reflect on their past team experiences to identify what they will bring to the clinical experience and what they would like to get out of it (Carnegie Mellon University, 2014). Completed ahead of time, the self-assessment prepares students to discuss and negotiate how they will work together as a team to meet the goals of the community clinical experience.

A **team agreement** identifies the goals for the community clinical experience in three areas: (1) team process, (2) professional accountability, and (3) professional attitude and behavior. Each area includes questions to stimulate discussion based on team members' experiences and resources such as this text, together with course outlines, clinical policies, and guidelines. Once the team has decided on an approach for each item, the decisions are documented and the draft team agreement is submitted to the clinical instructor.

In most cases the team agreement can be completed during weeks one and two of the clinical experience. It is a working document that helps guide and monitor progress and evaluation throughout the community clinical experience. As the team gains experience, they may modify the document to incorporate new learning on what works well for the team.

Completing the team agreement together is a good way to start the team's collaborative learning experience. Each person first shares his or her own perspective from the pre-clinical assessment. Each person then participates actively in the give and take of the discussion. Finally, the completed agreement is a concrete example of shared knowledge creation. The document is different from anything any one member could have done alone.

The **weekly report** is a brief form used to detail and inform relevant people of what the team accomplished during the week and what they expect to do the following week. It is the most important tool for team organization and communication. Consistent use of the weekly report is key to demonstrating accountability for the community project.

Box 2.6 lists the items included in the weekly report. This concise report, summarizing the work of the team, is prepared jointly and sent by email to the team members, clinical instructor, community advisor, and others, such as a manager or community members, as necessary. The clinical instructor uses the weekly report to monitor team progress and provide feedback. An upcoming scenario includes an example of a completed weekly report.

The report guides the team through the items that need to be discussed and reported each week and provides an alternative to communication methods usually found in institutional settings, such as end-of-shift reports. The

---

**BOX 2.6**

**Weekly Report**

Distribution List:

Date Completed and Sent:

Team Members Present:

A. Purpose of Activities This Week [Linked to project work plan/timeline (see Chapters 3 and 4)]

B. Activities, Decisions, Results, and Timing for the Week:

C. Plans for Next Week, Meetings, and Upcoming Activities:

D. Comments or Questions:

E. Team Evaluation:

weekly report should generally be one-half to one page in length and take no more than 15 to 30 minutes to complete once the team is familiar with what is expected in each section. More details and explanations related to the project will be included in other forms introduced in later chapters.

The report provides the means for the team to document, practice, and provide professional accountability to each other, to the clinical instructor and community advisor, and indirectly to the community group. The weekly reports are working documents for the team and provide content for the project report. Weekly reports are not included in the final project report attachments.

## Overview of Teamwork during the Three Periods of the Project

Once the student team meets, learns about the assignment, and has discussed team roles and responsibilities, teamwork on the project can begin. From experience, we find the projects fit into three periods: getting organized, getting things done, and finishing up. The next sections discuss team development during these periods, and the use of the team forms. We mention other forms, such as the project timeline/work plan and project report, but leave discussion of those project forms to later chapters. Chapter 8 expands on this for the final period of the project—finishing up.

In each period, we consider three areas: (1) team organization, (2) team rapport, and (3) evaluation of self and team. Consistent attention to these aspects of team development, combined with determined efforts to harness the knowledge, skills, and abilities of the team members, will help you build a team and complete a project that makes a difference.

### Weeks One and Two: Getting Organized

When the team first comes together, members will be motivated to clarify expectations and organize themselves. Table 2.3 outlines the tasks and tools related to team functioning in the first two weeks.

At the first meeting, the team might choose to address the three areas of teamwork in any order. For example, your team might find it easier to start to build team rapport by sharing information, drawing on the pre-clinical assessments (see Appendix A.2.1) in a round-robin and allowing 2 to 3 minutes for members to introduce themselves. Prior completion of the self-assessment form means that everyone is prepared and the process will go more smoothly. On a second turn around, each person might identify one thing he or she wants to get out of the experience.

Determining an initial team leader and recorder will provide structure to the team and help to make sure that the team speaks with one voice. The team needs to revisit the team roles and responsibilities at regular intervals and during evaluation to clarify roles and sharing, or rotating, responsibilities.

Another primary organizing task is to lay the ground rules on how the team is to function. The team agreement form (see Appendix A.2.2) provides some questions to guide the discussion on how the team will work together to complete the community project. In some ways, the completed form resembles a contract, a commitment to

Sharon, the clinical instructor, supervises three student teams, each with four students. The teams are in different organizations not far from each other: a women's drop-in center, a high school, and a public health nursing infant immunization program provided through well-baby drop-ins. Only the team working with public health has a Registered Nurse as an advisor/preceptor. During the weekly clinical hours, the students work as a team with a variety of people: (a) the advisor or contact person assigned by the placement organization, (b) a community group, (c) the clinical instructor, and (d) other staff or organizations as needed. The locations where the teams interact with people in the community vary for each placement.

Sharon explains that she is particularly interested in teams learning team and collaboration skills. Not only will this help to ensure that their community work makes a difference, but the students will then feel they have accomplished something worthwhile as well as having developed leadership skills to benefit their future career.

All three teams feel overwhelmed when they first start to organize. They feel that they are juggling two different aspects of nursing, working both in the community and on a team.

Sharon informs the teams that they need to complete four tasks: (1) determine a team leader, (2) decide how the team will make decisions, (3) decide how and when members will communicate with each other and the instructor, and (4) draft a team agreement. She explains that after orientation she will not be so specific but will expect the team to keep up with requirements on their own.

The team working with public health begins by discussing how they will get around to the different well-baby drop-ins to identify common issues related to immunizations. They soon realize they need more information and will wait until their placement orientation at public health. After they review their pre-clinical individual assessments, they are quickly able to identify who has the necessary experience and is willing to be the first leader and recorder. As well, the group agrees that they want everyone to participate in making the decisions and carrying out the work. The recorder leads the team in completing the first weekly report with him.

In the second week, the team feels the resolve to work on things together has really been paying off. The public health nurse advisor and clinical instructor tell the team they are pleased with their work, which was complete and on time.

**Discussion Topics and Questions**

5. Discuss the advantages and disadvantages of working in the community both with and without a community or public health nurse as advisor in the placement.

6. Why is documentation in the form of a weekly email report especially important in a community clinical experience?

# First Weekly Report

Distribution List: (students) Helen, Jennifer, Carry, Geoff (recorder), Sharon (instructor), (preceptor/advisor to be added at public health orientation)

Date Completed: Sept. 12, 2015

Team Members Present: Students listed above present all day

## A. Purpose of Week's Activities (give number and step in timeline—see Chapters 3 and 4):

- Organize team by deciding on leader, decision making, communication, and drafting a team agreement (Step 1).

## B. Activities, Decisions, Results, and Timing for the Week:

- Team activities—2 hours
- Completed the four assigned tasks: Identified Carry as leader and Geoff as recorder and agreed to use consensus decision making. (In future, the team will follow the weekly report format.) Team will communicate with each other by email. Drafted team agreement that included importance of weekly team evaluation for review by clinical instructor, and prepared weekly report to get feedback from instructor (and the advisor next week when we have her email). We will submit our weekly report by 16:00 hours at the end of clinical.

- Open discussion on what we want to learn at orientation. We decided that each member would bring two questions to public health orientation. Sent weekly report in body of email and draft agreement as an attachment to clinical instructor at 16:00.

## C. Plans for Next Week, Meetings, and Upcoming Activities:

- Orientation (tomorrow) at public health, 1414 Health Benefits Street, Room 400, at 08:30.
- Meet with preceptor/advisor to obtain details of next two weeks—each member to ask prepared questions if information not provided.

## D. Comments or Questions:

- Will we go together as a group to the well-baby drop-ins, or will we go in pairs or individually?

## E. Team Evaluation:

- At the end of our meeting, we used a round-robin to ask each member about their first impressions: how they had contributed to the group, what they liked, and what they wanted changed. Each person identified a role and seemed pleased with their contribution. Two people concurred that the members were being especially "nice" to each other, rather than a more natural give and take. The leader commented that in the weeks to come we will likely want to have more "niceness"!

**Table 2.3: Tasks and Tools for Weeks One and Two**

| Focus | Tasks | Tools and Location |
|---|---|---|
| Team organization | Identify initial clinical expectations and guidelines (e.g., clinical days, links with clinical instructor, assignment/reports).<br>– determine team leader and recorder<br>– discuss expectations for each role<br>– complete team agreement using information from the pre-clinical assessments<br>– complete weekly report | Clinical expectations and guidelines (course documents)<br>Tools in text (see Appendix A.2):<br>– pre-clinical self-assessment<br>– team agreement<br>– weekly report |
| Team rapport | Share experience and interests:<br>– Identify what you can contribute to team.<br>– Identify what skills/experience you would like to gain from teamwork.<br>– Discuss what the team would like to accomplish by the end of the project. | Tools in text (see Appendix A.2):<br>– pre-clinical self-assessment<br>– team agreement |
| Evaluation | Evaluate team functioning:<br>– Evaluate team functioning in forming team and preparing weekly reports.<br>– Take all members' views into account.<br>– Conduct formal evaluation if required by course requirements. | Clinical expectations for evaluation (course documents and appendices)<br>Tools in text (see Appendix A.2.2):<br>– team agreement<br>– weekly report |

working together in a certain way to meet objectives and satisfy member needs and preferences. It is a working document and can be adapted as necessary. Your organization or the educational institution may specify some items for the agreement; your team discussions will yield further items.

Completing the first and second weekly reports is another team task that will help the team put in place a daily routine that will likely change over time. A routine that the authors have found to be effective is for the team to complete the report at the end of each clinical day or week of work on the community project. You can use the items in the weekly report to form the team meeting agenda. The weekly report refers to linking activities to the steps you will be covering in the project work plan and timeline. You will learn about these tools in Chapters 3 and 4 and can review them in sections A.3.1 and A.3.2 of the Appendix.

It is important for team members to reflect on and evaluate progress. This requires the team to consider the progress of the team project and to determine if the team is working together in a supportive and satisfying way to meet both team and individual goals. In other words, the team must evaluate tasks and morale. Review the evaluation forms and expectations to ascertain when they are to be completed.

## Weeks Three to Eight: Getting Things Done

By week three, the team will have established relationships with the clinical instructor and community advisor and acquired a working knowledge of the neighborhood. As team members make connections with a community group and the project takes shape, they will have a clearer idea of where they are going. Assessment of the community will become a major focus. They should be starting to feel part of a team and be addressing the tasks and tools in Table 2.4. The table refers to forms related to planning and completing the project that will be introduced in upcoming chapters.

In this six-week period, the team has been together long enough for the relationships to mature or perhaps show signs of strain. This is the time to reflect on the forming, storming, and norming stages of team development and on the knowledge and skills acquired by team members. Recognizing the need for conflict resolution and dealing with conflict is a worthwhile team skill to develop. While few people enjoy confrontation, it is unwise to ignore concerns. For example, if you are reluctant to go to a team meeting, this could be a sign that the team is experiencing conflict. Sometimes you can identify what is making you uncomfortable, but often the tension comes from feeling that you cannot express your views openly. It is likely that if you are feeling tense or stressed over goals and priorities, other members will be feeling the same. To move your group toward becoming a team, you must bring your feelings out in the open in a way that the team can deal with constructively. Being open and honest about how you are feeling can help others to do the same, thereby triggering a release of tension.

To open up the discussion, your team may decide to role-play conflict resolution using a silly or relevant example (e.g., what would the team do if one member came to clinical

**Table 2.4: Tasks and Tools for Weeks Three to Eight**

| Focus | Tasks | Tools |
|---|---|---|
| Team organization | Review and possibly reassign the team roles and responsibilities at some time during this period to give everyone an opportunity to try the leadership roles. | Clinical expectations and guidelines in course documents |
| | Update team agreement as necessary. | Tools in text (see Appendix A.2 & A.3):<br>– weekly report<br>– timeline/work plan<br>– final report |
| | Complete weekly reports. | – team agreement |
| Team rapport | Share learning and identify what skills you are gaining and would like to gain from remaining experience. | Tools in text (see Appendix A.2.2):<br>– team agreement |
| | Reflect on team rapport. | |
| Evaluation | Reflect on the progress of the project and team performance, including feedback from the clinical instructor. | Clinical expectations for evaluation<br>Tools in text (see Appendix A.2 & A.3):<br>– team timeline/work plan<br>– self-/team assessment forms |
| | Complete individual and team midterm evaluations as indicated in course documents. | |

Rumblings that started at the third meeting of the public health team erupted at the fourth meeting. Two team members feel the recorder is bugging them too much about what goes into the weekly report; the others feel it is important for everyone to be involved. The team goes through the conflict resolution process, described above, and eventually agrees that it is time to clarify their roles.

Geoff explains that, as team recorder, he feels he should keep track of the decisions made by the team and distribute the finished weekly report. He is finding it difficult to get team members together to make the decisions necessary to complete the report. While listening to his frustration, the others come to realize and accept that the whole team is responsible for the decisions that go into the report. They use brainstorming to identify what is important to them: being a well-functioning team, recognizing the contribution of members, and sharing the load. Moving on, they decide on a consistent time and place to meet

at the end of the day to work on the report, thank Geoff for his work, and agree to rotate responsibilities for the leader and recorder roles. The outgoing leaders will work with their replacements until they feel comfortable. Two team members volunteer to update the team agreement and bring it back the next week for review by the team and clinical instructor.

By the fifth week, everything seems to be on track again. People are smiling and commenting that they are glad that they made the effort to "clear the air." They feel the discussion helped them learn more about each other and develop trust. Geoff jokes that he has "battle scars," but he really is feeling quite proud of being able to speak up and having the team listen to him.

**Discussion Topics and Questions**

7. What is beneficial and challenging about dealing with conflict?

8. What are the benefits of mentoring someone to take over the recording role?

covered with paste-on tattoos, or if a member was consistently late or unprepared). Effectively dealing with conflict is a great excuse to celebrate your team development. Humor is really helpful.

When conflict emerges, the team roles and responsibilities may require clarification. An important team skill is sharing the workload and learning to delegate tasks to individuals or subgroups. When delegating responsibilities, team decision making and documentation becomes even more important to ensure that communication and accountability is maintained. Rotating the leadership roles will give team members the opportunity to take on responsibility and develop skills and to experience different leadership styles.

Your educational program or placement organization may provide you with a required team evaluation form for midterm and final evaluations. If other forms are not available, the team or instructor may choose to ask members to complete the Self-Assessment of Functioning on Team (Appendix A.2.6) and Individual Assessment of Team Functioning (Appendix A.2.7). A tool for self-reflection of an event is also available (Appendix A.2.5). By discussing the results, your team can consider different ways to improve your team functioning.

## Weeks Nine to Twelve: Finishing Up

In the final weeks of the project, the team concentrates on bringing the project and the clinical experience to a satisfactory conclusion. Table 2.5 indicates a shift toward completion of the project and the preparation of final reports. The scenario in Chapter 8 provides more details on team development during this phase.

**Table 2.5: Tasks and Tools for Weeks Nine to Twelve**

| Focus | Tasks | Tools |
|-------|-------|-------|
| Team organization | Reconsider team roles and responsibilities in preparation for completing the project. | Clinical expectations and guidelines<br>Tools in text (see Appendix A.2 & A.3):<br>  – weekly report<br>  – timelines/work plan<br>  – final report<br>  – team agreement |
| Team rapport | Reflect on team morale.<br>Share learning and identify what skills/experience you have gained from teamwork and can use elsewhere.<br>Celebrate success. | Tools in text (see Appendix A.2 & A.3):<br>  – pre-clinical self-assessment<br>  – team agreement |
| Evaluation | Assess self and team functioning.<br>Evaluate relevance of the project to team, clinical instructor, community advisor, and community group. | Clinical expectations for evaluation<br>Tools in text (see Appendix A.2 & A.3):<br>  – team agreement<br>  – self-/team evaluation forms |

## Building a Sense of Accomplishment

As you develop skills as a community health nurse, you will come to realize that opportunities to get feedback from clients and instructors are often limited in the community. Reasons for this involve working on a team in a complex environment where change occurs over a long period. The team can address this lack of or limited feedback by making a particular effort toward building a sense of accomplishment for each other and the team. A **sense of accomplishment** means that a person or the team feels that they are achieving or have achieved what they set out to do. Each member can contribute to the sense of accomplishment by taking the time and effort to acknowledge the small things that occur each day, such as when someone comes up with a new idea, helps someone understand an issue, finds the information you need, runs a good meeting, or prepares a complete and timely report. Thanking a team member or instructor can become contagious!

Another activity that provides a sense of accomplishment is working with community members to create an enjoyable activity that they feel will improve health. Enjoyable activities greatly improve the experience for everyone. Music and food are multinational and intergenerational and bring people together. You can capitalize on activities that are already in place, such as church meetings, sports events, club meetings, and other community events, to provide opportunities to contact people where they live and play, and determine what interests them and what they enjoy.

A sense of accomplishment is also necessary for the effective functioning of your team. This comes from regularly looking back on your work to identify what you have learned from both your failures and your successes. You will probably find that you develop inside jokes that deal with behaviors that are disruptive to the team. For example, in one of my team experiences, I had a habit of giving out orders until one of my team members started responding with "Aye, Aye, Captain!" When the team is under a lot of stress, try to insert some humor. Humor allows people to relax and view things differently. Remember to plan social events, as minor as "toasting" with a coffee cup to a full party, when you have reached a milestone in the project.

The effectiveness of the community project depends on team members who are committed to following a process of working with each other and with the community. A sense of accomplishment may evolve quickly when both tasks and moral functions work well, or can take more time because of issues beyond the control of the team. A sense of accomplishment and enjoyment is the lubricant that smoothes the process.

## Summary

Chapters 1 and 2 introduce community health concepts, theories, and a process to follow when learning how to practice as a community health nurse. This chapter explains two foundational components of community health nursing: community health nursing projects and team development. Two scenarios based on actual team projects illustrate the overall idea of working on a project. Team development begins by providing theory related to teams, moves through the development of team roles and skills, and ends by providing procedures and tools to fulfill team responsibilities to both the project and each member's professional development. Table 2.6 summarizes the five stages of team development in relation to the three required team functions.

Although the theory, knowledge, and skills are important, one factor that will make a difference in what the team, team members, and community gain is developing a sense of accomplishment. Taking time to recognize successes, deal fairly with issues, and actively involve the community and organizations will help you develop a sense of accomplishment.

## Classroom and Seminar Exercises

1. Identify a conflict situation from previous teamwork and apply the conflict resolution process.
2. Using team situations you have been involved in, describe and discuss each of the five stages of development reached by the team.
3. Develop a team agreement for your team using the form in Appendix A.2.2.
4. Prepare a weekly report after your orientation to the clinical setting, or one that the public health team in the scenario might have sent after the conflict resolution meeting.

**Table 2.6: Summary of Effective Team Development**

| Stage | Team Organization | Documentation and Communication | Self- and Team Evaluation |
|---|---|---|---|
| Forming | Set up team procedures and assign tasks to individual members. | Initiate team agreement and weekly report. | Share skills and resources brought by team members. Document evaluation of team in weekly report. |
| Storming | Identify differences and resolve to find common ground and develop rapport. | Identify and discuss issues related to documentation and communication based on feedback from clinical instructor and advisor. | Evaluate ability to identify and deal with conflict in weekly report. |
| Norming | Revise group process as the project evolves. Include opportunity to perform new roles. | Revise procedures for documentation and communication following discussion of issues. | Evaluate team functioning in terms of team agreement and program requirements, revising team agreement as necessary. |
| Performing | Monitor tasks for fairness and completion. | Monitor and adjust based on feedback. | Evaluate completion of tasks and rapport in weekly report. |
| Ending | Ensure equitable completion and show appreciation to advisors and placement site. | Communicate final plans and results. Submit final reports. | Evaluate team functioning in terms of team agreement, team learning, and program requirements. |

# References

American Association of Colleges of Nursing. (2008). *The essentials of baccalaureate education for professional nursing practice*. Retrieved from www.aacn.nche.edu/publications/position-statements

Bacon, D., Stewart, K., & Silver, W. (1999). Lessons from the best and worst student team experiences: How a teacher can make the difference. *Journal of Management Education, 23,* 467–488.

Baker, D. (2001). The development of collective efficacy in small tasks. *Small Group Research, 32*(4), 451–474.

Barker, J., Tjosvold, D., & Andrews, I. (1988). Conflict approaches of effective and ineffective project managers: A field study in a matrix organization. *Journal of Management Studies, 25*(2), 167–177.

Bender, P., Tanner, C., & Chesla, C. (2009). *Expertise in nursing practice: Caring, clinical judgment, and ethics* (2nd ed.). New York: Springer Publishing.

Brickell, J., Porter, D., Reynolds, M., & Cosgrave, R. (1994). Assigning students to groups for engineering design projects: A comparison of five methods. *Journal of Engineering Education, 7,* 259–262.

Brower, A. (1996). Group development as constructed social reality revisited: The constructivism of small groups. *Families in Society, 77,* 336–344.

Carnegie Mellon University, Eberly Centre. (2014). *Group projects*. Retrieved from www.cmu.edu/teaching/designteach/design/instructionalstrategies/groupprojects/index.html

Caruso, H. M., & Wooley, A. W. (2008). Harnessing the power of emergent interdependence to promote diverse team collaboration. *Diversity and Groups, 11,* 245–266.

Chinn, P. (2012). *Peace & power: Building communities for the future* (8th ed.). Sudbury, MA: Jones & Bartlett.

Collins, J., & Porras, J. (2002). *Built to last: Successful habits of visionary companies.* New York: HarperCollins.

Diem, E., & Moyer, A. (2010). Development and testing of tools to evaluate public health nursing clinical education at the baccalaureate level. *Public Health Nursing, 27,* 285–293. doi:10.1111/j.1525-1446.2010.00855.x

Drinka, T. (1994). Interdisciplinary geriatric teams: Approaches to conflict as indicators of potential to model teamwork. *Educational Gerontology, 20,* 87–103.

Ellis, D., & Fisher, B. (1994). *Small group decision making: Communication and the group process* (4th ed.). New York: McGraw-Hill.

Engleberg, I., & Wynn, D. (2000). *Working in groups: Communication principles and strategies* (2nd ed.). Boston: Houghton Mifflin.

Feichtner, S., & Davis, E. (1984–85). Why some groups fail: A survey of students' experiences with learning groups. *Organizational Behavior Teaching Review, 9,* 58–71.

Gibbs, G. (1988). *Learning by doing: A guide to teaching and learning methods.* Oxford, UK: Further Educational Unit, Oxford Polytechnic.

Keagan, S. (1998). *Teams of four are magic!* Retrieved from www.kaganonline.com/free_articles/ dr_spencer_kagan/ASK03.php

Kezsbom, D. (1992). Re-opening Pandora's box: Sources of project conflict in the 90's. *Industrial Engineering, 24*(5), 54–59.

Kozar, O. (2010). Towards better group work: Seeing the difference between cooperation and collaboration. *English Teaching Forum, 2.* Retrieved from http://americanenglish.state.gov/ files/ae/resource_files/48_2-etf-towards-better-group-work-seeing-the-difference-between-cooperation-and-collaboration.pdf

KU Work Group for Community Health and Development. (2013a). Building teams: Broadening the base for leadership. *Community Tool Box* (Chapter 13, Section 4). Retrieved from http://ctb.ku.edu/en/tablecontents/sub_section_main_1123.aspx

KU Work Group for Community Health and Development. (2013b). Styles of leadership. *Community Tool Box* (Chapter 13, Section 3). Retrieved from http://ctb.ku.edu/en/table-contents/sub_section_main_1122.aspx

Lassiter, P. (2000). Group approaches in community health. In M. Stanhope & J. Lancaster (Eds.), *Community & public health nursing* (5th ed., pp. 458–473). St. Louis, MO: Mosby.

Mannix, E., & Neale, M. A. (2005). What differences make a difference? The promise and reality of diverse teams in organizations. *Psychological Science in the Public Interest, 6*(2), 31–55.

Matteson, P., & Zungolo, E. (2000). Educating nursing students in the neighborhoods: Lessons learned. In P. Matteson (Ed.), *Community-based nursing education: The experience of eight schools of nursing* (pp. 224–228). New York: Springer.

Michaelsen, L., Knight, A., & Fink, L. (2002). Getting started with team learning. Chapter 2 in *Team-based learning: A transformative use of small groups.* New York: Praeger.

Mind Tools. (2014). *Conflict resolution.* Retrieved from www.mindtools.com/pages/article/ newLDR_81.htm

National Survey of Student Engagement. (2006). *Engaged learning: Fostering success for all students.* Retrieved from http://nsse.iub.edu/NSSE_2006_Annual_Report.pdf

Ontario Healthy Communities Coalition. (2002). *From the ground up: An organizing handbook for health communities.* Retrieved from www.ohcc-ccso.ca/en/from-the-ground-up

Oxford Brooks University. (2011). *Reflective writing: About Gibbs reflective cycle.* Retrieved from www.brookes.ac.uk/services/upgrade/study-skills/reflective-gibbs.html

Pieterse, V., & Thompson, L. (2006). *A model for successful student teams.* Proceedings of the 36th SACLA Conference (p. 195). Retrieved from www.cs.up.ac.za/cs/vpieterse/pub/ PieterseThompson.pdf

Robbins, H., & Finley, M. (1995). *Why teams don't work: What went wrong and how to make it right*. Princeton, NJ: Peterson's/Pacesetter Books.

Salas, E., Rozell, D., Mullen, B., & Driskell, J. (1999). The effect of team building on performance: An integration. *Small Group Research, 30*(3), 309–329.

Sampson, E., & Marthas, E. (1990). *Group process for the health professions* (3rd ed.). Albany, NY: Delmar.

Schon, D. (1983). *The reflective practitioner: How professionals think in action*. New York: Basic Books.

Schubert, P. (2003). Caring communication and client teaching/learning. In J. Hitchcock, P. Schubert, & S. Thomas (Eds.), *Community health nursing* (2nd ed., pp. 219–248). Clifton Park, NY: Delmar Learning.

Spector, N. (2010). Collaboration: A nursing perspective. In B. Freshman, L. Rubino, & Y. Chassiakos (Eds.), *Collaboration across disciplines in health care* (pp. 107–132). Sudbury, MA: Jones & Bartlett.

Strom, P., Strom, R., & Moore, E. (1999). Peer and self-evaluation of teamwork skills. *Journal of Adolescence, 22*, 539–553.

Tanner, C. (2006). Thinking like a nurse: A research-based model of clinical judgment. *Journal of Nursing Education, 45*(6), 204–211.

Tuckman, B., & Jensen, M. (1977). Stages of small group development revised. *Group and Organizational Studies, 2*(4), 419–427.

Woods, D. (1994). *Problem-based learning: How to gain the most from PBL*. Waterdown, ON: Donald R. Woods.

Yalom, I. (1985). *The theory and practice of group psychotherapy* (3rd ed.). New York: Basic Books.

## Website Resources

KU Work Group on Health Promotion and Community Development, *Building Teams: Broadening the Base for Leadership*: http://ctb.ku.edu/en/tablecontents/sub_section_main_1123.aspx

These KU web pages discuss teams and team building, advantages and disadvantages of teams, what makes a good team, and how to build a team.

KU Work Group on Health Promotion and Community Development, *Training for Conflict Resolution*: http://ctb.ku.edu/en/tablecontents/sub_section_tools_1164.aspx

This KU web page provides a series of questions to guide you in determining your interests and those of your opponent to help you deal with conflict.

Registered Nurses of Ontario, *Healthy Work Environments Best Practice Guidelines: Collaborative Practice among Nursing Teams*: http://rnao.ca/sites/rnao-ca/files/Collaborative_Practice_Among_Nursing_Teams.pdf

*Embracing Cultural Diversity in Health Care: Developing Cultural Competence*: http://rnao.ca/sites/rnao-ca/files/Embracing_Cultural_Diversity_in_Health_Care_-_Developing_Cultural_Competence.pdf

The RNAO Best Practice Guidelines provide recommendations related to a topic for individual nurses, the organization, and external context. The recommendations for individual nurses for cultural diversity are provided in three categories: self-awareness, communication, and new learning.

Part 2

# The Community Health Nursing Process and Community Health Nursing Projects

Part 2 of the text engages students in learning community and public health nursing practice by completing a community health project. The six chapters in this section are organized around three interrelated themes: (1) gaining knowledge and skill in applying the community health nursing process, (2) learning about community health nursing by completing a community project, and (3) teamwork. Each chapter immerses the reader in a realistic team-based community project and examines the concepts and skills appropriate to successive phases of the nursing process.

The first three chapters orient students and new practitioners to the community and to community health assessment: Chapter 3 addresses the establishment of relationships within a project and community, and the assessment of secondary data; and Chapters 4 and 5 discuss approaches for gathering primary data from community groups, and working collaboratively with a community group to interpret data and identify health issues. Chapters 6 through 8 are concerned with planning, taking action, evaluating, and bringing the project to a satisfactory conclusion. This completes the cycle of assessment, planning, action, and evaluation within a community project. Teamwork, as discussed in Chapter 2, evolves throughout the project phases. (The following box provides an outline of the chapters in Part 2.)

You will find that the chapters weave together relevant theories, concepts, and principles, building on each other to illuminate the knowledge, skills, and attitudes to support community health nursing practice and teamwork. The numerous case studies provide insight into the various ways that community health nurses engage with community partners, build partnerships, and promote community health as they practice in a variety of community settings and with diverse populations. At the end of this section of the book, you will have acquired basic knowledge and skills for practice and teamwork and come to appreciate the potential of community projects for learning about community health nursing.

## Overview of Part 2

### Chapter 3
Starting well: Beginning a community project starts the assessment process with orientation to the team, the project, and the collection of secondary data.

### Chapter 4
The assessment of the neighborhood and community group expands the assessment with the collection of primary data.

### Chapter 5
The analysis of assessment data draws together primary and secondary data sources to identify priorities for action and conclude the assessment process.

### Chapter 6
Planning the action involves examining the theoretical frameworks for intervention and describing the planning process.

### Chapter 7
Taking action provides the practical considerations for carrying out a planned intervention.

### Chapter 8
Ending well addresses the evaluation of a community project, preparation of a summary report, and drawing community relationships to a satisfactory conclusion.

# Starting Well: Beginning a Community Health Nursing Project and Assessement— Steps 1 and 2

· · · · · · · · · · · · · · · · · · · · · · · · · · · · · · · · · · · · · · · · · · · · · · · · · · · · · · · · · · · · · · · · · · · · · · · · · · · · · · · · · · · · · ·

Applying the community health nursing process within the context of a community project provides the framework for this chapter. For student teams, getting started involves developing collegial relationships, becoming oriented to the community project and the sponsoring organization, and taking the first steps toward learning about the community through an assessment of secondary data. The steps are expanded in Box 3.1 below.

Entering the community and learning how to practice nursing in this new and what may appear to be relatively unstructured setting can be unnerving for students and new practitioners alike. What challenges might you anticipate? Even though you know what it is like to live in a community, you require an orientation to the world of community health nurses. This involves many new relationships—with the student team, mentors in the community organization, and community members. Getting to know the community and learning about the place and the people in order to promote healthy communities is an important focus. Learning how to conduct a community needs assessment introduces the skills and knowledge that will prepare you for practice. In this chapter, students are introduced to the epidemiological constructs used to describe the health of populations. They are directed to essential information resources such as policy documents and learn how to draw the information together to guide practice. This chapter draws on the themes of teamwork outlined in Chapter 2 and provides students with strategies for organization, decision making, and evaluation. The scenarios in this chapter feature students in a community health center learning how to include activity in a health promotion program for older adults.

## Learning Objectives

· · · · · · · · · · · · · · · · · · · · · · · · · · · · · · · · · · · · · · · · · · · · · · · · · · · · · · · · ·

After reading this chapter and answering the questions throughout the chapter, you should be able to:

1. Establish working relationships within a community project.

### Key Terms and Concepts

census data • epidemiology • gatekeepers • incidence rate • morbidity data • mortality data • preferred health situation • present health situation • prevalence rate • primary and secondary data • sociodemographic data

Today, the students will meet their community advisor at the Summertown Community Health Center (SCHC) for the first time. In preparation for the assignment, their faculty clinical instructor advised them that their project concerned health promotion with older adults and directed them to the organization's website. The students feel excited and a little apprehensive when they report to their advisor, Jeanine, the nurse manager of health promotion services.

After making introductions, Jeanine explains her role and gives the students a brief orientation to the health center before reviewing the expectations for the clinical placement. The students learn that SCHC is the lead organization in a community coalition of health services and community groups to promote active living. The coalition is well organized and has coordinated several community projects over the past five years. Currently, the coalition is developing a project to increase the participation of older adults in community groups that promote active living as a way to prevent chronic disease. The steering group for the project includes a member of the SCHC board, two representatives from the Council on Aging (COA), a fitness instructor from the city Recreation Department, Jeanine, and a nurse practitioner from the health center. The COA has compiled recent research about the evidence of strong links between activity and the prevention of chronic disease, such as type 2 diabetes. Knowing there is a high prevalence of diabetes in older adults, they plan to discuss prevention in the project proposal to increase the possibility of obtaining support from agencies that fund diabetes prevention.

As part of their orientation, the students will review the existing data on the population and the health issue. Further details of the project will be worked out over the next two weeks. After orienting themselves to the health center, the students leave feeling they have jumped in at the deep end but are eager to get started. On their next clinical day they will meet with the nurses who lead a health and wellness group for older adults at the health center.

**Discussion Topics and Questions**

1. As a member of the student group in the above scenario, what information would you seek out at the orientation to the community organization?
2. Discuss the role community members might play in developing programs on priority health issues.

For suggested responses, please see the Answer Key at the back of the book.

2. Understand the different perspectives of the community and appreciate the relevance of community assessment to community projects.
3. Identify the theories, concepts, and components of a comprehensive community health assessment.
4. Appreciate the responsibility of the community health nurse to involve communities in health assessment.
5. Explain how to locate and analyze sociodemographic and epidemiological data and key policy documents.
6. Conduct a document review and organize information according to the community health nursing process.

## Orient to the Community Project (Step 1)

The first steps of a community assessment—getting oriented to the community and developing the knowledge and skill for community assessment—are foundational to all community projects. These first two steps are expanded in Box 3.1 below. Subsequent

**Steps 1 and 2 in Completing the Community Health Nursing Project**

ASSESS
1. Orient to community project
   a. Establish relationships
   b. Define the project, population group, and issue
2. Assess secondary data
   a. Review sociodemographic data
   b. Review epidemiological data on health status
   c. Review previously conducted community surveys and program statistics
   d. Review national and local policy documents
   e. Review literature and best practice guidelines
   f. Summarize secondary data

3. Assess physical and social environment
4. Assess primary data
5. Analyze assessment data

PLAN
6. Plan action

ACT
7. Take action

EVALUATE
8. Evaluate results and complete project
9. Evaluate teamwork

steps in the community health nursing project are emphasized in later chapters as you learn more about community health promotion.

A community project, as conceived in this text, is sponsored by a community organization and conducted with community members. The projects, which are designed to enable students and new practitioners to learn about community health nursing, provide an entry to a complex world. Since these projects take a considerable amount of time, resources, and coordination, it is important to prepare well. Advance planning provides direction for the project and, if done with community input, allows you to draw on the experiences of others. As well, talking things through ahead of time helps to ensure that the resulting action will be relevant, supported, and sustained. A systematic approach is essential.

The majority of student projects are embedded in broad community health initiatives and relationships that extend beyond the timelines of a student clinical experience. Usually, health providers and/or members of a community group or organization have done some preliminary work on their own before they consult with the nursing faculty to identify settings and topics that student projects might address. Therefore, learning about the history of your project and the context of practice is an important aspect of orientation. In addition to becoming familiar with the placement or sponsoring agency at this first meeting, students will be initiating work relationships and finding out how to establish contact with the community group. These activities will help to clarify the focus of the project so that it can be shaped to meet the needs of both the community and student learners.

## Establish Relationships (Step 1a)

The faculty clinical instructor responsible for your student group will link you to the community organization and to your community advisor. A primary consideration is to clarify roles and relationships. You may find that the advisor will supervise the project as part of his or her workload as a public or community health nurse. Or, in settings where an experienced community health nurse is not available, your instructor may co-supervise with a responsible person from the organization, considered an advisor, mentor, or community contact. For example, if you were working with a class of students learning English, the teacher and instructor might share supervision. In this way, your student group has access to nursing expertise as well as community "know-how."

Plan to learn as much as you can about your community organization. Although your community advisor is your main resource, you will probably have contact with others within the organization. As well, certain aspects of your work may require you to follow organizational procedures, which can take time. For instance, in health organizations, activities involving community members will probably be governed by protocols and may require managerial approval. Getting to know the organization, its mandate, and how it functions will help you to understand the working environment and help to make your community experience run smoothly.

Effective communication is crucial to the success of community projects, so start out by scheduling regular face-to-face meetings with your team and advisors. Frequent meetings are needed initially. Later on, meetings can be shorter or more spread out, but are still necessary to monitor progress and to plan. If meetings are not prescheduled, you may find that you lose valuable time trying to have a decision approved. Meeting face-to-face provides the opportunity for the advisors and team to establish relationships, develop trust, and learn from each other. Such opportunities may be limited in community settings where practitioners work independently and are not always on-site, so it is better to arrange regular meetings from the start.

You are likely to meet many new people in different settings in the first few days in the community, which can be confusing. Keep track of all those involved in the project and understand your responsibility to them and their responsibility to you. For example, at organization meetings, record the names and positions of people who are present, or who are identified, by name, contact information, and their relationship to the project (see example in Table 3.1 below). People do not mind signing a sheet or telling you who they are and how you can contact them. Your advisor can help you to do this. Since changes often occur, keep the list up to date.

As discussed in Chapter 2, patterns of communication and documentation systems vary from organization to organization. From the outset, it is important to clarify expectations regarding the usual methods of communication, for example, face-to-face meetings, email, or telephone, and the expected response time to messages. As well, confirm the process for submitting weekly reports, which summarize progress and flag future direction, at this time. Regular, timely, and relevant communication is basic to maintaining good relationships with everyone concerned with the project.

### Identify Community Contacts

Some student teams will work directly with a community group, while others will be based in an organization such as a public health department or community health center that has ongoing links with a number of groups in the community. If there is no opportunity to meet with community contacts at orientation, the student team needs to explore how to engage with community members in the first weeks of the project. This requires some forward planning. Your advisor can facilitate entry to the community, for example, by providing contact information and by introducing students at a meeting. These early meetings with community members will assist in your team's orientation to the community and are a first step toward building relationships that can progress into collaboration with a community group.

Keep in mind that this process takes time. It is important to keep track of your interactions with community members to identify people who can help your project in some way, sometimes called gatekeepers. **Gatekeepers** are people in formal or informal positions who control access to the community group. Examples of gatekeepers are school principals, teachers, the manager of a business or firm, or volunteers active in community organizations such as tenants' associations. Remembering names and learning "who's who" helps in the orientation to any work setting.

## Define the Project, Population Group, and Issue (Step 1b)

At the orientation meeting with the community organization, it is customary to discuss the rationale for your project and to reach agreement on the specific goals. Usually, this will include a review of the historical perspective and key events that led to the initiation of the project. For example, you may find that the project is addressing an emerging health issue or that the organization has initiated the project in response to requests from a community group. Although this may not seem significant at the time, it will help you to understand the broad influences on community health.

Additional background information will be uncovered over time. Since student projects are not usually fully defined at the outset, ask questions to clarify your purpose. You may feel uncomfortable doing this, particularly when taking on a new role in an unfamiliar setting (and perhaps not wishing to appear inexperienced). Although these feelings are understandable, remaining silent does not give the project organizers or community contacts an indication of your interests, or of what you know and what you want to know. One method to get past any awkwardness is for each team member to prepare one question for meetings with different groups. Questions can encourage a discussion and lead to greater understanding while demonstrating the team's interest in the project.

As well as learning specifically about the project, you need to learn about other community organizations or agencies involved in the project and their particular interests. The mission statement or mandate of the lead and other organizations and the priority for the project are usually well documented, and it would not be unusual to find that many community agencies have a long history of working together. Although mandates tend to be written in broad terms, they provide context and direction. For example, if an organization is funded to provide health promotion services for a defined geographical area and the goal of your project is to increase mobility in older adults, then the project will have to be relevant to all older adults in the area, not just those who attend a particular health center.

The steering group meeting starts promptly. There is a printed agenda, and the nurse practitioner volunteers to record the minutes. After introductions, Jeanine provides a brief overview of the coalition for the students' benefit. Members from the Council on Aging (COA) talk about their organization and the importance of mobility for healthy aging. Clearly they are very excited about the student involvement and provide four copies of physical activity guidelines for older adults (Canadian Society for Exercise Physiology [CSEP], 2012; US Department of Health and Human Services, 2008; World Health Organization, 2010a) for the students to take away and read.

Jeanine leads a discussion on roles and responsibilities. She explains that under her guidance the students will begin by reviewing previously collected demographic data and existing information on the health status of older adults in the community. This will help to inform the proposal. The working group developing the project proposal would like to include these statistics in the first draft, which is due in four weeks. They invite the students to attend the meeting where the draft will be discussed. Other committee members will read and comment on draft reports and attend meetings every other week to discuss progress.

The students are eager to start. They feel they will have time to contribute some of the necessary statistics, which they need for their own project. Acting on a recommendation from the health center board member, the dates for the steering group meetings are set before they adjourn. After the meeting, the students arrange weekly meeting times with Jeanine and start to put together the contact list, as shown in Table 3.1.

On the way to the bus, the students agree that Jeanine is very well organized, and they feel confident in her ability to guide their project. Darren says, "I can't believe it; they really were pleased to have us helping." Lise agrees, but says, "This increases the pressure to do well. I know I will feel better once we get started, but right now, I wish I felt more certain about what to do. What if we gather the wrong information?"

**Discussion Topics and Questions**

3. Think about the community where you live, and identify what community groups might be interested in participating in a coalition to promote active living.
4. The students have been asked to contribute to the presentation of statistics at the coalition meeting. Identify what skills they might bring to this task.

## Community Health Assessment

Assessment refers to the process of gathering information from a variety of sources to understand the present situation of a community group and its preferred health situation to generate information for health planning. The **present health situation** includes community assets or strengths, such as people with skill in solving community problems, or other resources, such as an unpolluted environment. As well, it includes barriers to good health, or potential areas for improvement. The **preferred health situation** refers to the changes or improvements in health desired by the community group. Health providers often use the term "needs assessment," but this term tends to focus attention on problems to be solved, rather than on abilities that might be strengthened (Heaven, 2014; McKnight & Kretzmann, 1997). Both perspectives are important.

As with the assessment of individual and family health status, community assessment is an iterative process, although considerably more time-consuming and complicated. Communities are complex social systems when compared with individuals and families. There are many different aspects of a community that the team needs to consider, and there are many different sources of information to draw upon. Gathering

**Table 3.1: Project Contact List**

| Project Contact List | | | |
|---|---|---|---|
| **Name** | **Position** | **Email and Phone/Reporting Frequency** | **Relationship to Project** |
| Jeanine Roger | Community health nurse; manager of health promotion services | jroger@work 555-6666 ext. 226 Include in weekly summary. | Clinical Advisor Provides direction for project (in person and by email). Chair of community coalition. |
| Jan Surrey | University faculty | jsurrey@university 444-3333 ext. 123 Include in weekly summary. | Faculty Clinical Instructor Provides direction in person and by email. Responsible for student evaluation. |
| Jean Morrow | Manager of community programs | jmorrow@work 444-3333 ext. 345 (ext. 346 Exec. Assistant Simon) Fax 333-4444 | Approves staff time for student project. Reports to executive. Approves questionnaires. |
| Kerri Czabo | Fitness instructor, Recreation Department | kczabo@city | Director of fitness programs in city apartment buildings. Developed chair exercises for less active older adults. |
| Rita Valli | Nurse practitioner | rvalli@work 555-6666 ext. 543 Works 2 p.m. to 8 p.m. weekdays. | Runs fall prevention clinic. Knowledgeable about physical activity and older adults. |
| Ruth Hemliner | Executive Director, Council on Aging | rhemliner@agency 456-7890 ext. 456 Works Monday–Thursday. Steering group only. | Founding member of community coalition. Knows everyone! Contact for information on coalition. |
| Ed Jones | Member of SCHC Board | ejones@home Steering group only. | Chair of planning committee (retired city planner). Contact for copy of last community needs assessment. |

this information provides the opportunity for community members to engage in a collaborative process and thereby increase the relevance of health planning. In turn, this is expected to improve health outcomes, as noted in a comprehensive introduction to the key principles in planning, designing, and implementing community engagement efforts (see McCloskey et al., 2011).

Community participation is a key principle of primary health care; however, health providers report that it is not easy to engage communities in the assessment, planning, and evaluation of health programs. This is consistent with the evidence that the nature and level of community involvement varies widely (Rifkin, 2009). Putting resources into building knowledge and skills so that individuals and communities can participate in decision making about health is arguably a necessary step toward improving health equity (Brennan Ramirez, Baker, & Metzler, 2008; Edwards & Moyer, 2000; Rissel & Bracht, 1999). In this text, collaboration with the community is seen as an essential part of the community health nursing process. At the same time, we acknowledge that the potential for collaboration can vary considerably from one community to another. To be effective and achieve results, collaborating with the community requires sustained effort.

## Conceptualizing Community for a Community Health Assessment

Perspectives of community and community health help to frame a community assessment. While there is no universally accepted definition of "community," the term usually refers to a group of people who live within a geographical area, or who have a common interest, and are part of a complex system of networks and associational ties (Hampton & Heaven, 2014; Israel, Checkoway, Schultz, & Zimmerman, 1994). Two different perspectives of community and community health that underpin community health practice are the community as social setting and the community as client.

Originally explicated by Hawe (1994), these two perspectives are not easy to untangle. The first perspective views the community as a social setting with a powerful and incompletely understood influence on individual and group health and health behavior. According to Hawe, the social setting encourages or rewards certain behavior. By implication, when seeking to change health behaviors, like smoking or activity levels, it is not sufficient to ask individuals to change behavior; rather, it is necessary to change the social and physical environment that supports the behavior. For example, laws against smoking in public places, increases to the price of cigarettes, and bans on the sale of tobacco to adolescents combine to create an environment that discourages the initiation of smoking in youth. By changing the environmental cues, in a phrase coined by Milio (1976), the healthy choices become the easy choices. Working within this perspective of community as social setting, health providers encourage community participation with a view to changing the social environment. Following community organizing principles, they gain entry to the community, engage residents, and harness community resources to achieve professionally defined health goals, such as smoking cessation and active living.

The second perspective described by Hawe (1994) is the community as a complex human system in dynamic and mutually influencing interaction with its environment. From this perspective, community health refers to the ability of the community as a social system to take control, solve problems, and adapt to change (Goodman et al., 1998). Building on earlier work by Bronfenbrenner (1979), ecological models of health acknowledge that human subsystems—individuals, families, groups, and organizations—form an integral part of the whole, but view the community as greater than the sum of its parts (McLeroy, Bibeau, Steckler, & Glanz, 1988; Sallis, Owen, & Fisher, 2008; Stokols, 1992, 1996). This is the same as viewing an individual as more than his or her physiological, psychological, social, and spiritual systems and a family as more than the sum of its individual family members. The overarching goal of health action from this perspective of community is to strengthen the capacity of the community to function effectively as an integrated whole and to be healthy. From this perspective, the health status of individuals, families, and groups is just one measure of the health of the community.

Clearly, the way you think about community and community health provides a framework for determining what data is collected in the community assessment and how it is collected. In the first model described, the community assessment process is more likely to be professionally driven and focus on identifying the resources for, or need for, specific evidence-based health promotion and prevention interventions. Capacity building may be seen as a means to an end. In the second model, capacity building is the central aim. Community assessment is used as a means to engage the community in a capacity-building or problem-solving process that will identify opportunities for mobilizing resources and building community capacity (Labonte, Woodard, Chad, & Laverack, 2002). Approaches such as CHANGE—Community Health Assessment aNd Group Evaluation (Centers for Disease Control and Prevention [CDC], 2010), and the Community Health Needs Assessment for Canadian First Nations and Inuit communities (Health Canada, 2000)—seek to be more community-driven. However, health providers are usually involved and can take advantage of the opportunity for capacity building. More and more, both approaches are entwined.

## Components of a Community Health Assessment

Community health is a multidimensional concept, and, traditionally, a community assessment contains the following components: a demographic profile of the population; a description of the patterns and variations in health status; and information on the physical, sociocultural, and political aspects of the community that impact health (Anderson & McFarlane, 2010; CDC, 2010; Rissel & Bracht, 1999). These socioenvironmental factors, commonly referred to as the determinants of health, or social determinants of health, were introduced in Chapter 1.

A comprehensive community assessment is a large and costly undertaking and is usually facilitated by professional teams. Fortunately, much of the information that is required to inform health planning can be assembled from a range of existing data sources; for example, data collected by government on an ongoing basis, such as births, deaths, records of childhood immunization; census data; and data collected routinely by health authorities to inform planning. Often referred to as **secondary data**, because the data were originally collected for other purposes, they may not answer specific questions that are of interest to you. **Primary data**, on the other hand, is collected directly from community residents and health service providers to provide specific information.

Gathering secondary data is not unlike the inquiry a community health nurse might undertake when starting a new position, or the process that a community group might undertake before developing an agenda for health action. Gathering information is a learning process, and knowledge is power.

# Assess Secondary Data (Step 2)

The purpose of assessing secondary data is to learn what is already known about the population and health issues of interest, and about the determinants of health relevant to that population. The following list provides the six substeps of this component of the community assessment. The order of the first five is not significant and may be adjusted according to need:

a. Review sociodemographic data
b. Review epidemiological data on health status
c. Review previously conducted community surveys and program statistics
d. Review national and local policy documents
e. Review literature and best practice guidelines
f. Summarize secondary data

## Review Sociodemographic Data (Step 2a)

**Sociodemographic data** includes characteristics of the population and information on social patterns, especially age structure, which are crucial for health planning at national, regional, or provincial and local levels. The census, which is conducted on a regular basis, is a key source of this data. **Census data**, collected by household, includes the number of people in the household by age, sex, marital status, occupation, and other variables, such as income and ethnicity. Census reports provide a profile of the population as a whole at one point in time and allow comparison between and within different regions of the country (see US Census Bureau and Statistics Canada in "Website Resources" for this chapter). The census can also be used to identify trends and make projections about what the population will look like in the near future. When reviewing demographic data, remember that some groups, for example, the homeless and illegal immigrants, are not accurately represented in the census. In addition, some numbers are based on self-identification and therefore may be unreliable for health planning. For instance, there is reliable evidence that Aboriginal peoples may not self-identify or are incompletely enumerated (Smylie, 2000).

It is much easier to assemble sociodemographic information when the community or population of interest is identified geographically using the commonly accepted boundaries defined by the census. Census information is aggregated from the census divisions to provide community-level data. Usually these boundaries correspond to recognizable neighborhoods, but it is essential to check. There is easy access to aggregated census data for cities and planning regions in the United States and Canada, but it may not be necessary to consult these sources. Departments of public health, regional health authorities, or local planning groups compile community profiles routinely to guide decision making.

When beginning a community project, knowing the boundaries of your community of interest is important. Planning a search strategy and documenting it accurately saves time in the end. Once you identify what data will be useful to your project and where to find it, develop a set of questions to guide your search for sociodemographic data. Box 3.2 provides a sample set of questions that can help to structure the search and provide a framework for collating the information that you find.

## Review Epidemiological Data: Measuring Health Outcomes, Risk Factors, Health Practices, and the Social Determinants of Health (Step 2b)

Reading and interpreting health surveys and reports to gather information on the health status of your population of interest and health determinants is a key part of the community assessment. This requires a working knowledge of epidemiology, the science concerned with the patterns of health and illness in the population. According to Last, **epidemiology** is "the study of the distribution and determinants of health-related states or events in specified populations and the application of this study to the prevention and control of health problems" (as cited in Bonita, Beaglehole, & Kjellström, 2006). You may find it useful to consult a basic epidemiology text (e.g., Bonita et al., 2006) if you are not familiar with epidemiological concepts and methods. The self-study courses listed in "Website Resources" at the end of this chapter are another option.

A basic method of epidemiology is to count the frequency of health outcomes, or events such as live births, and to estimate proportions or rates in populations. By comparing the rates between different people, places, and times, it is possible to identify the patterns of health and illness and look for trends. The two most commonly used rates, which all nurses should understand, are the prevalence rate and the incidence rate.

The **prevalence rate** is a measure of the number of persons with a condition in a group or population at a given time. This is expressed as a rate per unit of population (K), for instance, the number of cases per 100,000:

$$\text{Prevalence} = \frac{\text{Number of existing cases in place at point in time} \times K}{\text{Number of persons in place at midpoint of year}}$$

Prevalence rates provide a useful snapshot of chronic health conditions, such as diabetes. Applying the rate to a population of interest gives a working estimate for the purpose of planning health resources. In order to make comparisons, prevalence rates have to be adjusted for age because the prevalence of disease varies by age. For example, in 2010, the prevalence of diabetes in US residents, 20 years and older, was 11.3 percent, compared to a prevalence rate of 26.9 percent in people 65 years and older (National Diabetes Information Clearinghouse, 2013). The higher rate reflects that type 2 diabetes is a disease associated with aging. Standardization of the rates, usually by age, enables comparison across place and time. For instance, a report from a national surveillance system, using age-standardized data, shows the prevalence of diagnosed diabetes in Canadians 1 year of age and older has increased by 70 percent, from 3.3 percent in

BOX 3.2

**Sample Questions on the Community and Population**

- What are the boundaries of my community of interest?
- What groups in the community are of particular interest to me (e.g., men and women aged 65 years and older; new immigrants)?
- What is the profile of this subgroup (e.g., by gender, language, education, income, housing, and living conditions)? How does this profile compare with the community as a whole?
- Will the size of this subgroup increase or decrease in the next 10 years?
- Where does this subgroup live in the community? Are members spread evenly throughout the community, or do they tend to settle in some areas rather than others?

1998/99 to 5.6 percent in 2008/09 (Public Health Agency of Canada, 2011, p. 17). This comparison confirms that the burden of diabetes in the population, and on the health care system, is steadily increasing.

**Incidence rate** is a measure of all new cases arising in a population at risk during a defined period, usually one year.

$$\text{Incidence} \quad = \quad \frac{\text{Number of new cases in place during time of observation} \times K}{\text{Population in place at midpoint of time}}$$

Incidence provides information about the rate of development of a condition in a population, that is, the increase in new cases over a specified period of time. Birth rates and death rates are special cases of incidence referring to the number of people being born or dying in a specific place and at a specific time.

Measures of morbidity, mortality, and well-being provide a snapshot of health and disease in the population. **Mortality data** are compiled from death certificates and have long been used as a proxy measure of health or life expectancy. When standardized for age, the data can be used to pinpoint the primary causes of death by life stages. Other measures, such as untimely death or potential years of life lost (PYLL), are calculated from mortality data. This tells you how many years of life a person has lost, compared to the average for the population (usually taken as 75 years). PYLL can be used to compare the benefits of different types of interventions to extend life.

**Morbidity data** provide information on the major burden of illness in the population. For example, incidence data on common communicable diseases such as measles and chickenpox and seasonal influenza (flu) is collected locally and aggregated to inform health service planning, locally, nationally, and internationally. National public health surveillance systems, such as the US Centers for Disease Control and Prevention (CDC) and the Public Health Agency of Canada (PHAC), compile the information, track the incidence rates, and submit to the World Health Organization as part of a global tracking system. Monitoring the trends provides advance warning of outbreaks. Data on the incidence and/or prevalence of conditions such as sexually transmitted infections (STI) and chronic disease, symptoms of ill health, and risk behaviors (e.g., smoking or engaging in unprotected sex), together with indirect measures of ill health, such as days of work lost, provide comparative measures of ill health in a population. Similarly, information is collected on indicators of health and wellness, such as perceived health and health practices (e.g., regular visits to a doctor or midwife during pregnancy), together with information on lifestyle behaviors known to promote or pose a risk to health (e.g., eating habits, daily exercise, social relationships). Together, these measures of health and illness provide a comprehensive picture of the health of a population.

### Gathering Information on the Social Determinants of Health

Data on the social determinants of health, such as poverty, gender, and the environment, are constructed from census data and routine household surveys. When using the data to compare populations, it is important to understand how the constructs were conceptualized and measured. For example, the United States has an official measure of poverty (US Census Bureau, 2014). However, in Canada, as in most countries, poverty is measured in a variety of ways; no one measure is used consistently (Canadian Council on Social Development, 2001). As an example, one study exploring the relationship

**Figure 3.1: Activity Limitations in Adults 65 Years and Older by Socioeconomic Status (SES)**

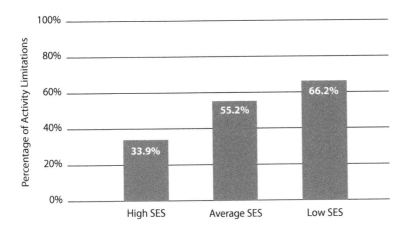

*Source*: Adapted from Predy, G. N., Edwards, J., Fraser-Lee, N., Ladd, B., Moore, K., Lightfoot, P., & Spinola, C. (2008, November). *Poverty and health in Edmonton* (p. 26). Edmonton, AB: Public Health Division, Alberta Health Services (Edmonton Area). Retrieved from www.albertahealthservices.ca/poph/hi-poph-surv-hsa-poverty-and-health-in-edmonton-2008.pdf

between poverty and health in an urban population (Predy et al., 2008, p. 26) uses socioeconomic status (SES) to examine the impact of poverty on the health of adults, 65 years and older. In the population studied, approximately two-thirds of the respondents with low SES had activity limitations, compared with only one-third of adults with high SES (see Figure 3.1). Although the relationship was not statistically significant, the figure graphically illustrates that poverty is an important determinant of health, measured here as activity limitations.

There is abundant evidence that health is strongly influenced by social factors but the pathways are not self-evident. Understanding the mechanisms underlying the relationship between socioeconomic status and other social determinants of health is the subject of intense study. The World Health Organization framework for action on the social determinants of health (Solar & Irwin, 2007) summarizes the competing arguments used to explain the relationship between the unequal distribution of income and health in Table 3.2.

### Sources of Secondary Data

There are many sources of routinely collected data pertinent to health. As previously noted, the census, vital statistics, and national disease surveillance systems monitor health and illness. In addition, national agencies, such as Statistics Canada and the US Centers for Disease Control National Center for Health Statistics monitor a broad range of social, economic, and environmental topics (see "Website Resources" at the end of this chapter). Some important sources and types of data are summarized in Table 3.3 below. Becoming familiar with key data sources is essential learning for community health nurses.

Departments of public health, regional health authorities, or local planning groups often have responsibility for assembling and publishing regional or community profiles to guide health policy and decision making. The reports usually draw together information on health and the determinants and on a broad range of risk and protective health behaviors from national, regional, and local health surveys. These reports may be

**Table 3.2: Explanations for the Relationship between Income Inequality and Health**

| Explanation | Synopsis of the Argument |
|---|---|
| Psychosocial (micro): Social status | Income inequality results in "invidious processes of social comparison" that enforce social hierarchies, causing chronic stress and leading to poorer health outcomes for those at the bottom. |
| Psychosocial (macro): Social cohesion | Income inequality erodes social bonds that allow people to work together, decreases social resources, and results in less trust and civic participation, greater crime, and other unhealthy conditions. |
| Neo-material (micro): Individual income | Income inequality means fewer economic resources among the poorest, resulting in lessened ability to avoid risks, cure injury or disease, and/or prevent illness. |
| Neo-material (macro): Social disinvestment | Income inequality results in less investment in social and environmental conditions (safe housing, good schools, etc.) necessary for promoting health among the poorest. |
| Statistical artifact | The poorest in any society are usually the sickest. A society with high levels of income inequality has high numbers of poor and, consequently, will have more people who are sick. |
| Health selection | People are not sick because they are poor. Rather, poor health lowers one's income and limits one's earning potential. |

*Source*: Solar & Irwin, 2007, Table 1, p. 31, attributed to Macinko, Shi, Starfield and Wulu, 2003.

organized by population group—children; pregnant women; adults, and seniors (Chief Provincial Public Health Officer, 2011)—or by social determinants, such as poverty (Predy et al., 2008).

More and more health information is available online from interactive databases. For example, the Illinois Project for Local Assessment of Needs (IPLAN) database assembles county- and community-level reports based on a health assessment and planning process that is conducted every five years by local health jurisdictions (Illinois Department of Public Health, 2009). IPLAN reports can be displayed for a single health indicator, or a range of indicators, by state or county or community. Similarly, the Canadian Community Health Survey (Statistics Canada, 2013) collects data at the sub-provincial level on health status, health care utilization, and health determinants. A core questionnaire on over 300 topics enables comparison across reports. Summary tables and reports on the various topics, by health region(s), can be accessed on the Canadian Institute for Health Information (CIHI) website.

Online health information databases are increasingly being used to identify priorities and support health planning at the community level. Having access to such data enables community participation. For example, the websites of the US Department of Health and Human Services *Community Health Status Indicators* (2009) and the Robert Wood Johnson Foundation and Wisconsin Population Health Institute (2012) provide access to county health rankings, together with tools to design a roadmap to health planning. (See "Website Resources" in this chapter.)

## Review Local Surveys and Program Statistics (Step 2c)

Local public health units, community health agencies, and health and social planning departments periodically assess community needs and resources to inform planning.

**Table 3.3: Sources of Readily Available Health Data**

| Type of Data | Data Source | Comments |
|---|---|---|
| Sociodemographic variables (e.g., age, gender, by geographical area) Some data on health determinants (e.g., income and education) | Census data | – Census uses standard questions<br>– Data are available for the whole population |
| Mortality by cause of death, age, and gender | Vital statistics (e.g., registry of deaths) | – Comprehensive<br>– Not a sensitive measure of health but provides information on ill health and preventable causes of death |
| Morbidity data<br>– Incidence and prevalence of specific conditions | Communicable and Notifiable Disease Reports (e.g., Influenza surveillance; Cancer Register) | – Disease registries are limited to a few conditions |
| Proxy measures of morbidity | Hospital discharge data<br>Drug utilization data<br>Workplace injuries | – Emphasis on conditions requiring medical treatment |
| Health behavior and practices (e.g., type and level of exercise and activity; patterns of mammography uptake) | National or regional health and social surveys | – Provides a profile of the population as a whole, but the sample sizes may not be large enough to provide details for a specific area |
| Physical, social, and environmental determinants of health | National data on Education, Housing, and Employment<br>Air pollution index<br>Crime statistics | – Relevant to population/ community as a whole |
| Needs assessments of communities and population groups | Local surveys and research reports | – Can be tailored to a specific focus<br>– Data may not be comparable |

These assessments are tailored to local needs and thereby provide more detailed information on a community, or particular segments of it, than national reports. Consultation with the community is a key part of the assessment process, and the resulting reports are rich repositories of up-to-date health information that may not be available elsewhere. Routinely collected data on the utilization of health services and program evaluations are another valuable source of community data.

The collection of health and wellness data presents many methodological difficulties, which should be kept in mind when reading health reports. For instance, when the presence or absence of illness is determined through self-reporting, as in many community studies, it may contain inaccuracies. As well, health behavior may be overestimated or underestimated, perhaps because of a desire to present a good picture, or because it is difficult to remember accurately. For these reasons, well-designed national and regional surveys with large samples and standardized approaches are required to ensure reliable and valid data. Smaller-scale surveys may provide equally valid and reliable data, but the measures may not be comparable to those used in previous studies or in other regions. All this is to say that it is important to review data collection methods to know what questions were asked in a study and how the data were processed.

Before initiating any costly data collection process, it is wise to review the existing

After the steering group meeting, the students begin to draw together the secondary data that will inform their project. They intend to have it ready for discussion at the next meeting. Following advice, they familiarize themselves with a recent report that includes demographic and health data on adults 65 years and older for the health region, which includes both the city where the Summertown Community Health Center is located and the surrounding rural area. This will provide a sufficiently large population for obtaining meaningful health statistics. After a lively discussion on the best way to proceed, the students develop questions to guide their search and then split up to work in pairs. Robin and Darren choose to review the demographic information, leaving the review of health data to Lise and Mika. At the end of the second week on the project, the students report that there are 73,520 adults, 65 years and over, in their region. They put together a population pyramid and numerous tables to show a further breakdown of the population by 10-year intervals, gender, income, living arrangements, and other characteristics. A key find is a report classifying city neighborhoods by socioeconomic status (see example in Predy et al., 2008, Appendix A).

**Discussion Topics and Questions**

5. Identify your community. In a small group, discuss the boundaries and explain what community means to you.

6. Using your own community as an example, discuss ways in which the community reinforces healthy or unhealthy behavior, such as physical activity.

data. Not only does a systematic analysis of what is already known save time and avoid duplication of effort, but it also helps to focus the inquiry. Since secondary data were collected for other reasons, it will be necessary to think carefully about what information you need. Formulate questions to guide your search. Then identify and locate suitable data sources, extract pertinent information, and assemble it in such a way as to tell a story. The "story" you want to tell will comprise the summary of secondary data referred to in Box 3.1, which will be used to inform your project. Think of it as building a jigsaw puzzle. The order in which you retrieve the information is not crucial; you can start at any point and gradually fill in the pieces until, at the end of this exercise, you have as complete a picture as possible and understand how the pieces fit together. A thorough examination of existing data will help you to understand the patterns of health and illness in your community or population.

## Review Policy Documents (Step 2d)

National and regional governments provide broad direction for health through public policy documents and strategic plans that direct funding. These policy frameworks ensure a common understanding and promote consistent approaches toward achieving health goals. A review of policy documents relevant to your population of interest and health focus will help to situate your project in relation to the broader community health concerns.

Becoming familiar with these key documents is important because they are likely to contain the most pertinent and up-to-date research on the topic. The World Health Organization (WHO) pursuit of the goal of "Health for All" (WHO, 1978), with its emphasis on health promotion, is a good example. Over the last 30 years there has been a shift in emphasis from the provision of health services to the provision of a broader range of resources for population health. Compelling evidence, such as the fact that globally, a quarter of all preventable illnesses are the result of the environmental conditions in which people live, later underpinned the *Adelaide Statement on Health in All Policies* (WHO, 2010a). In this statement, all sectors of government are encouraged to include health and well-being as a key component of policy development. In this way, policies, based on evidence and grounded in common values, facilitate decision making about health across different sectors.

In recent years, governments in Western countries have produced a number of policy documents that endorse a population health approach. Typically, these documents acknowledge the need to invest in improving living and working conditions, as well as health services, for a healthy population. They also signal the intent to use comprehensive and collaborative approaches to improve health outcomes through action on the determinants of health. For example, a population health framework and action guidelines can be found on the Public Health Agency of Canada (2012) website, and the concepts are carried forward in collaborative federal, provincial, and territorial government initiatives, such as the Integrated Pan-Canadian Healthy Living Strategy (Secretariat for the Intersectoral Healthy Living Network, 2005) and in health planning documents (British Columbia [BC] Office of the Provincial Health Officer, 2010, p. 21).

The United States and England take this planning a step farther. In addition to articulating national population health strategies, they identify priority areas, and set national goals or targets with timelines for achievement. For example, the recently updated US *Healthy People 2020: Framework* (US Department of Health and Human Services, 2010) identifies four overarching goals that are intended to inform national and state health planning. Similarly, in England, the most recent public health strategy, *Healthy Lives, Healthy People* (Secretary of State for Health, United Kingdom, 2010), commits to protecting the population from serious health threats; helping people live longer, healthier, and more fulfilling lives; and improving the health of the poorest, fastest. These approaches build on the framework for addressing health inequities in the final report of the WHO Commission on Social Determinants of Health, led by Sir Michael Marmot (Commission on Social Determinants of Health, 2008).

In turn, the international and national strategy documents provide direction for state, provincial, and territorial planning authorities. For example, *Healthy People 2020* encourages states, cities, and communities to set health goals based on national objectives. In Canada, federal, provincial, and territorial Ministers of Health agreed to a set of broad health goals in 2005, which are expected to inform provincial and territorial public health objectives (PHAC, 2006a). The next steps are being examined (Chia & Phillips, 2010). As noted above, health goals guide the development of some health policy frameworks (BC Office of the Provincial Health Officer, 2010, p. 21).

Other useful sources of health policy documents are the World Health Organization and the Pan American Health Organization (PAHO). Voluntary and nongovernmental organizations, special interest groups, and professional bodies also produce health policy documents for their own ends and to influence government policy. Nowadays, many of these documents are available on the Internet. At the local level, most organizations have policy documents, and strategic and operational plans that guide planning decisions. It is not realistic to try to provide a comprehensive list of data sources because the production of health information is an iterative process. At the end of this chapter, you will find a list of key national websites, which will provide an entry point for locating health strategy documents.

These health strategy documents and work plans are a valuable resource. Not only do they articulate the conceptual models of health that are guiding decision making, but they also present up-to-date analyses of the epidemiological and experimental evidence on which population health needs and priorities are based. Considerable work has gone into putting together this evidence base to guide health planning and policy. In addition to identifying priorities, and providing detailed and specific direction on effective interventions, the documents also guide funding allocations. Understanding policy frameworks and aligning new programs with priority areas increases the probability of gaining support for community health initiatives.

**Determining a Population-Based or Issue-Based Direction for Community Projects**
At this point it is useful to reflect on the many different starting points for community health projects. Sometimes a project starts with questions about a geographically defined population, for example, the residents of a rural community, perhaps further defined by age (e.g., all adults older than age 65 living in the rural area of a community) or by developmental stage (e.g., adolescents, or pregnant women and their families). A variation of this approach is to focus on community settings such as workplaces and schools that provide access to certain populations and, like communities, provide an environment that influences health and well-being. Alternatively, projects might take as their starting point a population group such as single parents or Aboriginal men thought to be at high risk because of lifestyle or other risk factors, or through inequitable access to the social determinants of health.

Other starting points are a health issue or concern, such as homelessness, a disease, or a condition such as diabetes, or health-related practices, such as the use of family planning methods. Within these categories, you may also define the population by age, as in teenage smokers. Regardless of whether your project starts with a people-based or issue-based question, you will need to clarify the geographical boundaries of your population and its defining characteristics, such as age or gender, to focus your inquiry and gather pertinent sociodemographic and epidemiological data.

## Review Literature (Step 2e)

It is not usually necessary to conduct an exhaustive review of the literature on a health issue as part of a community assessment, other than to fill in any gaps in your knowledge. However, to appreciate the meaning and importance of health data, it is necessary to understand the complex relationships that contribute to wellness and illness. Epidemiologists have long used a model of the interaction of genetics and the environment to explain the natural history of disease development and understand causation, which is essential for prevention (Bonita et al., 2006, p. 4). A web of causation (Brunt & Sheilds, 2000) uses the metaphor of the spider's web to conceptualize the multiple interacting factors, social and biological, that influence health and wellness. Although such models are used to explain disease causation, they can also be used to visualize the relationships that support health.

The conceptual framework underpinning the work of the WHO Commission on Social Determinants of Health provides a more complicated view of the dynamic interplay of the multiple factors that influence health inequities (Blas & Sivasankara Kurup, 2010). Broadly speaking, inequities in health are conceptualized as arising from the social context interacting with individuals/populations throughout life, resulting in differential

The search for health data takes longer than anticipated but is productive. Following a link provided by their advisor, Lise and Mika find a WHO policy document related to older adults and active living (WHO, 2010b). The document summarizes global recommendations for physical activity to enhance health and prevent non-communicable disease for three age groups, one of which is adults 65 years and over. Just what they want! The paper provides links to many other resources and includes definitions of key concepts used in the activity guidelines: frequency, duration, intensity, type, and total amount of physical activity. This they find particularly useful.

Additional finds are detailed national reports on the state of aging and health (CDC, 2013; PHAC, 2006b). The US resource has an interactive database; the Canadian resource includes a demographic profile and health assessment, complete with tables and graphs. They forward the references to their colleagues. During their search they come across a guide to creating cities that support active aging (WHO, 2007), which could prove useful later on. Mika says, "At least we know how to navigate the WHO site now and have links to specific US and Canadian resources. Plus, we have identified some keywords to describe physical activity."

**Discussion Topics and Questions**

7. Complete Table 3.4 to show the connections between one or two social determinants of health and the ability to maintain age-appropriate physical activity levels (see Wilkinson & Marmot, 2003).

8. Obtain a community needs assessment from a community clinic, public health department, or regional health authority in your area. Locate information in the assessment pertaining to one of the social determinants of health examined in Question 7, and discuss how the information is or might be used to inform a health promotion program.

**Table 3.4: Determinants of Health and Physical Activity**

| Determinant of Health | Rationale |
| --- | --- |
| Social Support (support from family, friends, and social relations) | Helps give people the emotional and practical resources they need to solve problems, deal with adversity, and maintain a sense of mastery and control over life circumstances. This has a powerful protective effect on health and may act as a buffer against health problems. Supportive relationships may also encourage healthier behavior patterns, such as participation in regular physical activity. |
| Education and Literacy | |
| Social Environments | |
| Physical Environments | |
| Personal Health Practices and Coping Skills | |
| Healthy Child Development | |
| Biology and Genetic Endowment | |
| Health Services | |
| Gender | |
| Culture | |

BOX 3.3

**Sample Questions on Health and the Determinants**

- What are the indicators of wellness in the community of interest?
- What is the prevalence/incidence of preventable ill health and disability in this population? How do the rates compare with other like communities?
- How does the health problem or issue impact on other problems identified as a priority in the community?
- Are some population groups affected more than others?
- Select an indicator of wellness/ preventable ill health. How is it influenced by socioenvironmental determinants?

exposure, vulnerability, outcomes, and consequences in health. To be fully informed about these causal links, you will need to become familiar with the models and review the medical and nursing evidence, including best practice guidelines that guide interventions (see Chapter 7). Sometimes you will find that the information on a particular health topic has been critically reviewed in national and regional strategy documents. The questions listed in Box 3.3 can be used to guide your inquiry.

### Managing Information and References

A systematic process will facilitate the review of existing information. As you locate and read the numerous documents, reports, and Web-based materials, you will accumulate a lot of information. Keeping track of your findings will be easier if you keep a complete record of all the written and Web-based resources you consult, with notes. Any photocopies or printed material should be clearly marked with full reference information in case you need to return to the source. Similar to any academic paper, the information must be referenced. This is no different from keeping study notes or conducting a review of the literature. However, because this is a group effort, you will need to agree to a process that works for all members of the group and avoids unnecessary duplication. Reference management software can be used to record references, including personal notes. If linked to a word processor, the references can be inserted into a document or generated as a bibliography.

Time management is important to consider when seeking and reviewing secondary data. For some issues, such as smoking, there will be an overwhelming number of studies and reports. In those cases, look for a review of studies (meta-analysis) or best practice guidelines (see Chapter 7). For other issues, a considerable amount of time can be spent with few results. To use time efficiently, seek advice from the project organizers on key words, data sources, and an approximate amount of time to spend searching.

### Summarize Secondary Data (Step 2f)

The most difficult part of a review of the secondary data can be summarizing the information. Aim for a short paragraph of four or five sentences for the student projects. One way to help condense the information is to identify and combine those references that have the same or similar information. For example: "Several sources identify that people over 65 are $x$ percent less active and have a greater number of illnesses related to immobility than people 55 to 64 (list of references to support this data)." As well, it is important to identify data, such as high levels of need, that provide a compelling reason for working with the community group or issue. Also important is research-based evidence from best practice guidelines that recommends a specific approach. A helpful way to sort through the information is to ask if a piece of information is interesting to know or important to know in working with the community group. It may be necessary to go through a couple of revisions to shorten the summary.

Mika and Lise share information on the different patterns of physical activity with aging, shown in Table 3.5. The table generates a lot of discussion. Kerri, a fitness instructor, comments that the findings fit with her experience with exercise groups in apartment buildings. She wonders if it would be useful to look more closely at the 65–74 year age groupings to see whether the decline in intensity of physical activity is the same for men and women. They speculate on what factors might be influencing the large drop in physical activity at the end of the teenage years. As well, they start to identify what factors in the physical and social environment might be influencing physical activity in older adults.

Mika and Lise quickly scan the websites and locate information on physical activity and chronic disease, as well as a number of policy documents on chronic disease prevention. One of the most comprehensive identifies disease prevention and health promotion as major elements of the strategy (Haydon, Roerecke, Giesbrecht, Rehm, & Kobus-Mathews, 2006). Looking at their results, Jeanine mentions that interest in diabetes prevention has increased rapidly since the presentation of the results of two international intervention projects, which provided strong evidence that type 2 diabetes might be prevented through lifestyle interventions that include physical activity. Mika agrees to locate the papers at the university library. The group is pleased to find that so much information is available. They feel better prepared to move forward with the community project. They discuss how the situation would be quite different in the case of emerging health issues, such as the environmental impact of pesticides on health or severe acute respiratory syndrome (SARS), when the evidence base for diagnosis and treatment is lacking and few policy documents are in place.

After reviewing their work, they identify one gap because they have no information on the ethnic composition of their population. They have learned that certain subpopulations are identified as being at high risk for type 2 diabetes, know that their health center serves many different ethnic groups, and feel certain that they will be able to provide this information. As well, the team will keep ethnicity in mind as they begin to plan the next steps of their project, steps 4 and 5 of the assessment, the collection of primary data (to be discussed in Chapter 4).

The group members agree that efforts to date have been successful beyond their wildest dreams. "Maybe we have been too successful," says Darren. "How are we going to keep track of this information?"

**Discussion Topics and Questions**

9.  Identify factors in the social and physical environment that might explain the decreasing rates of activity in the age groups presented in Table 3.5.

10. The Commission on Social Determinants of Health (CDSH, 2008) advocates for urban planning to create "healthy places." Recommendations include the following: "design urban areas to promote physical activity through investment in active transport; encourage healthy eating through retail planning to manage the availability of and access to food; and reduce violence and crime through good environmental design and regulatory controls, including control of the number of alcohol outlets" (p. 202). Thinking about the neighborhood around your school or workplace, discuss how it might be improved to create a healthy place using the CDSH recommendations.

**Table 3.5: Intensity of Leisure-Time Physical Activity by Age, Canada, 2005**

| Intensity | Age Range | | | | |
|---|---|---|---|---|---|
| | 12–17 | 18–24 | 45–54 | 55–64 | 65+ |
| Active | 50.9% | 38.3% | 22.0% | 22.6% | 18.5% |
| Moderate | 22.6% | 23.5% | 25.6% | 26.3% | 24.5% |
| Inactive | 26.5% | 38.2% | 52.4% | 51.1% | 57.0% |

*Note:* Broken line between "18–24" and "45–54" age groups indicates break in data.
*Source:* Gilmour, 2007, p. 46.

**Table 3.6: Simple Reference Tracking Method**

| Topic | Reference Tracking Information | |
|---|---|---|
| | Reference | Key Ideas |
| National diabetes statistics | Public Health Agency of Canada. (2011). *Diabetes in Canada: Facts and figures from a public health perspective*. Available from www.phac-aspc.gc.ca/cd-mc/diabetes-diabete/pub_stats-eng.php | The report offers the most recent diabetes statistics in Canada, giving rates of disease by age group, sex, place, and time. The health consequences of diabetes, health care utilization, and statistics on risk factors for developing diabetes and its complications, including obesity/overweight, unhealthy diet, physical inactivity, and smoking, are provided. |
| Physical activity guidelines for Americans | US Department of Health and Human Services. (2008). *2008 physical activity guidelines for Americans*. Washington, DC: Secretary of Health and Human Services. | The report summarizes research findings on the health benefits of exercise and provides activity guidelines for different age groups (children and adolescents, adults, older adults); for safe physical activity; and for groups with special needs (pregnant women, adults with disabilities, and people with chronic medical conditions). |
| Guidelines for creating age-friendly cities | WHO. (2007). *Global age-friendly cities: A guide*. Geneva, Switzerland: WHO. Available from www.who.int/ageing/publications/Global_age_friendly_cities_Guide_English.pdf | The report presents the concept of healthy aging and provides guidelines for creating age-friendly cities. The guidelines are informed by discussions with older adults, caregivers, and service providers in 33 cities across the world. |
| Cooperative survey of diabetes education centers | Local survey. | Utilization of diabetes clinics by city. |

## Teamwork during Steps 1 and 2 of a Community Project

The orientation to the community project and to the student team happen simultaneously. By necessity, students have to agree, in a relatively short space of time, how they will function as a team and begin the assessment on which to base their community project. This critical period for developing morale, or in other words, the relationships and team spirit, will help the team prosper and succeed. It is useful for students to meet as a group before the first visit to the placement organization. This provides an opportunity to get to know each other and make initial decisions about how the team will present itself and function as a unit at the orientation to the organization. This "warm-up" session provides opportunity to share first impressions, air views, and start organizing the team, including the selection of a group leader. Team members may prefer to appoint a temporary leader and defer the final decision about leadership until they have a better understanding of each other and the project requirements. The time can be considered well spent if it helps to establish a positive impression of the whole team right from the beginning. First impressions are important.

As described in Chapter 2, team members have to decide on roles and responsibilities during the first few weeks of the community experience. During this formative phase of team development, members of the team are also becoming oriented to the project and placement. Typically, in the first few weeks of the community experience, the team will have to accomplish the following tasks:

1. Team Organization and Decision Making
   - Negotiate the roles and responsibilities of team members.
   - Consider the initial work plan and timelines, including a strategy for involving community members.
   - Set up a routine for completing the weekly report.
2. Team Rapport
   - Get to know each other and develop a trusting relationship.
3. Evaluation
   - Reflect on and evaluate team performance, as an individual and group, as set out in the course requirements.

## Team Organization and Decision Making

One of the first steps is to establish a base and decide how you will communicate, by phone or email. Regular meeting times are important, so set a schedule from the start. This will provide time to organize and time to develop an effective working relationship. It is also important to think through how the team will accomplish its work. One approach is to draft a list of tasks, based on preliminary guidelines, to provide a common road map of activities and timelines for the community project and a framework for reporting on progress. Compiling the routine reports will encourage the group to reflect on progress in relation to the plan. In effect, these reports summarize team activities, the decisions made, and the rationale behind them. Your advisor and instructor should be able to follow your progress by reviewing the documentation and give feedback.

Familiarizing yourself with the community organization and the different ways of working in the community can be challenging at first, especially when you have responsibilities as a new team member. Keeping track of who is doing what and the different lines of inquiry by team members is essential. A work plan, sometimes termed "action plan," is a useful tool for summarizing the collective goal and planned action. In its simplest form, the plan lists the goal-related activities, indicating responsibility for each activity, with timelines for start and completion. Sometimes the activities are displayed in a Gantt chart or timeline, a type of bar chart (to be described in Chapter 4). Having the overall plan in mind provides a benchmark for monitoring progress. Progress toward the goals can be briefly summarized on the work plan, or detailed in the weekly report, as required by clinical instructors and advisors. Plans are bound to change, given the great many factors that influence them. These changes are much easier to accommodate without losing sight of the goal when documented in a work plan with timelines. Table 3.7 illustrates a simple work plan (more structured examples are provided in Chapter 4 and in Appendix A.3.1).

**Table 3.7: Draft Work Plan**

| Assessment Work Plan for Project: Physical Activity and Older Adults<br>Revision Date: September 10, 2015 | |
| --- | --- |
| **Steps, Activities, and Time Frame** | **Results Summary, with Completion Date** |
| 1.  Establish relationships within project and community, Sept. 8–21 | Complete Sept. 21 |
|    a-1.  Establish relationship with project organizers | Sept. 8: Met Jeanine, the project leader, and reviewed the project proposal. Roles and responsibilities discussed and agreed upon. We will meet face-to-face every second week and correspond by email weekly. |
|    a-2.  Meet community contacts | Sept. 8: Met SCHC staff and coalition members at orientation. Next meeting: Sept. 14 at 2 p.m. Coalition communication method is by email. |
|    b.  Define the project, population group, and issue, Sept. 8–16 | Sept. 8 and 9: Reviewed background documents provided by SCHC and COA. The project will focus on activity levels of adults, 65 years and older, living in the city. |
| 2.  Assess secondary data, Sept. 8–Oct. 10 | Will submit summary on Oct. 10. |
|    a.  Review sociodemographic data, Sept. 8–16 (Robin & Darren)<br>   –  develop guiding questions<br>   –  locate sources<br>   –  review, extract information | |
|    b.  Review national, regional, and local policy documents, Sept. 8–16 (Lise & Mika) | Sept. 9: On hold until after the review of health status. |

## Evaluation

A debriefing session after the orientation to the organization will allow the team to share first impressions and reflect on the experience. In addition to bringing the team together as a unit, it paves the way for thinking ahead and planning in a more informed way. One hour should be enough. As the team moves on, evaluation is a continuing item on the agenda and in the weekly report. Initially, team members may find it useful to reflect on how the team is familiarizing itself with people in the placement setting and community. All team members should be encouraged to contribute impressions, both positive and negative. When team members routinely share perspectives, they develop a team identity, a sense of accomplishment, and create an environment where concerns can be addressed as they arise. Over time, the approach to evaluation will evolve as the team matures, and in relation to course requirements.

# Summary

Community assessment is the first step in understanding community needs and resources, and an essential component of community health planning. The assessment also serves other, less tangible purposes, such as raising awareness of health issues and building community participation. By providing an entry point for citizen involvement, community assessment creates an opportunity to engage citizens in identifying health needs and potential solutions. The examination of secondary or existing data lays the foundation for community assessment. Gathering sociodemographic and epidemiological data on the population of interest and examining relevant policy documents and other sources of evidence provides a well-grounded basis for a shared understanding of community health issues. Achieving this shared understanding is a good start to the project and prepares you for assembling your own primary data in the community, which is the focus of Chapter 4.

Contributing as a team member is key to getting started on a community project. The first few weeks are crucial for team development: appointing a leader, defining team structure, and establishing effective modes of communication are all necessary for effective team decision making and morale. Early investment in team building sets the stage for interactions with the community and provides a good start for your project.

## Classroom and Seminar Exercises

1. With two or three other students, compare two communities using one of the following two definitions of community capacity:
   a. Labonte and Laverack (2001, p. 113) say, "Community capacity is not an inherent property of a particular locality, nor the individuals or groups within it, but of the interactions between both. It is also a function of the resource opportunities or constraints, such as the economic, political and environmental, of the conditions in which people and groups live."
   b. Goodman et al. (1998, p. 258) use the following definition of community capacity to guide their work: "The characteristics of communities that affect their ability to identify, mobilize, and address social and public health problems."
2. You have been selected to present findings to the steering group. From the data presented in this chapter, prepare key messages for three overheads.

## References

Anderson, E. T., & McFarlane, J. M. (2010). *Community as partner: Theory and practice in nursing* (6th ed.). Philadelphia, PA: Lippincott Williams & Wilkins.

Blas, E., & Sivasankara Kurup, A. (Eds.). (2010). *Equity, social determinants and public health programmes*. Geneva: World Health Organization. Retrieved from http://apps.who.int/iris/handle/10665/44289

Bonita, R., Beaglehole, R., & Kjellström, T. (2006). *Basic epidemiology* (2nd ed.). Retrieved from http://whqlibdoc.who.int/publications/2006/9241547073_eng.pdf

Brennan Ramirez, L. K., Baker, E. A., & Metzler, M. (2008). *Promoting health equity: A resource to help communities address social determinants of health.* Atlanta, GA: US Department of Health and Human Services, Centers for Disease Control and Prevention.

British Columbia [BC] Office of the Provincial Health Officer. (2010, August). *Investing in prevention: Improving health and creating sustainability.* The Provincial Health Officer's special report. Vancouver: BC Office of the Provincial Health Officer. Retrieved from www.health.gov.bc.ca/library/publications/year/2010/Investing_in_prevention_improving_health_and_creating_sustainability.pdf

Bronfenbrenner, U. (1979). *The ecology of human development.* Cambridge, MA: Harvard University Press.

Brunt, J. H., & Sheilds, L. E. (2000). Epidemiology in community health nursing: Principles and application for primary health care. In M. J. Stewart (Ed.), *Community nursing: Promoting Canadians' health* (2nd ed., pp. 564–583). Toronto, ON: Saunders Canada.

Canadian Council on Social Development. (2001). *Defining and re-defining poverty: A CCSD perspective.* Retrieved from www.ccsd.ca/index.php/policy-initiatives/policy-statements-briefs-submissions/112-defining-and-re-defining-poverty-a-ccsd-perspective

Canadian Society for Exercise Physiology. (2012). *Canadian physical activity and sedentary behaviour guidelines handbook.* Retrieved from www.csep.ca/english/view.asp?x=804

Centers for Disease Control and Prevention (CDC). (2010). *Community health assessment and group evaluation (CHANGE) action guide: Building a foundation of knowledge to prioritize community needs.* Atlanta, GA: US Department of Health and Human Services. Retrieved from www.cdc.gov/healthycommunitiesprogram/tools/change/pdf/changeactionguide.pdf

Centers for Disease Control and Prevention (CDC). (2013). *The state of aging and health in America 2013.* Atlanta, GA: CDC. Retrieved from www.cdc.gov/aging/help/DPH-Aging/state-aging-health.html

Chia, M., & Phillips, K. (2010). *Next steps in the development of health goals for Canada: Objectives, indicators and targets.* Retrieved from carolynbennett.liberal.ca/files/2010/07/ACF11F.doc.

Chief Provincial Public Health Officer of Manitoba. (2011, November). *Priorities for prevention: Everyone, every place, every day.* Retrieved from www.gov.mb.ca/health/cppho/pfp.pdf

Commission on Social Determinants of Health (CSDH). (2008). *Closing the gap in a generation: Health equity through action on the social determinants of health.* Final Report of the Commission on Social Determinants of Health. Geneva: World Health Organization. Retrieved from http://whqlibdoc.who.int/publications/2008/9789241563703_eng.pdf

Edwards, N. C., & Moyer, A. (2000). Community needs and capacity assessment: Critical components of program planning. In M. J. Stewart (Ed.), *Community nursing: Promoting Canadians' health* (2nd. ed., pp. 420–442). Toronto, ON: Saunders Canada.

Gilmour, H. (2007). Physically active Canadians. *Health Reports, 18*(3), 45–65. Retrieved from www.statcan.gc.ca/pub/82-003-x/2006008/article/phys/10307-eng.pdf

Goodman, R. M., Speers, M. A., McLeroy, K., Fawcett, S., Kegler, M., Parker, E., & Wallerstein, N. (1998). Identifying and defining the dimensions of community capacity to provide a basis for measurement. *Health Education and Behaviour, 25*(3), 258–278.

Hampton, C., & Heaven, C. (2014). Understanding and describing the community. *Community Tool Box* (Chapter 3, Section 2). Retrieved from http://ctb.ku.edu/en/table-of-contents/assessment/assessing-community-needs-and-resources/describe-the-community/main

Hawe, P. (1994). Capturing the meaning of "community" in community intervention evaluation. *Health Promotion International, 9*(3), 199–210.

Haydon, E., Roerecke, M., Giesbrecht, N., Rehm, J., & Kobus-Mathews, M. (2006, March). *Chronic disease in Ontario and Canada: Determinants, risk factors and prevention priorities*. Toronto, ON: Ontario Chronic Disease Prevention Association & Ontario Public Health Association. Retrieved from www.ocdpa.on.ca/publications/chronic-disease-ontario-and-canada-determinants-risk-factors-and-prevention-priorities

Health Canada. (2000). *Community needs assessment*. Retrieved from www.chssn.org/en/pdf/networking/aboriginal%20health%20assessement.pdf

Heaven, C. (2014). Developing a plan for assessing local needs and resources. *Community Tool Box* (Chapter 3, Section 1). Retrieved from http://ctb.ku.edu/en/table-of-contents/assessment/assessing-community-needs-and-resources/develop-a-plan/main

Illinois Department of Public Health. (2009). *IPLAN— Illinois Project for Assessment of Needs*. Retrieved from http://app.idph.state.il.us/

Israel, B. A., Checkoway, B., Schultz, A., & Zimmerman, M. (1994). Health education and community empowerment: Conceptualizing and measuring perceptions of individual, organizational and community control. *Health Education Quarterly, 21*(2), 149–170.

Labonte, R., & Laverack, G. (2001). Capacity building in health promotion. Part 1: For Whom? And for what purpose? *Critical Public Health, 11*(2), 111–127. doi:10.1080/09581590110039838

Labonte, R., Woodard, G. B., Chad, K., & Laverack, G. (2002). Community capacity building: A parallel track for health promotion programs. *Canadian Journal of Public Health, 93*(3), 181–182.

Macinko J., Shi, L., Starfield, B., & Wulu, J. (2003). Income inequality and health: A critical review of the literature. *Medical Care Research and Review, 60*(4), 407–452.

McCloskey, D. J., McDonald, M. A., Cook, J., Heurtin-Roberts, S., Updegrove, S., Sampson, D., … & Eder, M. (2011). Community engagement: Definitions and organizing concepts from the literature. In Clinical and Translational Science Awards Consortium (CTSA) Community Engagement Key Function Committee Task Force on the Principles of Community Engagement (Ed.), *Principles of community engagement* (2nd ed.). Washington, DC: US Department of Health and Human Services. Available from www.atsdr.cdc.gov/communityengagement/

McKnight, J. L., & Kretzmann, J. P. (1997). Mapping community capacity. In M. Minkler (Ed.), *Community organizing and community building for health* (pp. 157–172). New Brunswick, NJ: Rutgers University Press.

McLeroy, K. R., Bibeau, D., Steckler, A., & Glanz, K. (1988). An ecological perspective on health promotion programs. *Health Education Quarterly, 15*(4), 351–377.

Milio, N. (1976). A framework for prevention. *American Journal of Public Health, 66*(5), 435–439.

National Diabetes Information Clearinghouse. (2013). *National diabetes statistics 2011*. Retrieved from http://diabetes.niddk.nih.gov/dm/pubs/statistics/dm_statistics.pdf

Predy, G. N., Edwards, J., Fraser-Lee, N., Ladd, B., Moore, K., Lightfoot, P., & Spinola, C. (2008, November). *Poverty and health in Edmonton*. Edmonton, AB: Public Health Division, Alberta Health Services (Edmonton Area). Retrieved from www.albertahealthservices.ca/poph/hi-poph-surv-hsa-poverty-and-health-in-edmonton-2008.pdf

Public Health Agency of Canada (PHAC). (2006a). *Public Health Agency of Canada sustainable development strategy 2007–2010*. Retrieved from www.phac-aspc.gc.ca/publicat/sds-sdd/sds-sdd2-app-ann2-3-4-eng.php

Public Health Agency of Canada (PHAC). (2006b). *Healthy aging in Canada: A new vision, a vital investment, from evidence to action*. Briefing paper prepared for the Healthy Aging and Wellness Working Group of the Federal/Provincial/Territorial (F/P/T) Committee of Officials (Seniors) by Peggy Edwards and Aysha Mawani, The Alder Group. Ottawa, ON: PHAC. Retrieved from www.phac-aspc.gc.ca/seniors-aines/publications/public/healthy-sante/vision/vision-bref/index-eng.php

Public Health Agency of Canada (PHAC). (2011). *Diabetes in Canada: Facts and figures from a public health perspective*. Ottawa, ON: PHAC. Retrieved from www.phac-aspc.gc.ca/cd-mc/diabetes-diabete/pub_stats-eng.php

Public Health Agency of Canada (PHAC). (2012). What is the population health approach? Retrieved from www.phac-aspc.gc.ca/ph-sp/determinants/index-eng.php

Rifkin, S. B. (2009). Lessons from community participation in health programmes: A review of the post Alma-Ata experience. *International Health, 1*, 31–36.

Rissel, C., & Bracht, N. (1999). Assessing community needs, resources and readiness. In N. Bracht (Ed.), *Health promotion at the community level: New advances* (2nd ed., pp. 59–71). Thousand Oaks, CA: Sage.

Robert Wood Johnson Foundation and University of Wisconsin Population Health Institute. (2014). *County health rankings and roadmaps*. Retrieved from www.countyhealthrankings.org/

Sallis, J. F., Owen, N., & Fisher, E. B. (2008). Ecological models of health behavior. In K. Glanz, B. K. Rimer, & K. Viswanath (Eds.), *Health behavior and health education: Theory, research, and practice* (4th ed., pp. 465–485). San Francisco, CA: Jossey-Bass.

Secretariat for Intersectoral Healthy Living Network, F/P/T Healthy Living Task Group and the F/P/T Advisory Committee on Population Health and Health Security (ACPHHS). (2005). *The integrated pan-Canadian healthy living strategy*. Ottawa, ON: Canadian Minister of Health.

Secretary of State for Health, United Kingdom. (2010). *Healthy lives, healthy people: Our strategy for public health in England*. London, UK: Department of Health.

Smylie, J. (2000). A guide for health professionals working with Aboriginal peoples: The socio-cultural context of Aboriginal peoples in Canada. *Journal of Society of Obstetricians and Gynaecologists of Canada, 100*, 1–12.

Solar, O., & Irwin, A. A. (2007). *A conceptual framework for action on the social determinants of health*. Social Determinants of Health Discussion Paper 2 (Policy and Practice). Geneva: World Health Organization. Retrieved from www.who.int/sdhconference/resources/ConceptualframeworkforactiononSDH_eng.pdf

Statistics Canada. (2013). *Canadian Community Health Survey—Annual component (CCHS)*. Retrieved from www23.statcan.gc.ca/imdb/p2SV.pl?Function=getSurvey&SDDS=3226&Item_Id=50653&lang=en

Stokols, D. (1992). Establishing and maintaining healthy environments: Toward a social ecology of health promotion. *American Psychologist, 47*(1), 6–22.

Stokols, D. (1996). Translating social ecological theory into guidelines for community health promotion. *American Journal of Health Promotion, 10*(4), 282–298.

US Census Bureau. (2014). *How census measures poverty*. Retrieved from www.census.gov/how/infographics/poverty_measure-how.html

US Department of Health and Human Services. (2008). *2008 physical activity guidelines for Americans*. Washington, DC: Secretary of Health and Human Services.

US Department of Health and Human Services. (2009). *Community health status indicators [CHSI] 2009*. Washington, DC: Secretary of Health and Human Services. Retrieved from wwwn.cdc.gov/CommunityHealth/HomePage.aspx

US Department of Health and Human Services. (2010, November). *Healthy people 2020: Framework*. Retrieved from www.healthypeople.gov/sites/default/files/HP2020Framework.pdf

Wilkinson, R., & Marmot, M. (Eds.). (2003). *Social determinants of health: The solid facts* (2nd ed.). Copenhagen, Denmark: Regional Office for Europe of the World Health Organization.

World Health Organization (WHO). (1978). *Declaration of Alma-Ata*. Report from the International Conference on Primary Health Care, Alma-Ata, USSR, September 6–12. Retrieved from www.who.int/publications/almaata_declaration_en.pdf

World Health Organization (WHO). (2007). *Global age-friendly cities: A guide*. Retrieved from www.who.int/ageing/publications/Global_age_friendly_cities_Guide_English.pdf

World Health Organization (WHO). (2010a). *Adelaide statement on health in all policies.* Adelaide: Government of South Australia. Retrieved from www.who.int/social_determinants/hiap_statement_who_sa_final.pdf

World Health Organization (WHO). (2010b). *Global recommendations on physical activity for health.* Retrieved from www.who.int/dietphysicalactivity/factsheet_recommendations/en/


## Website Resources

There are many useful Web resources for health data. A few key sites are listed in this section. Many of the national and international sites are interconnected on particular topics, such as flu surveillance. Be aware that websites are frequently restructured to meet changing needs. If you are unable to gain access to specific pages within a website, go to the main site and either follow the links or try to locate the information by using the appropriate keywords. If you have the title of a publication, you can enter it in a search engine to search the Web.

### Health Indicators

Centers for Disease Control and Prevention, *Community Health Status Indicators*: wwwn.cdc.gov/CommunityHealth/HomePage.aspx

This site provides access to key community health status indicators for public health professionals and community members interested in the health of their community. The indicators are available by year, state, and county. A mapping function is planned.

The home page provides a link to a 2009 report by the Community Health Status Indicators Project Working Group, *Data Sources, Definitions and Notes for CHSI 2009* (Washington, DC: Department of Health and Human Services).

Public Health Agency of Canada (PHAC), *Canadian Best Practices Portal*: http://cbpp-pcpe.phac-aspc.gc.ca/

Under "Resources" you will find links to "Evidence-Informed Decision-Making: Information and Tools," "Health Indicators," "Public Health Competencies: Information and Tools," and "Planning Public Health Programs: Information and Tools." All but the last connect to a further network of links. For example: under "Health Indicators" you will find links to Canadian Health Indicators, Provincial/Territorial, International Organisations, and Health Indicators from Other Countries.

To give you an idea of what this means, under "Canadian Health Indicators," there are several links, each briefly described: PHAC, Statistics Canada and the Canadian Institute for Health Informatics (CIHI), Health Canada, The Pan-Canadian Public Health Network, Aboriginal Affairs and Northern Development, and the Federation of Canadian Municipalities (FCM). Of note, the last three sites have links to measures of health inequalities, well-being, and quality of life, respectively.

National Center for Health Statistics: www.cdc.gov/nchs/

"FastStats" provides quick access to statistics on topics of public health importance, including diseases and conditions, injuries, life stages and populations, and health care and insurance.

US Census Bureau: www.census.gov/
   The census bureau is the leading source of data on the people and the economy of the US. For quick facts about people, business, and geography, go to "Data/Data Tools and Apps" and follow the links.

World Health Organization, *Health Statistics and Health Information Systems: Country Measurement and Evaluation*: www.who.int/healthinfo/systems/en/
   This site provides links to a range of population-based and health facility–based data sources for participating countries.

## Health Topics

The national and international sites listed above have an alphabetical link to resources on a vast number of health topics. For example, each topic included in the PHAC Best Practices Portal link to "Public Health Topics" offers further links to Data, Strategies, Guidance, and Systematic Reviews of the Literature.
   Similarly, the Centers for Disease Control and Prevention provide a link to the "Healthy People 2020" site at www.cdc.gov/nchs/healthy_people/hp2020.htm.
   As noted, the sites are embedded in a maze of interconnections and the "Healthy People 2020" site, which is interactive, can also be reached at www.healthypeople.gov/.

## Interactive Sites Providing Regional Data to Guide Community Action

Robert Wood Johnson Foundation and University of Wisconsin Population Health Institute, *County Health Rankings and Roadmaps*: www.countyhealthrankings.org/
   The County Health Rankings measure the health of nearly all counties in the US and rank them within states. The indicators are informed by a model of population health that links social and environmental determinants—influencing factors—and health. County health rankings are linked to elements of the model.
   The Roadmaps section provides an action model, tools, and resources that communities can use to improve community health by taking action on selected health indicators.

## Epidemiology Resources Online

Centers for Disease Control and Prevention, *CDC Learning Connection*: www.cdc.gov/learning/
   CDC TRAIN offers thousands of courses and requires log-in. The site also provides access to other learning resources, including e-learning products. For example, under "Epidemiology, Surveillance, Information and Statistics," there is a link to the Division of Scientific Education and Professional Development (DSEPD) website, which provides numerous educational resources for the training and development of the public health workforce.

Public Health Agency of Canada (PHAC), *Skills Online*: www.phac-aspc.gc.ca/php-psp/ccph-cesp/index-eng.php
   *Skills Online* is a continuing education program. The self-directed or facilitated modules available on this site are designed to strengthen the core competencies of public health practitioners in Canada.

The National Collaborating Centre for Methods and Tools: www.nccmt.ca/index-eng.html
   See the "Quick Link to Multimedia (videos)," where you will find 10 short videos on epidemiological concepts to help you understand research evidence.

# Chapter 4

# Assessing the Environment and Community Group—Steps 3 and 4

K nowledge of the community is fundamental to the practice of community health nurses. When community health nurses move to a new area of practice or begin a new project, they rely on their assessment skills to develop knowledge of the social, physical, and environmental dimensions of the community and identify the social networks and connections. Nurses gain this knowledge through spending time in the community, observing the physical environment, and interacting with community members and community organizations. They observe people in different age groups and cultures, and note how the people interact with facilities, services, and the neighborhood. They combine this knowledge with the secondary data they gather on the sociodemographic profile of the community and patterns of illness and health (epidemiology).

Chapter 4 provides the tools and approaches to interact with a community group and determine their strengths and concerns on a firsthand basis. The data collected directly from the community is called primary data and builds on secondary data provided by governments and organizations discussed in Chapter 3. As you learn to assess the community group directly, you will start to feel that the streets and doors of the community are opening to the team and providing a new, broader perspective of how people live, work, study, and play. This beginning knowledge provides meaning and context to the secondary epidemiological and sociodemographic data, and assists in selecting appropriate assessment methods. The understanding, selection, and use of assessment methods continue the development of the team's community health nursing knowledge and skills, and prepare you for analyzing the data, planning, and taking action in the following chapters.

In this chapter, the information from advisors and the secondary data is brought together as you learn how to explore and map both the physical features of a defined area on foot, by car, or on the Internet, and the social environment, by observing how and where people interact.

More in-depth information of the community is gained through interviews with people knowledgeable about the community, called "key informants." The process used in key informant interviews is a basic approach that is used in preparing and conducting other assessment methods. The three phases of the basic approach are: (1) initial preparation, (2) making arrangements and drafting and testing questions, and (3) conducting the assessment. The mapping and interviews contribute to developing the questions for two other basic assessment methods: progressive inquiry, which asks increasingly specific questions over time with the same group, and guided observation, which uses a checklist to collect data on certain activities. Two advanced assessment methods, focus groups and questionnaires, rely on data from earlier methods, those of mapping, key informant interviews, progressive inquiry, and guided observation.

The scenario includes two teams working with mothers with young children living in two low-income apartment buildings. The discussions and interactions among team members help to emphasize how to address both different characteristics of a community group and team dynamics. In this chapter, students learn how to directly assess a community group, use critical thinking to determine which assessment methods to use, and use a basic approach to design and implement selected assessment methods.

## Learning Objectives

After reading this chapter and answering the questions throughout the chapter, you will be able to:

1. Identify how assessment fits within the community project.
2. Understand how community health nurses come to know their community, including how community members interact with each other and their environment, how cultural groups work within their community and with others, the resources and services that are available and how they are used, and the community's interest in working together to improve their health.
3. Assess the physical and social environment of the community group by learning to use critical thinking with a team to make decisions and carry through with plans.
4. Compare the features of the assessment methods to the characteristics of the community group and choose the assessment methods that are appropriate for the community group.
5. Collaboratively plan and collect assessment data from the community group according to ethical practice and within timelines using the selected methods.
6. Consider the implications for teamwork during assessment of primary data.

> **Key Terms and Concepts**
>
> community mapping • cultural competence • culture • ethical practice • field notes • focus groups • guided observation • informed consent • key informant interviews • know your community • progressive inquiry • qualitative data • quantitative data • questionnaires • readability

## Assessment of Environment and Community Group

A fundamental part of community nursing practice is gaining knowledge of the community. Knowledge of the community builds through consistently and systematically observing the community, asking questions, listening to responses, and asking more refined questions until no new responses emerge. To **know your community** is when you can accurately predict what is important to the community and how the community is

Program managers of the Public Health Department in Old York (fictional), a city of almost 1 million people, decide that it is time to review their prenatal and postnatal programs. The city has grown rapidly in the last 10 years, and the statistics show that their services are reaching predominantly middle-income families. A review of the sociodemographic profile of the city neighborhoods helps them to identify where low-income, single-parent families are located.

One specific area, called Fairway, has a high percentage of single families living in subsidized public housing. The managers learn from the nurses working in the area that the newer buildings have a mixture of languages and cultures, while older ones have mainly English-speaking residents. Hospital statistics indicate that a higher proportion of the infants born in Fairway have a low birth weight, are not breast-fed, and are taken to the hospital emergency room more frequently than newborns in the rest of the city.

The managers recognize that they need to learn more about the families living in the low-income buildings and decide to offer community clinical placements on prenatal and postnatal health to two teams of nursing students. Each team will be placed in a subsidized housing building: one team in a building where residents speak a variety of different languages—the Multilanguage Project—and the other where residents are predominately English-speaking—the English Project. Each project team has four students and a public health nurse advisor/preceptor. A community health nurse clinical instructor from the educational institution will work with both teams. Both the public health nurse and clinical instructor are advisors to the team.

The community project begins with an orientation for the student teams. The public health nursing manager orients them to the Public Health Department, and staff explains the prenatal and postnatal programs and services. The students are given a list of references to refresh their knowledge on the neonatal period. After the general orientation, each team meets separately with their public health nurse advisor. The teams obtain statistical reports on the area and profiles of their buildings to get them started on a review of secondary data. The students realize that other teams in their class who are not working directly with public health nurses might not have this type of assistance. After the first day, the students are excited about getting started but feel a bit overwhelmed by all the information they have received. They are uncertain of their roles and what they will be able to accomplish, but feel that the community project will come together as they learn more.

**Discussion Topics and Questions**

1. What are some of the reasons why low-income women might not attend prenatal and postnatal classes?

2. Based on your responses to question 1, what questions would you want to ask low-income women who are pregnant or have a baby?

For suggested responses, please see the Answer Key at the back of the book.

likely to respond to different situations and issues, and know specific details, such as the community's sociodemographic and epidemiological makeup. Community health nurses use their community knowledge to make informed decisions about how the community group could be involved in improving their health. Maintaining the knowledge and links to community networks is part of their daily work.

An important part of knowing the community is being familiar with its cultural makeup. **Culture** is the blended patterns of human behavior that include language, thoughts, communications, actions, customs, beliefs, values, and institutions of racial, ethnic, religious, or social groups (Centers for Disease Control and Prevention, 2009). The sociodemographic data includes the cultural profile of the community and prepares you to watch for and ask about people from different cultures, such as how long different cultural groups have lived in the community. Raising your awareness of cultural groups is the beginning phase of developing cultural competence. **Cultural competence** is a set

**Steps 3 and 4 in Completing the Community Health Nursing Project**

ASSESS

1. Orient to community project
2. Assess secondary data
3. Assess physical and social environment
   a. Observe and map physical and social environment
   b. Interview key informants
4. Assess primary data
   a. Select specific assessment methods
   b. Collect data
5. Analyze assessment data

PLAN

6. Plan action

ACT

7. Take action

EVALUATE

8. Evaluate results and complete project
9. Evaluate teamwork

of congruent behaviors, attitudes, and policies that come together in a system, agency, or among professionals that enables effective work in cross-cultural situations (Centers for Disease Control and Prevention, 2009). Chapter 7 discusses culture in more detail.

This chapter continues with the next phase of the community assessment. The purpose of this phase is to gather primary data directly from people in the community in order to identify, with them, the core themes or issues that elicit their social and emotional involvement (Minkler & Wallerstein, 1997). Some of these people may become collaborators or partners on a community project. Community health nurses aim to reach the full range of people in the community group, not just those who are easily contacted.

There are two steps in the assessment of primary data. Step 3, the assessment of the physical and social environment, will give you a broad overview of the community. Step 4 is designed to obtain information on the health and concerns of your community group. These two steps require you to use your observational and interview skills.

Box 4.1 details the substeps of Steps 3 and 4 within the community health nursing project. The first three steps serve as a base or foundation for knowing the community. Step 4 provides information specific to the community group and health issue that becomes the focus of a community project.

## Assess the Physical and Social Environment (Step 3)

Gathering data on the physical and social environment helps you to gain an overall idea of the community and its resources. This step includes two basic assessment methods: (1) observation and mapping of the physical and social environment of the community group, and (2) interviews with key informants. You can use these methods concurrently or one at a time to gather the information you need to develop your project. However, both should be completed early in a project, along with the collection of secondary data (Chapter 2). The next section describes the skills you will need to gather the data.

The assessment methods used initially in the community may take some time to get used to because they are quite different from those used when working in an institution. However, they are not dissimilar to the process you use when entering a new environment, for instance, when moving to a new community. First, you need a map, hard copy or digital, and then you have to get out into the community to see, hear, and talk to people. By putting yourself in the shoes of a member of your community group, you will find it easier to identify what information you need and what questions you should ask to learn about this community. In addition to adding to your repertoire of skills, the assessment methods introduced in this chapter will help your team organize

**Multilanguage Project**

The students in the multilanguage building feel a little anxious about working with people who barely speak English. As they get to know one another, however, they learn that one team member speaks Spanish and another speaks Cantonese, languages used by many residents in the building. Obviously, the clinical coordinator has considered these attributes when putting the team together.

At the orientation, their advisor explains that they will be put in touch with a city support worker, who works in the building part time, and two older women, former residents of the building, who now volunteer by holding drop-in English language sessions in the building lobby. She tells them that her team has been developing these relationships for a couple of years.

As part of the preparation, the team reviews the statistics they received from their advisor and determines to add to them. They find more references to complete their assessment of what is known about the perinatal health of low-income women from diverse cultures. Their summary of the secondary data follows:

> Poor perinatal outcomes, such as low birth weight and death, are associated with many factors including smoking, drinking, low education level, and both young and older-age mothers (Public Health Agency of Canada, 2008; Maternal and Child Health Bureau, 2011), and poverty (Larson, 2007; Maternal and Child Health Bureau, 2011). Only 10 percent of non-English-speaking people in Old York attended prenatal classes in 2010 and 2011, compared to 20–50 percent for other population groups in the city. The multilanguage building is for those with a low income, and just over 30 percent of the residents are single mothers or families with a child under two.

Since the team wants regular feedback from both advisors, they book a weekly meeting with their advisor and instructor for the first month. At the meeting in the second week, they report that they have begun to record the names and contact information for key informant interviews and ask for feedback on their draft assessment goal: "Assess the prenatal and postnatal needs of women living in the multilanguage building." The team is starting to realize that the goal is too broad and think they should narrow the focus to some aspect of prenatal and postnatal health promotion or a specific group within the building. Their advisors agree.

**English Project**

The students working in the building where most residents speak English feel their work will be less stressful than that of the other student team because communication will be easier. From their advisor, they learn that the public health nurses have not established contacts within the building but have a beginning list of organizations in the area that provide services to low-income mothers.

At the first meeting, the student team decides to keep the meeting to half an hour because three members have other things to do. They decide they will not need to meet with their advisors right after the orientation but will arrange to meet later when they have something to talk about. After catching up on what they did in the summer, they chat for a while about the project. One student suggests that they conduct individual interviews with the women in the building. Another comments, "It must be hard to have a baby on your own when so young—younger than us." Another responds that even teenagers are used to looking after themselves, and pregnant women probably have lots of help from the health sector and social services. The student interested in conducting interviews leaves to look up more information on that method. The others start adding to the secondary data and find national statistics similar to those found by the multilanguage team.

**Discussion Topics and Questions**

3. What advantages and challenges did the multilanguage team have, and how could they deal with them?
4. What advantages and challenges did the English team have, and how could they deal with them?

your questions and consider how your community project is to develop.

Before moving into the community, team members need to consider how to present themselves and explain their purpose as part of ethical practice. Community nurses interact with people in the settings where they live and work and play. They need to become comfortable in introducing themselves and explaining who they are, where they work, and what they do. This is an important step toward gaining entry into the life of the community. For example, he or she could say, "I am the public health nurse and would like to visit you and your baby." Or, "I am a nurse working at your community health center and would like to learn more about the recreational opportunities for mothers in this area." As a student team, you might say, "We are nursing students working with (name of organization) to determine the health interests and concerns related to (specific topic if known) of people in this area." Usually a clear explanation of your purpose and an obvious interest in the people and community will inform people and encourage them to talk to you.

## Observe and Map the Physical and Social Environment (Step 3a)

This first basic assessment method provides an overview of the layout of the community where you will be working. **Community mapping** involves locating geographical features and landmarks on a map and identifying resources relevant to how the community or population group functions. At the outset, you need to establish the geographical boundaries for your community group and have preliminary thoughts on the issues and concerns that might be relevant to your project. This helps to set limits. If your community group lives in a defined geographical area or neighborhood, you can observe and map the area in person. If members of your community group are spread throughout the community—for example, adults living with a disability—you might concentrate on the services and resources available for that group in a community. Alternatively, you could concentrate on a location where your community group might be found, for example, a school or workplace, and map the surrounding area. The purpose of observation and mapping is to orient you to the community and its resources. In addition to providing a context for the project and identifying possible issues or factors relevant to the community group, it can offer the advisors a fresh view of the community and local situation.

Figure 4.1 shows an example of a neighborhood map with a legend identifying the symbols used to mark features relevant to mothers with young children.

### Preparation and Process

First define the neighborhood on a map (or use an Internet service such as Google Earth) and enlarge the map so there is room to include the symbols. Prepare a checklist of the features you wish to include on your map. This can be done in a brainstorming session or by consulting the guides in other sources (e.g., Anderson & McFarlane, 2014; Vollman, Anderson, & McFarlane, 2008). Focus on features that are particularly relevant to members of your community group. For example, if you are working with disabled people, you might look at the wheelchair accessibility of reasonably priced grocery stores and pharmacies. If working with teens, you might look for bicycle trails and sports arenas or clubs. Both groups would be interested in accessible public transportation.

Your sociodemographic data (Chapter 3) may indicate that a certain percentage of

**Figure 4.1: Example of a Neighborhood Map**

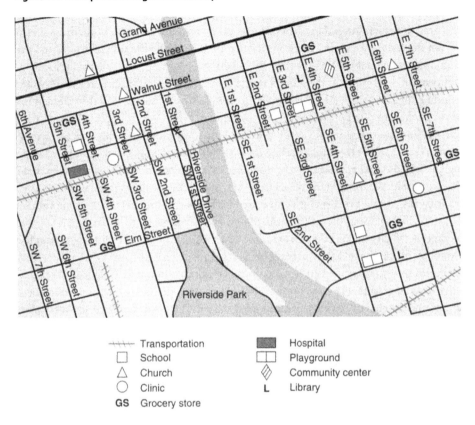

| | | |
|---|---|---|
| ┼┼┼ Transportation | ▢ (filled) | Hospital |
| ▢ School | ▢▢ | Playground |
| △ Church | ◈ | Community center |
| ○ Clinic | **L** | Library |
| **GS** Grocery store | | |

people from a different culture or speaking a different language live in the community. If so, watch for signs, stores, restaurants, or gatherings that indicate that facilities do or do not exist for certain cultures or languages.

The team can complete the neighborhood map by car, by bike, by bus, or on foot, augmented by Internet resources, as listed below in "geographical information." A map completed by motor vehicle is called a "windshield survey." The best approach is to choose the method of transportation used by most community members to understand their point of view. A good use of time is to locate your community on a map, expand and print it in sections, and distribute copies to team members. The maps and checklist will focus your observations, help to ensure consistency, and ensure that all areas are covered and not duplicated. You can assemble the map as you go or transfer the data from your observations in stages. For example, you could first locate key landmarks, then specific features. Use an agreed-upon set of symbols to mark churches, schools, grocery stores, and so on, and attach the legend to the map. If necessary, the symbols can be color-coded to grade them; for instance, to identify those used heavily or lightly by community members.

Explanatory details can be added as field notes. **Field notes** are detailed, concise, objective notes on an area of interest using a predetermined format. For instance, if you are observing how people get around in the neighborhood, you might make note of the road conditions, walking paths, amount and types of traffic, and public transportation. Be sure to include and explain unexpected features or events that could help with understanding the neighborhood. Systematic documentation of the information is a key part of the process. By sharing and reflecting on these notes, the team can develop a shared understanding of the community and its resources, or lack of them.

An important aspect of community mapping is observing how members of the community interact with each other, and where people gather and when. These observations will help you to understand how the community functions, where people work, conduct their business, and play. Similar to the physical features, view the interactions through the lens of a person from your community group, for example, a mother with young children. Ask what this mother would look for if moving to the area. She would want to know where to shop, what the transportation service was like, and how safe the neighborhood was. She would want to know what health services were close by, such as community health centers, physicians, dentists, public health nurses, hospitals, and pharmacies. As well as observing the features, find opportunities to talk to people and ask what it is like to live in the neighborhood and where people go for a particular service.

Another focus might be to locate resources specific to your community group; for example, finding wheelchair accessible exercise groups for persons with a disability, or health information for people who do not speak the dominant language. Use your advisors and resources like a municipal social services directory to find local associations and listings of relevant community services. Once you find one service, it can lead you to others. By locating information that has already been collected, the team will not repeat what has already been done. It is better to update information to make it current and, through the community project, to add more detailed information. Try to avoid recreating the wheel!

One important approach is to look for something in the area to admire, a feature that would make the area a good place to live. Positive features might be the cleanliness of the area, the number of people out walking, or the friendliness of people on the street. Commenting on these features is a great way to start a discussion with community members and leads you in identifying community strengths.

Later in the project, the team may choose to use a specific assessment method called guided observation to document certain actions or behaviors. For an example, see the observational assessment in the Appendix to Chapter 13.

The procedure for mapping is as follows:

1. Define the area and obtain relevant maps.
2. Prepare a checklist of physical and social features.
3. Walk, bike, or drive the neighborhood as a team or as delegated among members.
4. Mark features relevant to the community group on the map.
5. Attempt to discuss features with residents who are present in the area.
6. Compare and collate results with team members.

When time is short, use a vehicle, rather than walking or cycling, to complete a neighborhood survey. Another option is to use one of the resources indicated in the geographical information, and then make decisions about what information is necessary to gain the community's perspective and what is merely nice to know. Usually you will not have more than one session to conduct mapping; however, once you have the map, you can easily add to it.

**Multilanguage Project**

After their orientation, the students take a quick trip to the neighborhood. Their building is in a newly developed area, not close to stores and shops, but they do spot a couple of fast-food take-out restaurants featuring Spanish and Chinese food. They note a laundromat, elementary school, and several bus stops nearby. The visit helps them to prepare a list of features and services to include in their map and field notes.

After walking the neighborhood in pairs, team members transfer their information to an electronic copy of the map on a laptop. This comes in handy when they meet with the support worker and the two women volunteers at the building the following week. The volunteers, who immigrated some time ago, are intrigued by the map and call others over to look at it and pick out familiar places marked by the symbols. They point out where second-language classes are held and identify the least expensive grocery store on the map. The women seem really pleased that the students are taking such an interest in their neighborhood. The team plans to keep adding to the map and bring it to meetings with the residents of the building.

**English Project**

The students take a bus to their assigned building, which is one of several high-rise apartment buildings crowded into a fairly small area. First impressions are somewhat negative because of the litter blowing around the complex; however, the students are pleasantly surprised to find a busy and attractive playground for young children next to their building. Several young women are sitting on benches watching their children. A sign beside the playground states that the playground was completed that year by the building's tenants' association. The team members do not talk to the women.

**Discussion Topics and Questions**

5.  What neighborhood features might be important for pregnant women and women with small children, and what symbols (icons) could depict these features?
6.  What might you observe during your mapping that would indicate the lengthy presence of a large cultural group compared to a recently arrived group?

Observation and mapping

- is part of the initial assessment for every project;
- is conducted according the perspective of the community group needing services;
- can begin as soon as the population and issue are determined, a checklist is created, and resources are obtained; and
- helps to orient the team and indicates interest in the community.

## Interview Key Informants (Step 3b)

**Key informant interviews** are guided discussions with individuals who can provide credible advice on the health, experiences, and functioning of the community group. Key informant interviews are the second basic assessment method and are used in all projects. The procedure for key informant interviews involves determining what information you want, deciding who can provide the information and the questions that will elicit the required information, and how to arrange and conduct the interviews. This basic procedure applies to other assessment methods.

A key informant might be someone living in the community, a member of an organized community group, or a service provider. For example, possible key informants for a project involving vulnerable older adults living in an urban community, as in Chapter 3, might be members of an older adults' council or association, church leaders, and the home health nurses working in the area. Talking to an elderly man or woman who has lived in the area for years and is known and respected would give you an insider perspective; talking to a newcomer might give you a different one. The aim is to gain a broad understanding of the community from different points of view. For even larger projects or programs, other possible informants might be those with particular knowledge of the services used by older adults, for example, people working in the corner stores, pharmacists, and mail carriers.

The approach for preparing and carrying out these interviews is explained in detail below, because it is a basic method that applies to other assessment methods described in Step 4. The phases of the approach are: initial preparation, making arrangements, drafting and testing questions, and conducting the key informant interviews and meetings. Each phase discusses adaptations for interviews with community members, service providers, and small group meetings.

### Initial Preparation

Advisors and mentors can greatly assist your team with preparing and conducting effective key informant interviews. For example, they can help to focus the interviews and develop questions, participate in practice sessions, and identify potential participants.

With your project and purpose in mind, identify the information you need and who might have it. Generally, you want information about the community group that provides insight into health status or is relevant to a particular health issue. This includes such things as interests or concerns, resources, limits or barriers to health, and the way people like to do things in this community. Usually, you are seeking information on the following topics:

1. The community or location as a place to live/work/attend school/receive services, etc.
2. The availability and usefulness of community resources, such as social support systems, services, and activities
3. How people keep healthy
4. Limits or barriers on peoples' ability to keep healthy
5. Effective approaches to working with the community

The people who are likely to have the information you need are (a) individuals in, or closely associated with, the community group; (b) service providers or employees of organizations that provide services in the community; and (c) members of an organized group or association dealing with issues relevant to your intended community group. Your advisor can help orient you by providing background information on the community role of the key informant or group and their previous involvement with the placement organization and/or the topic. This preliminary introduction and preparation will help the team to gain confidence and learn to initiate contact with others. Key informant interviews are important for the information they provide and the connections they initiate with community members, as well as for providing the team with the first opportunity to introduce themselves and the project they are planning.

If you have the opportunity to meet with an organized group, expect to work in partnership with your advisor to prepare and conduct the meeting. Even community health nurses experienced in delivering educational sessions have difficulty leading group interviews at first. This partnership is important to build your skills and knowledge in a safe environment.

Next, consider how you will introduce your interview. The introduction for assessment methods where you are interacting directly with people always needs to begin with information on informed consent. Provide the introduction either at the beginning of the interaction or when initially setting up an appointment.

**Informed consent** for interactive assessment methods includes stating or writing (a) the purpose of the assessment method, (b) the time involved, (c) confidentiality, (d) how the team will use the information, and (e) the right of the person not to participate or answer a question. Informed consent is a part of ethical practice for all nurses (American Nurses Association, 2010; Canadian Nurses Association, 2008). **Ethical practice** means following the nursing code of ethics for your jurisdiction and the ethical values inherent in all codes, which are based on respect for human rights, including the right to life, to dignity, and to be treated with respect (International Council of Nurses, 2012). The information on informed consent also applies to the assessment methods in Step 4.

You are encouraged to write out your introduction so that everyone on the team can give the same information. Box 4.2 provides an example of an introduction, including informed consent, for an interview with a community member.

## BOX 4.2
### Introduction for Key Informant Interview with Community Member

*Introduction:* Hello, my name is _____. I am on a team working with _____ (name of person) from _____ (name of organization).

I want to talk to you because I feel you know people who are/have _____ (identify characteristics such as age, gender, attend a certain group, etc.). I would like to talk to you about this group of people so my team will have a better idea how to plan improved _____ (type of health service you are thinking about) and how best to approach them. I expect it will take us only 10 to 15 minutes. Your name or details about you will not be included. You can refuse to talk to me or skip questions you do not want to answer. Would you be willing to talk to me? If so, can we talk now or at a time that is better for you?

## Making Arrangements, and Drafting and Testing the Interview

In arranging for key informant interviews and meetings, the first decision is deciding whom to interview. Sources for key informant participants could be your list of contacts from your orientation meeting or community members you met during mapping. As stated above, your advisors often have a good idea of community members, service providers, and groups who would be approachable and knowledgeable participants.

Advisors can facilitate the process by letting people know that the team will be calling them to discuss a particular topic. In some cases, the advisor might think it best to make the first contact, or suggest co-conducting the interview or meeting. When approaching people for an interview or meeting, team members should explain that they are in the beginning phase of a community project, sponsored by the placement organization, and are open to advice.

Usually, you can conduct interviews with community members "on the spot," in a somewhat private place, or as both of you carry out your usual activities. The interview could also occur over a couple of encounters, depending on the situation. You may find that people will continue to seek you out to add more information.

Interviews with service providers take time to arrange. We suggest that you start booking these appointments as soon as possible since people usually need at least a week to find time to meet, and some are more difficult to reach. Face-to-face meetings are preferable, but interviews by phone, through email, or even Internet conference are also realistic for some situations. In formal interviews, you may want to have two team members or your advisor/mentor involved. Two people help to keep the conversation moving and log a thorough record of the interview. When two people are involved in the interview, use both of your names and the pronoun "we" when contacting the person.

To attend a meeting with a small group or committee, you need to know when they meet and who to contact. Usually you can get this information from your advisor/mentor or a key informant. If your advisor/mentor is in agreement with your contacting the group, determine who will make the contact and be involved. Try and do this as soon as possible to improve the chance of being included on the group's agenda, since many groups only meet once a month.

If the team is setting up the meeting with a group, introduce yourself to the contact person and provide a clear explanation of what you are hoping to gain from it and what involvement you would like from members. For example, you might say you will be asking two or three prepared questions about _____ (topic) to obtain feedback from the group. Indicate if your advisor/mentor will be attending and if that person will be initiating the discussion. Request 15 to 30 minutes and agree to the time that is offered.

At the same time as you are making arrangements, you need to draft and test the interview questions and process. Start preparing the interview questions as soon as possible using the list of topics given above. When drafting the interview questions, be clear about what it is you want to know and keep the questions simple. Box 4.3 features an example introduction and approach to interviewing a service provider.

Prepare material for both a community member and service provider interview. Both types of interviews are a necessary part of your assessment and the opportunity to conduct one type may arise before the other, depending on the availability of the participant. The interviews with community members are usually shorter (10–15 minutes) and have three or four general questions that will likely not cover all the topics. The longer interview (20–30 minutes) with service providers can include more questions and be more specific, such as asking about past and present experiences working with the community group or similar groups. Review the drafts with your advisor(s). Depending on your situation, one or both of your advisors must approve the questions and approach before you begin interviews.

Tailor the questions to the interviewee and the knowledge they are likely to have. For example, if your interest is a healthy active lifestyle, you would modify the questions depending on whether the interviewee is an active longtime resident of the community or a new resident with a disability, rather than a service provider, such as a home health coordinator, as shown in Box 4.3.

You will likely be surprised at how long it can take to come up with the questions that elicit the information you want from the interviews. Draft out the questions and try them out by practicing on each other. Then try them out with others outside your team. Think about what each question is asking and consider how people respond to it. Since key informant questions are verbal, you will be able to ask the person another question if they do not understand at first. You need to identify such a difficulty with the team and discuss other ways to word the question.

In a meeting with an organized group, expect to have a time frame of 15 to 30 minutes at the beginning or ending of their meeting. Limit the number of questions to encourage discussion from as many of the group members as possible in the short time that is available. You can either adapt the questions you have used in individual interviews, or be more specific if you have some idea of the issues. For example, if you were meeting with a parent-teacher association about smoking prevention, you might ask, "What do you see as the problems related to smoking in grades 7 and 8?" Depending on the response, you could follow with "What is being done or could be done to discourage smoking by these students?" and "What would be useful for our team to work on in this area?"

When new to community health, you will find it helpful to role-play the interviews, especially those with people in formal positions. As you practice interviews, and everyone on the team is clear about what information is needed, allow people to "ad lib" the questions a bit. This flexibility helps people to introduce the questions into the conversation using their normal language. Also, a pause after the first response allows time for the respondent to expand on what was said. The pauses and informal approach encourage conversation rather than giving the impression that the questions need to be answered quickly. With this approach, you will likely find that you have covered all the topics and have only asked a few direct questions.

Practice will help you to keep people on topic and deal with more difficult situations, such as informants who are impatient or unsupportive. After a role-play, debrief, review the questions, and revise the questions. Once you start feeling more comfortable, you may ask for feedback from an advisor. After this preparation, the team members are likely to feel more relaxed when they conduct the actual interview or meeting.

## Conducting Interviews and Meetings

The best approach for key informant interviews and group meetings is to initiate a conversation to learn about the community and recognize their contribution to the assessment. You can accomplish this by adopting a "listen to learn" approach to encourage them to relax and expand on the information they provide. Also, be aware of body language and adjust your approach to keep people engaged.

After conducting initial interviews with a few community members and service providers, review the responses you have received. If the responses are not providing the data you need, revise the questions and interview more, and possibly different, people.

At a key informant group meeting, the contact person usually introduces your team and advisor and indicates the relevance of your project to the group. Be ready at that point to give your prepared introduction, including the information on informed consent. You or your advisor/mentor may need to "ad lib" a bit to clarify your purpose, especially if it differs from that given by the contact person.

During the meeting, one team member needs to document the number of people present and record the responses to each question. One option is to write the responses on a flip chart, chalkboard, or computer so that the group members can see what is being recorded.

For all interviews and meetings, strive to have the meeting participants feel that their views are appreciated and will be considered when you take action, and that the information provided will be passed on. Finally, maintain interview etiquette by keeping to the time you indicated, and thank participants for their time and effort. When giving thanks, mention an item that you felt was particularly useful. If appropriate, also ask whether you might follow up with them.

There are no hard and fast rules to determine the right number of key informant interviews to conduct. You need to achieve a balance between making connections that will facilitate your project and having sufficient time to conduct a more focused assessment using other methods. At this point in the project, rely on the advice of your advisors to determine who and how many people to include. Later, if you identify other people and groups involved with the community and issue, you can conduct a key informant interview to bring them "on board," rather than run the risk of excluding an important resource.

In summary, key informant interviews are fundamental to getting to know the community and beginning a community assessment. Talking to key individuals about your community group orients you to the group, initiates relationships, and provides an entry to community networks.

This assessment approach contributes to the development of the project by involving key people in identifying the issues and strengths of the community group, developing assessment skills in team members, and providing a basis for developing and using more specific assessment methods.

**Multilanguage Project**

The students plan to conduct key informant interviews with the two volunteers who meet with the women in the lobby and a city support worker. The main purpose of the interviews will be to gather information about the building as a place to raise infants and children. They came up with two questions: "What is this building like as a place to raise young children?" and "What resources are there in the building for these families?" They draft the following list of questions:

1. Do women in the building find it difficult to raise infants and young children here?
2. Are there services that the women use to help them raise their children?
3. How do they keep themselves and their children healthy?
4. What makes it difficult for them to keep their family healthy?
5. What ways do you use to encourage the women to talk to you?

The public health nurse advisor suggests another key informant, the director of an agency who works with multicultural groups in the city. Setting up this interview is difficult. Eventually they talk to the woman's assistant, who suggests they submit their request in an email. They receive a prompt reply to the email.

Once the key informant interviews are almost complete, the team meets with their clinical instructor and advisor to consider the findings and discuss next steps. The team leader summarizes their progress by saying that with the help of the volunteers, they are starting to make connections in the building by meeting with women in the lobby. It has been a slow process: some of the women struggle to carry on a conversation in English, but they are interested in trying. From the community mapping, they have learned that there is a lack of low-priced grocery stores in the area, and key informants confirm that families have trouble finding and paying for some of the food they had in their home country. The advisors agree that the team has the start of a good relationship with the women in the lobby. They also feel that the team is pulling the data together and building an accurate picture of the lives of building residents.

By week four, the team has plotted out the assessment items of the project timeline (see Week Four Timeline in the Appendix at the end of this chapter). They feel reassured when they compare their progress with the flexible timeline provided in Table 2.1 in Chapter 2.

**English Project**

The students do not feel much further ahead at the third week. From census tract data, they have confirmed that Fairway has the third-highest proportion of low-income families and single mothers in the city. They have talked to a few people; however, they have not started the key informant interviews or completed the community map. Their main issue is that they cannot agree on the focus of their project and have difficulty coordinating schedules: one person wants to work independently, and another argues that teamwork is more efficient. Their clinical instructor is not happy with the lack of progress and sees gaps in the weekly reports, and provides this feedback to the team.

Team members feel frustrated and agree to use a conflict resolution strategy from Chapter 2 to identify how they can get back on track. When they meet, they find that everyone is dreading the meeting but wants to get things resolved. They decide to take a walk together to provide the opportunity to "air" feelings without having to face each other across a table. This works, and when they return, they are able to quickly review and allocate additional time and responsibility for the steps they had been missing. They cannot quite believe that their differences got resolved so quickly, but are happy to have a cooperative atmosphere for a change.

Their advisors commend them for dealing with their issues and their renewed energy and enthusiasm. The public health nurse advisor will contact public health nurses visiting mothers and infants in the apartment building to arrange key informant interviews. The team feels ready to work together. Now that they have a better sense of direction, they will consider different ways to engage the women in the building.

**Discussion Topics and Questions**
7. What information could the multilanguage team obtain from the key informants that might not be directly solicited by the questions?
8. Were the measures used to defuse the frustration of the English team members realistic, based on your own experiences?

## Summary of Steps 1, 2, and 3

The orientation to the community, assessment of secondary data, and assessment of the physical and social environment through community mapping and key informant interviews (project Steps 1 to 3) help to ensure that you will be working on relevant and feasible community issues. These three steps are, therefore, a beginning for all community projects and community practice.

As well as learning about the community, the team is gaining critical assessment skills that are fundamental to the progress of the project and to developing expertise in community health nursing practice. In particular, the three phases of the approach used in preparing for key informant interviews is a basic approach that carries through to other assessment methods.

The three phases of the basic approach are:

1. Initial preparation: determining purpose, topics, possible participants, informed consent
2. Making arrangements and drafting and testing questions
3. Conducting the assessment

The data collected during the initial steps of the project—orientation, assessment of secondary data, and assessing the physical and social environment—provide an overview of the community, how it functions, and its issues. In turn, this contributes to the progress of the community project by providing the team with the following information:

- How to work with the team and organization
- The issues that are important to the organization and community
- Sociodemographic information about the population from secondary data
- The people who know how to work with community members
- The features and resources of the community and setting

These first steps assist community health nurses in getting to know the community. In community health nursing, this is similar to developing a trusting relationship with individual clients/patients in institutions. Through multiple observations and interactions with community members and discussions with team members, you gain a perspective of the community that will develop and expand over the course of the project. Knowing the community includes knowing how to work in that community.

Knowledge of the community is a prerequisite to using tools and processes, including evidenced-based research, to bring about community change. Without this knowledge, health care professionals could introduce change but it would be difficult to sustain and could damage community relationships. Sustainable change occurs when you engage people in initiatives that are important to them.

## Assess Primary Data (Step 4)

The knowledge gained through community mapping and key informant interviews (Step 3) provides an orientation to the community and the people who live there. For example, the team will start to feel that they know their way around, where to buy a bottle of water or a coffee, where to talk to people, and will have gained an appreciation of some of the issues that concern the community. The issues might be mothers and older adults having difficulty dealing with poor sidewalks, lack of parks or play areas, or difficulty obtaining information on health services and programs. At the same time, they will have learned about community strengths, such as the efforts of the community group to start a community food box and kitchen, or to have signs to reduce speeding.

Moving from Step 3 to 4 entails a major shift in focus. From gathering data to obtain an overview of the community and a context for health care, you must now collect more specific information to investigate the health situation of the community group in greater depth. The assessment methods described below will build on the assessment skills learned earlier to observe community resources and conduct interviews. We describe four assessment methods in Step 4: two additional basic methods, progressive inquiry and guided observation, followed by the two advanced assessment methods, focus groups and questionnaires. Most teams will use one or both of the basic methods; a few teams involved in larger projects may use the advanced methods. Once you have an understanding of the different methods, you will use criteria to select the methods that fit best with the context and characteristics of the community group and the project purpose and timelines.

Each of the four methods helps to elicit data in greater depth and/or from a greater number of people or sources than the methods discussed earlier. The assessment methods follow the basic development process introduced in key informant interviews: initial preparation, making arrangements, drafting and testing questions, and conducting assessment.

Two basic assessment methods, progressive inquiry and guided observation, defined below, provide different ways to expand the depth and breadth of your knowledge of the community using methods suited to natural, informal settings. The use of one or both of these methods helps to focus your inquiry and is usually sufficient to determine an issue for action for a short-term project.

The use of the advanced methods of focus groups and questionnaires requires considerably more time, preparation, and organizational oversight than the basic methods. In some situations, the use of these advanced methods could be appropriate. For example, a team might be part of a large project preparing a questionnaire for a focus group. Or the team might be asked to work with an experienced staff member to develop and test a short, simple questionnaire based on the data from the basic assessment and example questionnaires. The decision to use one of these advanced methods is made by the advisors and the team, based on the requirements of the situation.

Community health nurses use the basic and advanced assessment methods to gather information in a systematic way to provide information on the present health situation and preferred health situation of a community group. They use the assessment information to guide community practice and develop programs, and for quality assurance.

The methods and experienced advisors guide students and new practitioners as they build expertise in gathering qualitative and quantitative data about a community. **Qualitative data** are word descriptions collected while asking open-ended questions or making observations. **Quantitative data** are numbers collected through closed-ended questionnaires or counting occurrences during observation.

## Progressive Inquiry

Progressive inquiry builds on key informant interviews and observations during mapping. **Progressive inquiry** is a cyclical process that involves an individual or team asking questions, analyzing the responses, and building on them to tailor more focused and specific inquiries, preferably with the same or a similar group of people. The aim is to engage community members in discussion to understand their health concerns and identify what they would like to change. The progressive nature of the inquiry makes it possible to validate findings as you go. Figure 4.2 depicts the repeating cycles in the process.

Starting with two or three general questions, team members pose the questions to individuals or small groups of two or three community members during one encounter. After analyzing the results, the team, which may incorporate community members, devises a more specific set of questions for the next session. The cycle of more and more specific questions continues until responses become consistent.

Progressive inquiry is a "gentle" approach and sufficiently flexible to accommodate a range of abilities to respond to questions. The method is particularly useful when communication is difficult, such as with people who are not fluent in the language spoken by team members, the visually or hearing impaired, and people who may be uncomfortable with formal procedures. There could be a variety of reasons for their discomfort: they may prefer to keep to themselves, rarely leave the home, and be somewhat isolated from society; they may mistrust new people; or they may not speak the dominant language. It would be unrealistic to expect such a person to speak up in a meeting or answer a questionnaire. Progressive inquiry allows you to proceed more slowly and develop a relationship that might eventually lead to further involvement.

**Figure 4.2: Cycles in Progressive Inquiry**

1. Team decides on 2–3 initial questions

2. Asks questions informally where people gather

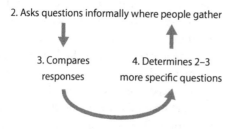

3. Compares responses

4. Determines 2–3 more specific questions

5. Cycle ends when consistent responses occur

Part 2: The Community Health Nursing Process and Community Health Nursing Projects

**Multilanguage Project**

Based on interviews with key informants and community mapping, the students decide to use progressive inquiry, thinking that the flexible and informal approach will help them get to know the women quickly. They prepare three questions: "How long have you been living here? How many children do you have? Do you like learning about food?"

When they visit the building, they find a few young mothers have gathered with the two older volunteers, and each team member asks the questions of at least two people. Although the volunteers answer the questions readily, the team members quickly realize that the younger women, who tend to be recent immigrants, are slow to respond and do not understand the question about food. They appear to find it difficult to answer questions on different topics. After discussing the results at their meeting with their advisors, they decide to ask two questions: "How long have you been living here? How easy it for you to shop for food?" They include the question about food because it came up as an issue in the key informant interviews and they found only one small convenience store in the neighborhood during mapping.

At the next visit to the building, and questioning three women each, they find that most women want to discuss food. They now feel ready to move to more specific questions: "What food do you like?" and "Where do you buy your food?"

The team is satisfied that the progressive inquiry approach works well for the women, and the data confirms that food is really a "hot" topic. Since nutrition fits well with healthy pregnancy and motherhood, the team continues to use this approach for a few weeks until no new issues emerge. If the topic of food had not engaged the women, the team had planned to ask about exercise or infant development.

**English Project**

The team feels more confident after completing the mapping, and conducting key informant interviews with the public health nurses who visit mothers in the building. They try to use progressive inquiry with women throughout the building but have little success; everyone seems too busy to stop and talk to them. They remember seeing women with children in the playground and decide to try the approach there. When they discuss other options with their advisors, both suggest interviewing the members of the tenants' association in the building or possibly interviewing the public health nurses in greater depth. The team needs to make decisions in the next week or two about how best to proceed and which other methods to use.

**Discussion Topics and Questions**

9. Explain how information gathered during mapping and key informant interviews informed the progressive inquiry questions for the multilanguage team.

10. What would the advantages and challenges be of using progressive inquiry with a group of people who have a culture that is different from your own?

---

Asking the same questions of community members allows the team to compare responses, validate themes, and identify trends. It is a systematic and gradual approach to collecting in-depth assessment information. The repeated questioning is a distinct advantage of the approach in that it promotes the development and maintenance of relationships.

Progressive inquiry is similar to the meaning of Freire's (1972) dialogue: questioning and challenging the issues to identify a limiting situation that can be changed. It is important to note that the term is being used differently in postsecondary and computer-based learning in Finland and, to a lesser extent, in North America. In those situations, progressive inquiry is based on cognitive research in educational practices and the development of new knowledge based on the philosophy of science, with emphasis on a systematic effort to advance shared knowledge (Lakkala, 2008). As used in this text, progressive inquiry is an approach to gather information systematically in natural settings for community health nursing practice. The purpose of advancing shared knowledge is the same in both situations.

### Initial Preparation

After agreeing on the initial purpose of the inquiry, the team decides how, when, and where to approach people, and develops two to three questions. As before, the questions should be reviewed with an advisor. Compared to the basic development approach, progressive inquiry repeats the two-to-three-question cycle after reviewing the responses and developing progressively more focused questions. Although the method has a short preparation time for each set of questions, the cycle needs to continue over a few weeks.

The team explains what informed consent means at the first meeting with the community group (see discussion on informed consent in key informant interviews, above). The explanation includes the information that the team will be asking questions during normal discussions to determine issues that are important to members of the community group and that they do not need to respond.

### Making Arrangements and Drafting and Testing Questions

Progressive inquiry is best suited to locations where the same or similar people gather on a regular basis. Therefore, arrangements for this method involve identifying a suitable location in the community setting, if necessary, with the help of the placement agency. For example, the location could be a school classroom, health center waiting room, an apartment lobby, or the cafeteria of an organization.

Each cycle of progressive inquiry involves drafting and testing questions and collecting data. The refinement of questions and quick turnaround helps to make the method particularly responsive to the needs and interests of the community group.

When you begin, ask general questions that allow people to tell you their story or talk about their experiences and the experiences of members of the community. Make the questions simple enough to be introduced into normal conversation. For example, you might ask: "What is it like to live here?" and "What activities can families and children do outside?" followed by "Do you find it is easy to walk in this neighborhood all year round?" Your goal is to identify the assets and strengths of the community group and learn how they do things together (Kretzmann & McKnight, 1993). In your subsequent contacts, and as you build trust and people seem comfortable with responding to questions, you can move into other areas, such as their barriers to health and desired health.

An advantage of this approach is that the questions can be tailored to the communication level of the audience. If you find there are difficulties, simplify the questions and use pictures or props. Your initial priority is to start a conversation.

Once the questions and approach are decided, each team member follows the directions and asks the questions in a nonthreatening manner during normal conversation with one or two community members. Use field notes after the interaction to record the number of people approached and to track the responses to each question; include comments on the usefulness of the approach. At the end of each contact period, the team meets to review and compare findings. With subsequent cycles, make note if the person has previously responded to questions.

Continue the cycle of questioning by developing and asking increasingly specific questions on the same topic. This allows you to validate the nature and level of concern about a topic. Repeat until all the pertinent questions have been answered and you have reached as many community members as possible. A team usually needs at least three or four sessions in the same setting with the same or a similar group of people to start obtaining consistent responses and progressively less new information. More sessions are needed for those who have difficulty communicating.

At any point in the questioning, the procedure may need to be changed. For example, if the team finds some members of a community group reluctant to respond to questions, they may decide to direct the questions to those who are interested in the hope that others will eventually join in. Over time, progressive inquiry may reveal issues you had not considered. As an example, one team working with new immigrants discovered that many participants spent considerable time boiling water because they did not have access to safe water from a tap in their home countries. The team decided to focus on this issue and part of their action was to offer a tour of a water treatment plant.

When time is short, concentrate on asking different people the questions during each cycle of the inquiry and reduce the number of people. Do not try to shorten the time taken to ask the questions and listen to the response. If you rush, community members will reduce the quality of their response, and you may damage the relationship that you have built with them.

## Guided Observation

**Guided observation** collects detailed information on defined interactions that occur in a designated public or private setting. A public setting could be a shopping mall; a private setting could be a building or location with restricted access, such as an exercise class or university cafeteria. Guided observation uses specific questions or a checklist to focus the observations. By systematically observing people in different places, your team can learn more about how settings influence the way people behave. For example, if your group is exploring the use of playgrounds, you might decide to observe and document safe or unsafe use of equipment, or bullying behaviors in a public park or a school playground. Other examples would be observing the services provided to older adults in stores and pharmacies, or the use of breast-feeding facilities in shopping malls.

### Initial Preparation
The basic development approach applies when preparing for a guided observation: determine the purpose of the data collection, or in this case, the items or interactions of interest. Similar to progressive inquiry, you need to identify appropriate locations for gathering the information you require.

In public settings, people may ask you what you are doing if they do not already know why you are there. Provide a simple explanation, such as "I am counting the number of students who are using the playground to prepare a report for the Recreation Committee," as part of informed consent. You could also show them the form you are using to reassure them that you are not collecting names or any identifying information.

### Making Arrangements, and Drafting and Testing Questions
In addition to selecting a location, in guided observation you need to decide on the most appropriate time of day to make the observations of interest. At shopping centers, for example, older people would probably be present in greater numbers during the day,

### Multilanguage Project

The team continues to use progressive inquiry with the women who attend the drop-in sessions in the lobby. More pregnant women and women with small children are starting to attend, and the women take turns in caring for the children in one corner of the room. Now that the women seem more comfortable with the team, they start mentioning other issues, such as how lonesome they feel without the support of their family. For instance, one woman explained that in her country, the family would gather around to care for the mother and baby when a new baby is born. The team makes a note of these concerns so they can pass them on to the public health nursing advisor.

The two volunteers who organize the drop-in gatherings in the lobby become more involved in the community project by participating in the development of the progressive inquiry questions, asking the questions, and analyzing the results.

### English Project

The team decides to observe child activity in the playground. Two team members draft a checklist; the other two check it over before they get input from their advisor. They test the checklist at a public park so they will be ready to use it on their next clinical day. They find it works well to record activities and events and that it provides opportunity to engage people in conversation.

Table 4.1 displays their draft checklist.

Luckily, the day is sunny when they start their observation. They find that women come to the playground throughout the day. One student focuses on the observations; the other uses the progressive inquiry questions on living in the apartment building. The information they gather supports what they have learned from the public health nurses: that many of the mothers they visit feel isolated and find it hard to connect with others. The women say they really appreciate the playground because they can get out and talk to other women. However, they really want a place to meet inside during poor weather. As well, the students hear negative comments about how the tenants' association does not do anything for women with little children.

Meanwhile, the other team members approach the tenants' association to see if they can attend their next meeting. They are given 15 minutes to speak at the beginning of the next monthly meeting, which occurs in two weeks. They plan to provide background information from their secondary data and an introduction to their project. They discuss with their advisor how to include their findings from the playground observations in the presentation. After viewing a rehearsal of the presentation, their advisor feels it will go well. She is unable to attend but has arranged for a colleague to be present and to introduce them.

**Table 4.1: Draft Checklist for Playground Observation**

Date:

Observer(s):

| Time | # Adults: Female/ Male | # Children: 0–5, 5–12, 12+ | Activities of Children | Comments (weather, events, comments from participants) |
|---|---|---|---|---|
| 8:30–9:30 | 3 F | –  1 baby in pushchair<br>–  1 toddler | –  Watching tree<br>–  Sitting on swing seat | One pregnant woman, not accompanied by child, talking and laughing with mother of baby. No interaction between two women and mother of toddler. Sunny. |
| 9:30–10:30 | | | | |
| 10:30–11:30 | | | | |

For the meeting, they bring a flip chart and markers to be sure that everyone can see the ideas recorded. Their advisor's colleague introduces them, and they thank the association for giving them time to speak, provide the rationale for their community project, and ask the group for help in identifying ways to support women in the building. They explain how they collected information from public health nurses and women in the playground, and data from their two days of observation. Association members are pleased to hear about the use of the playground because they needed that kind of information to report to the city parks department. The team reinforces the importance of the playground for reducing isolation and identifies that the women would like a place to meet in the building when the weather is bad.

On hearing that, the room falls silent. The atmosphere is a little tense, but then one person speaks up, saying that this has come up before. Apparently the tenants' association had started to look into it, but the issue got sidelined. This breaks the silence, and the meeting chair has to ask people to speak one at a time so the recorder can get everything down. When the flow of ideas slows, the chair asks for volunteers to investigate further and bring back a report for the next meeting. One person volunteers to work with a resident who was unable to attend the meeting, and the students agree to share their record of the meeting and remain in touch. The team leader thanks the person who volunteered. Their advisor's colleague tells the team that they did a very professional job. This feels like progress. Looking to the future, the team understands that public health can continue to build a relationship with the tenants' association when the community project is over.

**Discussion Topics and Questions**

11. How might the team in the multilanguage building use guided observation?

12. Explain why the English team feels that the meeting with the Tenant Association could result in the Association continuing a relationship with public health once the project is over.

and younger people, in the evening. If, for example, your team wants to observe the effect of smoking bylaws on teenagers, you might spend time outside a high school at lunchtime and a shopping center in the evening.

Often, community nursing projects occur in a setting with more limited access, such as a school, business, manufacturing plant, or meeting room. This will set bounds on what behavior you will be able to observe in relation to the focus of your inquiry. For example, if you are interested in school-age children and exercise, you might have to negotiate access to make observations in the classroom, the school gymnasium, and the playground. In a workplace, observations related to nutrition might be restricted to a cafeteria or lunchroom.

Once the purpose, topics/interactions, and location for the observation are determined, the team can draft an observation checklist. At a minimum, the checklist should record the time of day and number of people observed engaging in particular activities. Include a column to record unexpected events or comments made by people. Then, have different people test the draft on location and make revisions as necessary.

### Conducting Guided Observation

During the observation, try to be as unobtrusive as possible so people will behave normally. Once people are used to your presence and know what you are doing, you can ask questions to clarify your observations. If, for example, you notice that many girls just hang around and talk during recess at school rather than engaging in physical activity, you might ask questions to find out more. Because you are new to the situation, your observations can provide valuable insight for people who are familiar with the situation and take things for granted.

The following list details the procedure for guided observation:

1. Define what questions you want answered and prepare a statement to explain your presence for informed consent.
2. Arrange location and timing.
3. Draft a checklist of items, review it with advisors, and pretest in one location.
4. Revise the checklist if necessary and use it in the remaining locations.
5. At the end of the day, review and collate results.

It is possible to conduct guided observation at the same time as other assessment methods. For example, while other team members are using progressive inquiry, one person could be observing the interactions and recording what is happening in the room. The observer might notice that some participants are moving away from team members while others are moving closer, or that some people always stay on the edges of the group and rarely interact. You can compare both sets of data at the end of the day to obtain a more holistic perspective on how the group functions and determine ways to include more people if necessary.

## Focus Groups

**Focus groups** are small-group discussions guided by a trained moderator to learn more about opinions on a designated topic that will guide future action (KU Work Group for Community Health and Development [KU Work Group], 2014a). Focus groups are an advanced assessment method because they require lengthy preparation, tested questions, organizational review of the questions, and a trained moderator. The moderator introduces and leads the discussion using the prepared questions, encourages input from all participants, seeks clarification as necessary, and summarizes the discussion. The development process for focus groups described below assumes that the team is working under the close supervision of the advisor, who might also be the moderator.

Focus groups are most useful when program staff want to obtain in-depth opinions on a particular topic from people who have different perspectives on the subject and are comfortable in expressing their views in a group. For example, if they are seeking information on strategies for improving sleep in new mothers, they might talk to both experienced and new mothers as well as others with experience in supporting people during life transitions. If the focus were increasing exercise during adolescence, they might involve teenagers, the parents of teenagers, schoolteachers, and community recreation associations. Usually a program holds more than one focus group to gain different perspectives and to include people from different areas of the community.

The focus group demonstration in the Appendix to this chapter provides the format for conducting a focus group to reduce smoking by youth. The team can adapt the content in the example for different situations.

### Initial Preparation

Initial preparation follows the basic development approach, including defining the purpose of the questions and topics of interest, preparing to recruit people, providing informed consent information, and considering how many focus groups may be held. Plan to conduct a focus group for 30 minutes to an hour, with four to eight participants.

Also find out the timing and requirements of the organizational review. Organizations usually require a review for formal assessment methods, such as focus groups and questionnaires, to ensure that ethical practices are followed. An organizational review could take two to three weeks or more. In other situations, the organization may delegate the review to a manager or your advisor. If that is the case, it might be possible for an advisor to prepare the review in advance and to work closely with the team throughout the process and subsequent administration.

### Making Arrangements, and Drafting and Testing Questions

Consider who could provide insight into the topic, how to recruit them, and where to meet. Similar to previously mentioned methods of assessment, potential participants and meeting organizers usually need from two to four weeks to accommodate your request to meet with them.

Consult with your advisors to identify a suitable location for holding the focus groups. One option is to "piggyback" the discussion before or after a regular meeting or event, since it is usually very difficult to recruit participants one by one. Another option that may work in your situation is to hold an Internet teleconference. Scheduling two or three small focus groups with four participants has the advantage of providing training opportunities.

**Multilanguage Project**

The team working in the multilanguage building realized that a focus group would not be appropriate in their situation because the residents have limited ability in speaking English, especially in a group.

**English Project**

The public health nurses working in the Fairway area agree to participate in a 40-minute focus group one week following the tenants' association meeting. The team's advisor offers to moderate and suggests that the team adapt the questions and procedures from a previous focus group with nurses providing prenatal and postnatal care to women in another low-income area. She has learned that a full organizational review will not be required if her manager approves the questions, since the questionnaire had been used before.

The team decides to take advantage of the opportunity. The 10 questions from the previous focus group provide a good starting point, but do not address social isolation or women wanting a place to meet. Since this issue was identified in community mapping, key informant interviews, and progressive inquiry questions in the playground, they want it addressed. After deciding that five questions will be appropriate for the time available, the team chooses four questions from the list and adds question 3, related to support in the apartment building.

The manager approved the following questions:
1. What do you find rewarding about working with mothers in Fairway?
2. What do you find are the most important needs of mothers living in low-income buildings in the first few months after having a baby?
3. What could building staff and the tenants' association do to support these mothers?

4. What opportunities exist in the community or region that could support these mothers?
5. What ideas do you have about improving support for these mothers within the building?

They prepare the information letter and modify the guidelines. Since most of the questions have already been tested with nurses, they do not need another pretest, but they decide to role-play the focus group to get a better understanding of the process. One student is purposefully shy and another is very talkative in order to challenge the moderator. The talkative participant so flusters the moderator that she has difficulty covering the five questions. After the rehearsal, they explore different ways of dealing with the situation. Their advisor commends the team and proposes that team members share the recording and co-lead the discussion with her if things are going well. Two students volunteer to co-lead a question.

Just before the discussion is to start, the team finds the room has been double-booked. Luckily, they find another room with little delay. The six participants seem very aware of the time constraints and the students feel sufficiently confident to co-lead a discussion by the time they get to the last two questions. The participating nurses comment that the questions are very relevant, and that they enjoy having the opportunity to talk about how to improve the circumstances of new mothers. The team feels that they have had a great opportunity to learn about preparing and running focus groups.

**Discussion Topics and Questions**
13. What factors in the scenario made the focus group feasible?
14. What are the pros and cons of starting the focus group with the question "What do you find rewarding about working with mothers in Fairway?" What other initial question would you suggest?

For example, a trained moderator could demonstrate the moderator role with group one, and coach team members to moderate the remaining group sessions.

Additional requirements are to prepare and send out the focus group information/ invitations, put together a moderator and recorder guide (see example in the Appendix to this chapter), and select a moderator/facilitator and recorder.

While you are making arrangements, you need to draft and test the interview questions. As with other methods, the first step in developing questions is to clarify the purpose of the focus group. Ask: "What questions do we want answered and why is this information required?" Draft a maximum of 10 questions initially, with the expectation that you will reduce the number to five. Use the resources you have already collected, such as secondary data, key informant opinions, and progressive inquiry results, and consult with advisors.

Once you have five draft questions, pilot test them with people who have similar characteristics to those of the expected participants, debrief after the test, and reword or change the questions as necessary. The information regarding informed consent is included in the focus group invitation and at the beginning of the session.

### Conducting the Focus Group

After the introduction, the moderator can begin with a round-robin (introduced for the first team meeting in Chapter 2). Allow 2 minutes or so for participants to give their names and answer the first question (carefully chosen to break the ice) without interruption until everyone has spoken. This approach establishes the role of the moderator, gives everyone a chance to speak, and encourages the participants to share the speaking time with others. The recorder documents the comments in the order they are given, preferably verbatim. Participants are not identified by name, but may be numbered.

Plan to hold a debriefing session immediately following the focus group (see Appendix to this chapter for example questions). The debriefing helps you capture the mood or emotion of participants, which may be lost during the analysis, and allows you to make changes to improve the next session.

Focus groups work best with people who express themselves readily in public. To be effective, focus groups need advance preparation, tested questions, a trained moderator and recorder, and a topic that is interesting to participants. Focus groups with service providers can be particularly effective when participants have a common interest but work in different areas or disciplines.

## Questionnaires

**Questionnaires** are designed to collect consistent information using pretested questions from individuals at the same or different times and locations. Questionnaires are considered an advanced assessment method because they require considerable time and expertise to both develop and test questions that collect credible information in an ethical manner. In this text, we assume questionnaires are being used to identify the assets and needs of a community group, directly relevant to the development or evaluation of health services or programs, often called quality assurance. A further assumption is that the questionnaires will build on the primary and secondary data already collected as part of a community assessment. The KU Work Group for Community Health and Development (2014b) uses the term "concern survey" for this type of questionnaire. Similar to the use of focus groups, this is an advanced assessment method, and an experienced practitioner must work in partnership with the team to ensure that ethical standards regarding appropriate questions and approaches are met.

Questionnaires can vary in length and be structured in different ways. They may use open-ended questions, or closed-ended—yes/no, or multiple-choice—questions, or a combination. Usually they are self-administered. Although questions are also used to guide in-depth individual interviews, that application requires considerable time and expertise and is not included here.

Questionnaires collect information from people who can read, write, and respond to questions. Since the information or opinions provided are not openly shared with others, as they would be in a focus group, questionnaires are appropriate when gathering information on sensitive issues, such as sexual health issues or ways to reduce drinking and driving behavior, and service and program evaluation.

Relatively inexperienced teams may be involved in distributing questionnaires on risk behaviors if experienced practitioners have developed, tested, and received ethical approval for the questionnaires. They could also be involved in developing and delivering quality assurance or evaluation questionnaires to the people providing services or programs for people at risk.

### Initial Preparation

The development of questionnaires follows the basic development process discussed earlier. Your advisor will inform you if a review has been completed and whether or not further procedures are required. Ensure that a written introduction that includes informed consent is at the beginning of the questionnaire.

### Making Arrangements, and Drafting and Testing Questions

The questionnaire is designed to gather information on a certain topic, so your aim is to have it completed by as many people in your community as possible who are likely to have the information you need. Think about how you will get a representative sample of your community of interest. For a hospital or manufacturing plant, this would mean including people on all shifts. For people in a community program, such as a fitness class, this would mean including people who attend regularly as well as those who don't. For other situations, such as schools, you will need to find the appropriate location to reach the desired age range and gender.

You can distribute questionnaires in person at a community setting, send them out by mail or email, or make them available on the Internet. For example, questionnaires can be distributed and collected at a popular shopping mall; at work, they can be distributed with pay envelopes.

Once your purpose is clear, the first decision is in regard to what questionnaire format and delivery method is most appropriate. Questionnaires that people fill out themselves, called self-administered questionnaires, are the most practical but take considerable time to develop and test, especially if there are no previous versions. In some circumstances, you may need to read or explain the questions so that people who have difficulty reading or writing can participate.

The usual format is to structure the questionnaire with mainly closed-ended questions that require yes/no or multiple-choice answers. You can include one or two open-ended questions at the end. Not everyone will respond to the open-ended questions; however, they may reveal issues not previously considered. For example, in a survey conducted by the author with girls ages 11 to 14, 20 girls wrote in "to rebel against parents" when given the option to add to a list of reasons as to why girls might first engage in sexual intercourse.

Questions fit into one of two categories: sociodemographic or content. Sociodemographic questions on broad categories such as age, gender, family size, and language provide information on who completed the questionnaire and allow you to determine whether or not the overall response fairly represents the community of interest. Use content questions to explore the previously identified issues and strengths of the community. For example, questions on satisfaction with services and programs are consistent with quality improvement in community/public health. In relation to a well-baby clinic, you could ask respondents to indicate which services offered by the clinic are or would be used.

Both sociodemographic and content questions can aid in the development of services. However, the responses to sociodemographic questions such as age, language, and number of children might inadvertently reveal the identity of a person or family. Reviews of previous questionnaires and advice from advisors and experts will help keep the categories broad but still useful.

Limit the length of the questionnaire to one or two pages and ensure that it requires no more than 15 minutes to complete (KU Work Group, 2014a). This will also reduce the amount of time needed to prepare the questions and analyze the results. To achieve that length, each question must be weighed in terms of the information it will provide. For each question, ask "What will we do with this information?" If your response does not relate directly to the goal of the assessment, remove the question.

To ensure a good return for the investment, it is advisable for student teams to work with previously tested questionnaires, to keep the questions simple with "yes," "no," or "maybe" answers (see example questionnaire in the Scenario below), and to work closely with a person experienced in developing and using questionnaires. The KU Work Group for Community Health and Development (2014a) provides indices for developing properly worded items and examples of demographic questions. If there are no appropriate questionnaires available, a Web search may provide some useful prototypes. Involving community members in pretesting the questions is another way of greatly enhancing the relevance and readability of the questions.

The readability of the questions in a questionnaire is an important aspect to consider in self-administered questionnaires. **Readability** is the indication of number of years of education that a person needs to be able to understand the text easily at first reading. A study that tested written material for patients and clients using the most common readability scales found that most material was too difficult for many to understand (Ley & Florio, 2007). The readability scales used in the study were Flesch Reading Ease, Flesch-Kincaid Formula, Fog Index, Fry Readability Graph, and SMOG Grading (Ley & Florio, 2007). These findings emphasize the need to consider literacy and readability in all interactions with the community, especially with written material.

### Distributing the Questionnaires

As much as possible, encourage people to complete self-administered questionnaires immediately by providing tables, chairs, and pencils. Another option is to offer donated prizes, draws, and posters to prompt people to return their questionnaires. Email is an inexpensive way to reach people if you have access to email addresses. Above all, select a distribution method that is convenient for the people you want to reach in the community and have a backup plan if the first method does not work.

Questionnaires, compared to other assessment methods, can provide comparable data, quickly, from many people. Usually self-administered, they provide more confidentiality than assessments conducted in a group setting and can produce a good response rate if they are completed on the spot. The format can be adapted for those unable to read and

**Multilanguage Project**

Team members have developed a good relationship with the eight to ten women they see consistently and notice an increased confidence in the women's ease in speaking English.

Other women in the building are becoming involved, and the team discusses with the advisors whether they might get input from them using a questionnaire. The public health nurse advisor tells them that public health is very interested in having a questionnaire for use in similar situations. The requirements are as follows: (1) no more than one page in length, (2) a readability level of grade 4 or lower, and (3) the questions must be ready in one week for review by the organization review board.

The timelines are short, but the students feel confident they can produce a questionnaire in that time. Their advisor helps them to develop the introduction and the informed consent paragraph for the beginning of the questionnaire. The students use an online program to test the readability of the draft questions and are amazed to find it is at a grade 9 level. After working diligently to reduce the length of sentences and the number of words of three syllables, they finally get the reading level down to grade 3. The final questionnaire, entitled "Questions on Food for Women with a Baby," is provided below:

---

**Questions on Food for Women with a Baby**

We are nursing students from the Old York Nursing Program. We want to learn what questions you have about food. You can choose to answer the questions or not. Do NOT put your name on the paper.

Check ✓ the questions which interest you:
☐ What food is good for me?
☐ What food is good for a baby?
☐ Where can I shop for good low-cost food?
☐ How can I eat better when I feel sick?
☐ What could I eat in the morning?
☐ What could I eat at noon?
☐ What could I eat in the evening?
☐ What can I eat between meals?
☐ Please fill in other food questions _____.

Thank-you for your help!

---

The students consult the two volunteers on how to pretest the questionnaire and where and how it might be distributed. On their advice, they invite two women with moderate skills in English and two who are less fluent to complete the questionnaire in the lobby. The pretest goes well, and only minor changes are required.

As well, they follow up with the suggestion to distribute the questionnaire at a gathering in the lobby, where they will provide snacks. As soon as the questionnaire is approved, the team and volunteer women make the arrangements; the women personally invite other women with children to attend. At the beginning of the event, hardly anyone is present, and the team starts to feel anxious. Slowly more and more women show up. At the end, 10 women complete the questionnaire and five more hand it in the following week. Team members later learn that the women initially felt a bit shy and were worried about being able to understand the questions. Afterward, they were pleased that they could answer the questions.

**English Project**

The team working on the English project were involved in organizing focus groups and did not feel that a questionnaire would be appropriate in their situation. They made that decision because the residents rarely spoke to them inside the building and would therefore not be likely to complete a questionnaire for them.

**Discussion Topics and Questions**

15. What were the benefits and possible drawbacks of the team using a questionnaire after progressive inquiry questions?
16. If you were on the team in the scenario, how would you respond if the city worker in the building asked for the names of the women who completed the questionnaire so she could ask follow-up questions?

write, though this can introduce some bias. The responses to closed-ended questions can be summarized numerically; however, such questions are more time-consuming to develop and test.

Overall, questionnaires are a very valuable assessment tool in community health nursing practice for reaching people who can read and write. Additional methods would also be needed to reach people who are isolated or have difficulty with reading and writing.

## Select Specific Assessment Methods (Step 4a)

Once you become familiar with the specific assessment methods, you will realize that some methods will work better than others with certain groups. We have identified four criteria to use when selecting the appropriate assessment methods.

### Criteria for Selecting Specific Assessment Methods

Although the various assessment methods are used to collect data, they can also have a secondary purpose, such as developing relationships or facilitating communication. Think about which method or methods will work the best with your particular community and whether or not the method is feasible given your time and resources. Once you select a method, you will need to prepare and organize to carry it out while observing ethical practice. Your preliminary knowledge of the community will help you to decide which assessment method to use and when. For instance, it is more effective to use an assessment method that builds relationships with the community group before using other methods. By establishing a relationship first, you increase the chances of asking the right questions of the right people at the right time and location, using the right approach.

Because each method has advantages and disadvantages, the best choice with people who communicate well in English may be to combine two or more methods in what is called triangulation (Salazar, Crosby, & DiClemente, 2006). The methods are chosen to complement each other and reduce bias. However, combining the analysis from the methods can be more difficult.

Box 4.4 provides four criteria for using assessment methods. These criteria take into account both the characteristics of the community and the situation.

## Selecting Final Assessment Methods

At this point in the assessment process, your team has likely collected data on the community using mapping and key informant interviews. You will now use this information to consider what remaining assessment methods would work best. Each method provides different information and varies according to the four criteria outlined in Box 4.4.

For most teams, the choice is between using progressive inquiry, guided observation, or both. Progressive inquiry provides in-depth information when you have access to the same or similar people on a regular basis. Guided observation provides systematically collected information on the naturally occurring behavior of members of the community group in readily accessible settings. As mentioned previously, if both methods are appropriate, you could use them concurrently. One or both of these assessment methods will provide most teams with sufficient data to recommend a specific action

**BOX 4.4**

**Criteria for Selecting Appropriate Assessment Methods**

The criteria:

1. Builds relationships
2. Accommodates difficulty with communication
3. Fits with timelines
4. Provides numbers (statistics)

The criterion of *builds relationships* is inherent in the informal, basic assessment methods—community mapping, key informant interviews, progressive inquiry, and guided observation—and especially needs to be nurtured early in a project. Relationship building is fundamental for community health nursing practice and contributes to the effectiveness of the more formal assessment methods.

The criterion of *accommodates difficulty with communication* is also provided by the four basic assessment methods. For example, you can adjust your speaking speed and the complexity of your questions during key informant interviews and progressive inquiry when people do not understand your questions.

The criterion of *fits with timelines* is difficult to estimate. An overall "rule of thumb" is to complete the assessment data collection by the midpoint of your project, assuming you plan to carry through with action and evaluation. Figure 4.3 illustrates the midpoint in a typical student project. In addition, Table 2.1 in Chapter 2 provides more details for allocating time

for the substeps of the process. If your project focuses more on one part of the process, such as assessment or evaluation, you may have more time to devote to collect that specific data.

**Figure 4.3: Midpoint in a Short-Term Project**

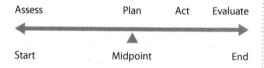

Table 4.2 in the following summary indicates the characteristics of each assessment method and can assist you in making your decisions. Also, be aware that opportunities can suddenly arise, such as being invited to a meeting where you could distribute a questionnaire or be involved in a focus group.

The criterion of *provides numbers (statistics)* may be needed to collect numerical data to substantiate the continuation or change in programs or services. Although developing and distributing questionnaires to a large number of people is not feasible in short-term projects, a pilot test of a questionnaire or taking part in the distribution of a prepared questionnaire may be appropriate. Methods such as guided observation and structured questionnaires provide information that can be summarized numerically.

(see Chapter 5). A few teams working with larger or longer term projects may also use one of the advanced methods as well, after discussions with their advisors.

## Collect Data (Step 4b)

Start using your selected basic assessment method(s) by following the procedures described above. If both progressive inquiry and guided observation are relevant, the procedures indicate how they might be used concurrently. If your team is using one of the advanced methods, you may use the two basic methods for a shorter period or involve fewer people to allow more planning time for the advanced method.

Once you start collecting data, you need to find a method to keep the data together and secure. Keeping data secure is part of confidentiality in ethical practice. As mentioned in progressive inquiry, keep field notes and a record to track your questions and responses. This information is necessary when analyzing your data and presenting results.

**Table 4.2: Comparison of Assessment Methods in Relation to Criteria**

| | Builds Relationships | Accommodates Difficulty with Communication | Fits with Timelines | | Provides Numbers |
|---|---|---|---|---|---|
| | | | Preparation | Duration | |
| Observation and mapping | Contributes | N/A | 1–2 weeks | 3 weeks | N/A |
| Key informant interviews or group meeting[1] | Yes | Yes | 1–3 weeks | 4 weeks | No |
| Progressive inquiry | Yes | Yes | 1–2 weeks | 4–6 weeks | Limited |
| Guided observation | Contributes | N/A | 1–2 weeks | 3 weeks | Yes |
| Questionnaire[1] | | | | | |
| 5–10 questions | No | No | 2–3 weeks | 4 weeks | Yes |
| 10+ questions | No | No | 3–4 weeks | 6 weeks | Yes |
| Focus groups[1] | Contributes | No | 2–4 weeks | 6 weeks | No |

*Note:* 1. Shorten time by having modifiable materials and prearranged processes.

## Teamwork during Assessment of Community Group

As teams work through Steps 3 and 4 of a community project, they are faced with certain challenges. Some result from the stage of development; others result from the different tasks that are required. Teams have to become organized, build team spirit, and keep morale high while they assess the physical and social neighborhood and resources (Step 3) and assess primary data (Step 4) to develop the community project.

## Team Organization

Five aspects of team organization become important during this time: (1) decision making, (2) documenting, (3) learning to delegate tasks, (4) maintaining or expanding collaboration with the community group, and (5) gaining experience in evaluating the team roles and functions.

### Decision Making

As the project begins to take shape, the team must think ahead and plan for future activities. Often, decisions have to be made with incomplete information, while other activities are still in process. For example, arranging a focus group requires preparation—setting dates and booking meeting rooms well ahead—in order to have sufficient time to recruit and notify participants. When making these arrangements, some things will be known, but others will not. For instance, you will likely know whom you want in the focus groups but not the questions you want to ask. When the dates are set, you then have to work backward to identify deadlines to be met for gaining approval, pilot testing, and so on. We call this planning process "backward mapping" and discuss it in more detail in Chapters 6 and 7. As well, you have to think ahead to data analysis. In order for things to run smoothly, team members have to consistently make timely decisions and coordinate activities.

Deciding among the different assessment methods is a particular challenge. Depending on the scope of the project, and the number and characteristics of the intended community group, most teams will use at least two data collection methods. Deciding on whether to use progressive inquiry or guided observation and focus group or questionnaires will depend on the nature of the project, the size of the community group, and how easy or difficult it is to make connections with the group. This requires the team to work through the various possibilities in a relatively short time and make decisions on necessarily incomplete information. While it can be stressful for some, making decisions and having a plan reduces uncertainty.

## Documenting

As the project evolves, the team needs to keep track of the process for the record. Working in subteams on different assessment methods and including community members in the project further increases the need for good communication. Team meetings and weekly reports become even more important.

Additional tools are provided to aid documentation. Chapter 3 introduced the project work plan (see also Appendix A.3.1) as a way to document activities and accomplishments according to the steps and substeps of the community project. Closely related tools, the project and assessment timelines (Appendix A.3.2), are Gantt charts that allow the team to plot out the timing of project steps over the course of the project in a one-page document. Refer to Table 2.1 in Chapter 2 to determine the approximate amount of time for each step and substep. Each step can be broken down in more detail as needed and checked off when completed. The estimated timelines can be entered in the chart to the end of the project, usually by the third or fourth week, even if it means making changes later. By checking and adjusting the timeline each week, the team has a record of accomplishments and is more likely to stay on track.

## Delegating Tasks

Developing the ability to delegate work in order to complete tasks on time and appreciating the importance of this for teamwork is a key learning for team members. With delegation, all members have to pay greater attention to decision making, documentation, and communication. For example, when tasks are allocated, the team needs a system for tracking who is responsible for meeting the deadline. This information can be documented in weekly reports to ensure that the lines of responsibility are clear. The responsible members are expected to complete their tasks by the due date or propose an alternative if they experience problems.

Delegation requires monitoring to ensure that assignments are completed and difficulties in fulfilling obligations are addressed. Two basic rules for dealing with issues are (1) deal with the issue, that is, discuss it within the team as soon as the problem is recognized; and (2) move the issue up to the next level quickly, to the clinical instructor and/or advisor, if the team cannot deal with it right away. An early fair and open discussion can lead to a quick resolution, in contrast to delaying or avoiding small issues, which can then grow. Since it is normal for all teams to have some issues, take the attitude that it is better to deal with situations immediately to prevent them from festering and becoming more difficult to resolve. Even if only one person is unhappy, take the opportunity to discuss it.

Another challenge to be aware of when members work separately is the potential to be diverted by interests in the community. For example, a community member may see the community project as a means to promote his or her own interests, for instance, obtaining a literature review on a topic not essential to the project. Such requests are difficult to ignore, especially when you want to continue to work with this person. You may find it helpful to include a statement in your team agreement that requests from the community will be dealt with by (a) listening carefully and recording the request, (b) explaining that requests have to be taken back to the team because you have a limited time to accomplish your project and need to consider each activity carefully, and (c) advising the person of the team decision. Although the request may not directly relate to your project, it could provide a way to meet with the community that might not otherwise have been available. Weigh the request in terms of time and possible contribution to the project.

### Increasing Collaboration
As you move through Steps 3 and 4 of the process, the team will be increasing collaboration with the community. The active involvement of the people in the community is important not only to encourage sustainability—ensuring that the community project will continue to be viable—but also to increase the capacity of the community to make plans and take action on their own. When you approach people with a "listen to learn" attitude and are prepared to start where the people are (Nyswander, 1956), they are reassured that their views and involvement are important. Another valuable way of thinking is to plan, as prescribed by the anonymous 1767 adage, "To stand in someone's shoes to see things from his or her point of view." For example, the English Project, in conducting a focus group with public health nurses to find out how they provide support, responded to the needs of community members and ensured the sustainability of efforts to increase support for women in the apartment building.

### Evaluating the Team
At the midpoint of the clinical, the team is encouraged or required to take time to review and evaluate the team and team agreement (see team evaluation tools in Appendix A.2.2, A.2.5, A.2.6, A.2.7). Suggestions are given in Chapter 2 on a process to follow.


## Team Rapport

Completing a community assessment requires teamwork, and working together effectively builds rapport. It also involves being sensitive to the morale of the team and learning to deal with the storming stage of development.

### Learning from Storming
Once the team has completed the orientation to the community project and started to collect secondary data, they have been together long enough to have faced some differences of opinion characteristic of the storming stage. As stated in Chapter 2, differences are a

normal part of human functioning. Consider storming as an opportunity to learn how to be receptive and creative with a group. Chapter 2 provides some helpful approaches to storming.

In the scenario, members of the English Project team were obviously having trouble, both personally and in terms of what the team was able to produce. Although they turned things around fairly quickly, not all teams are able to do so on their own. Some teams may find it useful to ask for assistance in going through a conflict resolution process with the clinical instructor or other experienced person.

### Evaluating Rapport

Storming can bring out negative feelings that can be challenging to address. Two short questionnaires, provided in Appendix A.2.6 and A.2.7, provide a means for team members to evaluate their own functioning and their view of their team's functioning. One scale is titled "Self-Assessment of Functioning on Team" and the other "Individual Assessment of Team Functioning." Both scales were developed by the authors and used in a survey of 459 nursing student in 2008–09. The internal consistency of both was high, at .80 for self-assessment and .88 for team functioning. Once the questionnaires are completed, the items can be used to guide a discussion on ways to improve team functioning and rapport.

## Summary

The assessment of primary data involves working directly with the people in the community group to determine their issues, strengths, assets, barriers to health, and desired health. Assessment requires careful thought and organization to select methods that foster a good exchange of ideas between the project team members and the community group. These methods are useful for building relationships, accommodating difficulty with communication (e.g., language and comfort speaking in public), fitting with preparation timelines, and obtaining numerical data if needed.

The basic assessment methods for all teams include community mapping, key informant interviews, progressive inquiry, and guided observation. Some teams may use one of the advanced methods: focus groups or questionnaires.

When you begin using the selected assessment method, you are entering another phase of the project. You have a clearer purpose and a narrower and more selective focus, and are placing greater emphasis on organization and keeping good records.

Teamwork during assessment is quite complicated because of the many different types of decisions that need to be made. The team leader and members need to hone their skills in decision making, communication, delegation, collaboration, and evaluation while maintaining their morale.

## Classroom and Seminar Exercises

1. Considering both the Multilanguage and English Projects in the chapter, discuss how the social determinants of health might limit women's attendance at prenatal classes and well-baby drop-ins.
2. Develop three questions on exercise for a group that interests you. Test out the questions using the readability link given in the reference list (ReadabilityFormulas.com, 2013). Simplify the questions and wording until the questions are at grade 4 level or below. What are the main differences between your first attempt and the final one?
3. Determine which assessment methods would be most appropriate to engage the highest number of participants and promote a relationship for the following community groups or issues:
   a. Workers in a small manufacturing plant
   b. Reducing smoking initiation in teens
   c. Participants at an older adults' drop-in center
4. Interacting with people in the community can create awkward situations that could conflict with ethical practice. Discuss the issues and explain how you would respond effectively to the following situations:
   a. You are introduced to a community group as "nurses from public health" when you are student nurses working on a project with public health.
   b. Community members make unfavorable comments about an agency or organization and expect you to pass on the comments.
5. Why would a focus group be preferred at a meeting over key informant questions or a questionnaire?

## References

American Nurses Association. (2010). *Code of ethics for nurses with interpretive statements*. Retrieved from www.nursingworld.org/MainMenuCategories/EthicsStandards/CodeofEthicsforNurses

Anderson, E., & McFarlane, J. (2014). *Community as partner* (7th ed.). Philadelphia, PA: Lippincott Williams & Wilkins.

Canadian Nurses Association (CNA). (2008). *Code of ethics for registered nurses* (2008 centennial edition). Retrieved from www.cna-aiic.ca/~/media/cna/files/en/codeofethics.pdf

Centers for Disease Control and Prevention. (2009). *Simply put: A guide for creating easy-to-understand materials* (3rd ed.). Retrieved from www.cdc.gov/healthliteracy/pdf/Simply_Put.pdf

Freire, P. (1972). *Pedagogy of the oppressed*. New York: Herder and Herder.

International Council of Nurses (ICN). (2012). *ICN code of ethics*. Retrieved from www.icn.ch/about-icn/code-of-ethics-for-nurses/

Kretzmann, J., & McKnight, J. (1993). *Building communities from the inside out*. Chicago, IL: ACTA Publications.

KU Work Group for Community Health and Development. (2014a). Conducting focus groups. *Community Tool Box* (Chapter 3, Section 6). Retrieved from http://ctb.ku.edu/en/table-contents/sub_section_main_1018.aspx

KU Work Group for Community Health and Development. (2014b). Conducting concerns surveys. *Community Tool Box* (Chapter 3, Section 10). Retrieved from http://ctb.ku.edu/en/table-of-contents/assessment/assessing-community-needs-and-resources/conduct-concerns-surveys/main

Lakkala, M. (2008). *Progressive inquiry*. Retrieved from http://wiki.helsinki.fi/download/attachments/41162207/Progressive+inquiry+model_introduction.pdf

Larson, C. (2007). Poverty during pregnancy: Its effects on child health outcomes. *Pediatric and Child Health, 12*(8), 673–677. Retrieved from www.ncbi.nlm.nih.gov/pmc/articles/PMC2528810/

Ley, R., & Florio, T. (2007, October). The use of readability formulas in healthcare. *Psychology, Health, & Medicine*. Retrieved from www.tandfonline.com/doi/abs/10.1080/13548509608400003

Maternal and Child Health Bureau, US Department of Health and Human Services, Health Resources and Services Administration. (2011). *Child health USA 2011*. Retrieved from http://mchb.hrsa.gov/chusa11/

Minkler, M., & Wallerstein, N. (1997). Improving health through community organizing and building. In M. Minkler (Ed.), *Community organizing and community building for health*. New Brunswick, NJ: Rutgers University Press.

Nyswander, D. (1956). Education for health: Some principles and their application. *Health Education Monographs, 14*, 65–70.

Public Health Agency of Canada. (2008). *Canadian perinatal health report: Key findings*. Retrieved from www.phac-aspc.gc.ca/publicat/2008/cphr-rspc/factsheet-fiche-eng.php

Public Health Ontario, Health Communication Unit. (2009). Situational assessment. Chapter 2 in *Health promotion planning workbook*. Retrieved from www.thcu.ca/infoandresources/resource_display.cfm?search=search&res_sub_topicid=32

ReadabilityFormulas.com. (2013). *Free text readability consensus calculator*. Retrieved from www.readabilityformulas.com/free-readability-formula-tests.php

Salazar, L., Crosby, R., & DiClemente, R. (2006). Qualitative research strategies and methods for health promotion. In R. Crosby, R. DiClemente, & L. Salazar (Eds.), *Research methods in health promotion*. San Francisco, CA: Jossey-Bass.

Vollman, A., Anderson, E., & McFarlane, J. (2008). *Canadian community as partner* (2nd ed.). Philadelphia, PA: Lippincott Williams & Wilkins.

Wass, A. (1999). Assessing the community. In J. Hitchcock, P. Schubert, & S. Thomas (Eds.), *Community health nursing*. Albany, NY: Delmar.

# Website Resources

### Community Forum, Public Forum, Listening Sessions

KU Work Group for Community Health and Development, *Conducting Public Forums and Listening Sessions*: http://ctb.ku.edu/en/tablecontents/sub_section_main_1021.aspx
  This KU web page provides practical guidelines for gathering systematic information.


### Focus Groups

KU Work Group for Community Health and Development, *Conducting Focus Groups*: http://ctb.ku.edu/en/tablecontents/sub_section_main_1018.aspx
  This page provides practical guidelines for conducting focus groups.


### Geographical Information

Google Earth: www.google.com/earth/index.html
  Google Earth provides 3D street views that can augment windshield surveys.

Wikipedia, *Geographical Information System (GIS) and Public Health*: http://en.wikipedia.org/wiki/GIS_and_Public_Health
  This Wikipedia page explains GIS in easy-to-understand terms.


### Questionnaires and Surveys

KU Work Group for Community Health and Development, *Conducting Concerns Surveys*: http://ctb.ku.edu/en/table-of-contents/assessment/assessing-community-needs-and-resources/conduct-concerns-surveys/main
  This KU web page provides practical guidelines for conducting concerns surveys.


### Search Strategy

To obtain information on the Internet about questionnaires or assessment methods, type the following into your search engine: "community questionnaire" or "community assessment." Other terms, such as "community needs assessment," "community asset assessment," or "survey" can also be used, as well as terms such as "health promotion," "food," "exercise," "immunizations," and "child care" along with "questionnaire" or "survey." See "Stategies for Using the Internet" at the end of Chapter 1 to limit your search to credible sites.

# Appendix to Chapter 4

**Project Timeline**

Project Title: Assessing and Supporting Multilanguage Mothers
Date: Week 4

**Week Four Timeline for Assessing and Supporting Multilanguage Mothers**

| Steps and Substeps in Process | 1 | 2 | 3 | 4 | 5 | 6 | 7 | 8 | 9 | 10 | 11 | 12 |
|---|---|---|---|---|---|---|---|---|---|---|---|---|
| ASSESS | | | | | | | | | | | | |
| 1. Orient to community project | | | | | | | | | | | | |
| Establish relationships | X | X | X | | | | | | | | | |
| Define the project, population group, and issue | X | X | X | | | | | | | | | |
| 2. Assess secondary data | | | | | | | | | | | | |
| Review sociodemographic data | | X | X | | | | | | | | | |
| Review epidemiological data | | X | X | | | | | | | | | |
| Review previously conducted community surveys and program statistics | | X | X | | | | | | | | | |
| Review national and local policy documents | | X | X | | | | | | | | | |
| Review literature and best practice guidelines | | X | X | | | | | | | | | |
| Summarize secondary data | | | | X | | | | | | | | |
| 3. Assess physical and social environment | | | | | | | | | | | | |
| Observe and map physical and social environment | | X | X | | | | | | | | | |
| Interview key informants | | X | X | | | | | | | | | |
| 4. Assess primary data | | | | | | | | | | | | |
| Select specific assessment methods | | | X | | | | | | | | | |
| Collect data: | | | X | X | X | X | | | | | | |
| progressive inquiry | | | X | X | X | X | | | | | | |
| written questionnaire | | | | | X | X | | | | | | |
| 5. Analyze assessment data | | | | | | | | | | | | |
| Assemble assessment data | | | | | X | | | | | | | |
| Analyze and validate data | | | | | X | X | X | | | | | |
| Develop action statements | | | | | | X | X | | | | | |
| Summarize assessment | | | | | | X | X | | | | | |
| PLAN | | | | | | | | | | | | |
| 6. Plan action | | | | | | | | | | | | |
| Select priority | | | | | | | | | | | | |
| Identify goal | | | | | | | | | | | | |
| 9. Evaluate teamwork | | X | | X | | X | | X | | X | | X |

## Focus Group Demonstration on Factors to Reduce Smoking by Youth

(Material can be adapted for different situations and used to prepare students in a classroom or seminar before, or in place of, being involved in a focus group in the community.)

### Moderator's Guide

(*The moderator reads the following*.) Thank you for agreeing to participate in this discussion. I would like you to introduce yourselves. (*Participants introduce themselves*.)

Statement of Purpose and Confidentiality:
In community health nursing, focus groups are one of the methods used to assess the community group's needs and interests. This experience will give us some idea of what it is like to be in and conduct a focus group. These focus groups are less formal than focus groups used in research and are often tape-recorded. The topic of discussion for today is smoking and what we could do to reduce smoking by youth.

We only have 40 minutes for our discussion, so it will be a much shorter version than most, which can take an hour to an hour and a half for a group of 10 to 12. However, we already know each other and have been working together before, so we can probably accomplish a lot in 40 minutes.

In the first part of this discussion, I will be asking for your experiences as smokers or nonsmokers and the different factors affecting this behavior. In the second half, we will be looking at the ways we can approach this problem, individually or as a group. In particular, I would like to know how you feel about

- the factors contributing to smoking and nonsmoking.
- the influence of the media and tobacco industry.
- the influence health professionals could have in decreasing smoking rates.

Your comments are completely confidential. Your name will not be associated with any comments you make during this discussion. This is an opportunity to be heard, and I encourage you to speak up. I also encourage you to speak about yourself and your experiences. There are no right or wrong answers. Please feel free to be totally honest.

_____ (recorder's name) will be taking notes using a number to represent each person.

I want everyone to have an opportunity to speak, so as moderator, I will start by using a round-robin, which means I will ask each of you in turn to speak with no interruptions. If you choose not to speak at that time, just shake your head. After everyone has spoken, I will open up the discussion. I will also end the same way. For the questions in between, the discussion will be open for everyone. I might sometimes call upon you to share your ideas, or, if you are speaking more than others, I may have to interrupt you to give other people an opportunity to comment. Please don't be offended. It is not that I do not want to hear what you have to say, it is just that we have only 40 minutes and I want everyone to have equal opportunity to comment. Are there any questions or concerns?

*continued on the following page*

*continued from the previous page*

**Focus Group Questions**

| Questions: Factors Affecting Smoking Status of Youth | Probes |
|---|---|
| 1. Thinking back as far as possible, what was your first experience with cigarettes? | As a child, were you exposed to advertisements, parents or siblings who smoked, ads on TV, or tobacco paraphernalia? |
| 2. Thinking of yourself and/or other people, what factors do you think encourage youth to start smoking and why do they continue? | Partying and smoking with friends, occasional or social smoker, smoking in family, wanting to belong, wanting to make choices independent of parents, stress, weight concerns, being "cool," fashion, addiction |
| 3. Consider mass media and advertising.<br>a. What messages encourage smoking?<br>b. What messages encourage nonsmoking? | Movies, TV, magazines, ads |
| 4. How does the tobacco industry influence smoking by youth? | Lawsuits, labeling, young models, smoking in movies, sponsorship or sports/cultural events—Are particular methods used to get youth to start smoking? |
| 5. As a group of future health care professionals, what could we do to<br>a. help youth refrain from smoking?<br>b. help youth quit smoking? | Increase awareness of the influence from media and the tobacco industry, cost of cigarettes, be supportive for those who are in the process of quitting, help people deal with stress and/or body image issues, be aware of the addictive nature of nicotine, refer person to a nicotine addiction clinic, advocate for smoke-free indoor air, "take it outside," offer "munchies" to quitters (celery, carrots) |

*(At the end of the questions, the moderator thanks the participants.)*

**Recorder's Guide**

Recording for focus groups:

1. Write each of the questions from the focus group on the top of a separate sheet of paper. Try to capture the essence of the conversation and important quotes. Write some observations about the nonverbal communication from group members.

2. Usually a recorder does not speak until the end. However, if you want to clarify a point or contribute to the conversation, do so. You need to remember to return to your note taking.

3. At the end of the discussion, clarify any questions you may have on what a person said.

**Information about the Focus Group**

| | |
|---|---|
| Date: | |
| Location: | |
| Number of participants: | |
| Name of moderator: | |
| Name of recorder: | |
| Name of facilitator to assist and lead debriefing (optional): | |
| Other comments: | |

## Debriefing Session

The debriefing can be led by the facilitator or another person in the group. You can use or adapt the following questions to guide the debriefing:

1. Did you feel that there was good discussion of the questions? Why or why not?
2. Advantages of focus groups are the depth and complexity of responses and the stimulation of new thoughts (KU Work Group, 2014a). Do you feel that these advantages were realized in this discussion? Why or why not?
3. Some of the disadvantages of focus groups are that the participants may influence each other's opinions, data are not quantifiable, a limited number of questions can be asked, the discussion is more difficult to analyze than answers to quantitative questions, and the quality depends on the skill of moderator (KU Work Group, 2014a). Did these disadvantages affect this discussion? Why or why not?
4. How did the size and location of the group affect the results?
5. Consider how easy or difficult it was for the moderator to meet the following characteristics of a good moderator: establish rapport, lead discussion without judgment, focus (return to questions), encourage discussion among all by controlling dominating speakers and encouraging quiet participants, and frequently summarize statements to ensure that appropriate meaning has been captured (KU Work Group, 2014a).
6. How easy or difficult was it to record the responses?
7. Is anyone planning to use focus groups in their projects? Was this demonstration useful to prepare you on what to expect?
8. What main points on smoking among youth were identified during the discussion?

## Focus Group Exercise

Conduct a focus group using the provided material above, or on a relevant topic, with 4 to 12 people. Debrief following the focus group.

1. What measures can you use as a moderator to ensure that everyone gets a chance to speak? (Start with a round-robin so everyone is encouraged to speak for a short time. Ask for other opinions, for example, "What do others think?" Basic approach for quiet people: Direct a specific question to them; if a person has not spoken much during the session, ask at the end what they feel were the important points. Talkative people: Explain before you start that if a person is speaking more than others, you may need to interrupt them and call upon others. If they are reminded about not talking too much, and continue to do so, do not respond to the content of what they said, rather state, "Thanks for your comment." (turn to another person) "_____ (name of another participant), what do you think?")
2. Why is the preparation and pilot testing of questions important for a focus group? (Since considerable time, effort, and cost is involved in bringing people together, the questions need to elicit the required data during the discussion. If the questions are confusing, or are not relevant, the data will not be useful and participants will likely not be willing to continue their participation. Although this same statement applies to all methods, by definition, the questions are "focused" to elicit the full range of opinions on a particular topic and may be used with more than one group.)

# Chapter 5

# Analysis—Step 5

A nalysis of assessment data is a transitional phase of the project; it is the end of assessment and the beginning of planning. During analysis, the assessment data is gathered together to first summarize it, and then to make comparisons among the data gathered by different assessment methods and between different participant groups. The team and community members will find it interesting to see if the ideas they have formed during the collection of data remain the same during analysis.

Collaboration and partnerships at this point are very important. Once there is assessment data, community members and organizations usually become more interested in the project. The challenging aspect is presenting the analysis to the community so that they understand why the assessment was done, how it was done, what preliminary results or evidence were found, and how the results could be interpreted. Your efforts are rewarded when the community validates your findings and helps to define relevant issues and actions.

The scenario from Chapter 4 involving the team working in the multilanguage building continues in this chapter. The scenes depict the team learning to assemble and summarize data from progressive inquiry and a questionnaire. The team works closely with the two collaborators to interpret the data, validate the results, and define issues for action.

## Learning Objectives

| Key Terms and Concepts |
| --- |
| action statement · collaborators · community of interest · concern · data analysis · evidence · gap analysis · issue for action · related-to clause · reliability · stakeholders · strength · validation · validity |

After reading this chapter and answering the questions throughout the chapter, you should be able to:

1. Use team decision making to analyze secondary and primary data collected from a variety of sources.
2. Identify and recruit collaborators from the community and stakeholders to determine a direction for the community project.
3. Validate assessment findings with the community and define the issues for action.
4. Develop action statements to address the issues for action.
5. Document the assessment.

**SCENARIO: Continuation of Prenatal and Postnatal Health Promotion with Women Speaking a Variety of Languages**

The two teams continue to work on community prenatal and postnatal health projects in the city of Old York under the supervision of their clinical instructor, Jessica. The Multilanguage Project involves working in a low-income building that houses families speaking a number of different languages to identify and act on issues related to prenatal and postnatal health. The team is now completing the assessment in order to move on to planning and action. The English Project team started with the same purpose, but the project changed to a more comprehensive assessment. This chapter will follow only the multilanguage team. Detailed information on each project for Steps 1 to 4 is available in Chapter 4.

The team of four students working in the multilanguage building has secondary data from their literature review, and primary data from mapping the area and key informant interviews with two volunteers, a city support worker, and the manager of a multicultural organization in the community. They used progressive inquiry with women meeting regularly in the apartment lobby and a questionnaire distributed over two weeks to other women in the building. They plan to sit down as a team this week and brainstorm about all the things that they need to do to complete the assessment and start moving on to planning. They are excited about the opportunity to present the information they have gathered to the women in the building.

**Discussion Topics and Questions**

1. How does the data from progressive inquiry add to the data gained through observation and key informant interviews?
2. How does the data from the questionnaire add to the data from progressive inquiry?

For suggested responses, please see the Answer Key at the back of the book.

## Moving from Data Collection to Analysis

The analysis of secondary and primary data is a crucial step in the development of a community project. **Data analysis** involves condensing, comparing, and interpreting data into information that people can comprehend quickly. You have gathered data from different sources during assessment, and you now need to consolidate and interpret the information and think through the implications of the findings to determine a direction for taking action. A systematic process makes analysis more manageable. The sequential steps of organizing and interpreting the collected information assist you in reaching conclusions supported by evidence from data and in fulfilling your obligation to the community, which is to identify their concerns and strengths or assets as a basis for action. **Concern** is the term used for an expressed or observed risk, problem, or issue of a community group that limits the achievement of the preferred health situation. A **strength** is an asset of the community, stakeholders, or environment that could be reinforced and help to address a concern. Without a logical process to identify the concerns and strengths, the analysis is likely to be incomplete or inaccurate.

In the initial phases of an analysis, you will likely work mainly with your team and advisors. This means reducing your involvement with the community group temporarily as you move from data collection to data analysis. Once you have some preliminary results, you can take them back to the group to check that you have an accurate picture and have identified their most important concerns and strengths. Giving feedback provides an opportunity for further community engagement.

Because of restricted time and resources, most short-term projects have small data sets that, although collected systematically, have limited reliability and validity. **Reliability** refers to the consistency of a measure in producing the same result over time (McKenzie, Neiger, & Thackeray, 2013). **Validity** refers to whether the data collection instrument is correctly measuring the concepts under investigation (McKenzie et al., 2013). Gathering reliable and valid data requires considerable time, expertise, and resources. However, if the approach is systematic, small data sets are likely to capture the prominent concerns and strengths of the community group to provide direction for action, especially since you will continue to collaborate with them. As well, the process of collecting and analyzing the data provides invaluable experience for teams and collaborators as a basis for future initiatives.

## Analyze Assessment Data (Step 5)

The purpose of analyzing the assessment findings is to identify health concerns and determine potential courses of action. The analysis completes the assessment process and provides a basis for planning.

The team needs to assemble the secondary and primary assessment data to analyze the information and determine the issues for action, from which concrete action statements are developed. To complete this step, you will summarize the findings in a project report. Box 5.1 lists the steps in the community nursing project with a focus on Step 5.

---

BOX 5.1

**Step 5 in Completing the Community Health Nursing Project**

ASSESS
1. Orient to community project
2. Assess secondary data
3. Assess physical and social environment
4. Assess primary data
5. **Analyze assessment data**
    a. **Assemble assessment data**
    b. **Analyze and validate data**
    c. **Develop action statements**
    d. **Summarize assessment**

PLAN
6. Plan action

ACT
7. Take action

EVALUATE
8. Evaluate results and complete project
9. Evaluate teamwork

**Assemble Assessment Data (Step 5a)**

As you begin to assemble the data, keep in mind that the secondary data sources you consulted—sociodemographic statistics, mortality and morbidity statistics, utilization data, and government and organizational policy statements—provide contextual information about the community and its key concerns in relation to the focus of your project. Further contextual information comes from mapping the community and key informant interviews. All these sources of information provided a basis for selecting and preparing questions for more specific assessment of the community group.

Assemble the data from each of the basic and advanced assessment methods you used. If different people gathered the information, provide an opportunity for everyone to give a short overview of the assessment process, tools, and data. This overview provides the team with a starting point for the analysis.

**Four Phases of Analysis of Assessment Data**

**1. Classification of Data into One of Three Areas Appropriate for the Project**
- Classify information as background or rationale for the project if it is based on secondary data sources, such as sociodemographic statistics, mortality and morbidity statistics, utilization data, and government and organizational policy statements.
- Classify data as concern if it indicates difficulties experienced by assessment participants, such as risks, issues, or barriers to health.
- Classify data as strengths if it indicates that community members and stakeholders have individual and group assets, such as previous initiatives, interest, and available resources.

**2. Summarization**
- Reduce data from each source.
- Identify main points.

**3. Interpretation**
- Compare with similar data, if available.
- Compare with objectives identified by the community or agency and government reports.
- Draw inferences or conclusions.
- Draft the main points and issues for action with supporting evidence—these points will facilitate decision making.

**4. Validation and Definition of Issues for Action**
- Present findings to advisors and collaborators for feedback.
- Validate the accuracy of the assessment with the community.
- Determine the present health situation (concerns and strengths).
- Determine the vision of where the community would like to be (preferred health situation).
- Define the issues for action by conducting a gap analysis between the present situation and the preferred state.

## Analyze and Validate Data (Step 5b)

The analysis process has four phases: "classification, summarization, interpretation, and validation" (Anderson & McFarlane, 2014), which are generic to analyzing data from both small and large projects and programs. The purpose of analysis is to clarify issues for action by identifying the health concerns and strengths that can help to address the issues. Box 5.2 illustrates the four phases.

### Classification
In this initial phase, group the data into one of three categories: background, concern, or strength. To determine whether the data is background data, ask "What information provides support for, or a reason for doing the project?" Alternatively, ask if the information indicates a concern or strength. At this time, look out for gaps in the data and possible reasons for them. It may be necessary to fill in these gaps before going further, depending on how significant they are.

### Summarization
Summarization has two parts: a summary of each source of primary data, and then a summary across data sources to identify the main points. You can use descriptive statistics, numbers, and percentages to summarize observation data and questionnaires. Categorize responses to open-ended questions from key informant interviews or focused discussions by grouping them according to topics or themes. Use broad categories at first, and then inspect the items in each category to pick out the nuances. For example,

under the topic "food," some responses might be concerned with availability, others with cost, and so on. Ask "What did most people say?" and "What are only one or a few people saying?" and cluster the topics and themes in order of frequency.

The summary of progressive inquiry is different from other methods because the questions to collect the data change over time. Similarly, the data evolve as you analyze responses after each cycle and use the responses to prepare new questions. You need to summarize how these cycles move from broader questions to more specific questions based on responses, as well as the summary of responses.

As you summarize the data and begin to get a sense of the content, think about how you might further organize the results. For example, with a short questionnaire you can use the questions as an organizer. Another possibility is to rank single yes/no or multiple-choice questions on a single topic, such as "preferred sources of information," from highest to lowest to quickly identify those with the most support. When working with data from small groups, include responses of less than five in questionnaires in the summary of your qualitative data.

Once you have summarized each source, write down the main points across sources. At this point, you just want to get the points down; you will discuss them in the next phase.

### Interpretation

The purpose of interpretation is to summarize what the data is telling you in terms of the concerns and strengths of the community group in order to identify the issues for action. An **issue for action** is the specific, documented concern or strength that, if addressed, will change the present situation to the preferred health situation.

Start by making comparisons to bring out key findings. Within the data, first consider the results by source and then compare across data sources, looking for similarities and differences. For example, it may be possible to compare information from secondary sources, such as on socioeconomic status and the use of health services by members of the community group, to those in a larger geographical area. Another approach is to compare data from two different groups, such as health professionals and community members.

The next step is to draw some preliminary inferences or conclusions that will help to focus your project. Prepare some simple questions to guide this work. The first question could be "What are the main findings related to health concerns/strengths in the data?" Next, "What other topics were apparent in the data?" and "Are any of the topics related?" Once the main and subsidiary topics are identified from the data, consider where the community group is now (present health) and where they would like to be (preferred health). Remember that the interpretation must be plausible and fit the data.

Keep track of your ideas and the supporting data on a flip chart or blackboard if possible. This will give everyone a chance to express his or her views and follow the process, thereby allowing a more objective and transparent discussion of conclusions. **Evidence** is the body of data that has been systematically collected and appraised to provide the basis for making decisions when planning a program (McKenzie et al., 2013). Everyone should be able to understand the logic of the process and feel that the conclusions are consistent with the evidence.

This approach helps you prepare to present your process and findings to others who have had less involvement, and possibly less understanding of the analytic process, than team members might have. You want to provide a clear explanation of your process and establish confidence in your evidence.

After again reviewing the secondary data, the multilanguage team assembles the primary data. They had decided to focus more directly on food after listening to the women and to key informants, and noting a lack of grocery stores on their community map. Progressive inquiry with the women who met in the apartment lobby allowed them to confirm that food was a common concern and helped them to understand the concern in more depth. They realized that they had been analyzing and validating the progressive inquiry data with the women and collaborators as they went along. They had used this to inform the development of a questionnaire, test it with some women in the lobby, and then distribute it to women in the building who had not been involved in the progressive inquiry in the lobby (see Chapter 4).

As they begin to classify the data, the first step of analysis, the team has no difficulty placing secondary data as background. Moving to the primary data, they realize that the information gathered from progressive inquiry and through the questionnaire relates to where the group is now, their strengths, and presumably what improvements they would like to see in the future. Observations reinforce this information. Team members saw how the women responded to challenges, and how they liked speaking to the volunteers and being involved with others in the building. From these observations, they feel confident in identifying two important

strengths: women in the building actively sought health information and took advantage of the support provided by the two volunteers and others in the building.

They use simple descriptive statistics to summarize the specific concerns around food from the questionnaires. Team members rank the topics by the number of women who expressed interest in learning about them. Table 5.1 summarizes the responses.

That leaves the responses to the open-ended question in topic #9. After reviewing them, they realize they can be grouped with other items. For example, "eating in the morning" fits with topic #5, "salty food" with #1, and "juice for baby" with #2. They decide to include topic #3, where to shop for healthy, low-cost food, as one of the key concerns because it was important to the women in the lobby.

**Discussion Topics and Questions**

3. Why would the team include the item on buying low-cost food as a concern when it did not elicit a high response on the questionnaire?
4. Do you agree that all the responses to the open-ended question fit with the questionnaire items? If not, what additional item could be added to the questionnaire, and why might that be important?

**Table 5.1: Summary of Responses to Questionnaire "Food for Women with a Baby" (Chapter 4)**

| Topic # | Question | Number Interested in Topic ($n = 20$) |
|---|---|---|
| 1 | What food is good for me? | 18 |
| 2 | What food is good for a baby? | 14 |
| 3 | Where can I shop for good low-cost food? | 8 |
| 4 | How can I eat better when I feel sick? | 6 |
| 5 | What could I eat in the morning? | 17 |
| 6 | What could I eat at noon? | 7 |
| 7 | What could I eat in the evening? | 6 |
| 8 | What can I eat between meals? | 16 |
| 9 | Please fill in other food questions. I don't like to eat in the morning—is that bad? (x 2) I like salty food. Is that okay? (x 1) Should I give my baby juice to drink between feedings? (x 2) When should I give my baby food on a spoon? (x 4) | 9 |

The final step in the interpretation is to conduct a gap analysis. **Gap analysis** is the difference between the present health situation and the preferred health situation. To conduct the gap analysis, you could discuss the differences first in groups of two or three. Ask each group, or individual, to identify the difference between the present and preferred situations. The common differences from the gap analysis become the issues for action. If there is no difference, the analysis has identified a strength that needs to be maintained.

If consensus is not immediately apparent, the best option is to allow time for reflection and for other ideas to emerge after team members have had a chance to consider different perspectives. This can help the team avoid jumping to premature conclusions.

Prepare a written draft of your results. Remember that these decisions are preliminary until validated by the community. Therefore, teams are encouraged to remain open to various conclusions.

### Validation and Definition of Issues for Action

Validation of the assessment results with the community is an important component of analysis because it allows the team to corroborate the interpretation and seek clarification on the findings and proposed action. **Validation** involves presenting and seeking feedback from the community on the interpretation of results. This involvement increases the engagement of the community in the project and, hopefully, future initiatives.

Up to this point, likely few community members or organizations have been involved in the project other than staff from the organization and the specific community group. However, once there are results from the assessment of a community group, more community members and organizations are likely to become interested in the project. If there is sufficient time, this interest can be encouraged by inviting more community

---

**SCENARIO: Interpreting the Data on Healthy Foods for Mothers and Babies**

After combining the responses in the open-ended question with the questionnaire responses, the team identifies the main concern as obtaining healthy foods for babies and mothers. Specifically, women want to know (a) about healthy foods for breakfast and snacks, and (b) where to obtain healthy, low-cost food. Thinking about these findings in relation to the secondary data, the team realizes that finding healthy food could be associated with low birth weight and increased illness in babies. Their two collaborators provide insight into why there is a discrepancy between the findings from the progressive inquiry with women in the lobby and those completing the questionnaire: many of the women who came to the lobby are new to the country and possibly have not yet figured out where to shop for low-cost food.

The team and volunteers identify that barriers related to obtaining healthy food for women and babies is the main concern coming from the data. The conclusions about preferred health were more diverse and often went beyond the data. For instance, one person said it was obvious that women did not have sufficient money to buy all the food they wanted. The team leader commented that although 8 of 20 women who completed the survey were interested in affordable food, they could not infer that this was due simply to a lack of money. After this explanation, everyone could agree that the preferred health situation was easy access to healthy food for mothers and babies.

**Discussion Topics and Questions**

5. How would combining data from different groups of people or using different methods make the analysis more difficult?
6. How would a team maintain confidentiality and anonymity while collecting, analyzing, and reporting assessment data? Why would this be especially important with small data sets?

members to be involved in the review of the findings. Additional community involvement provides a broader base for the project and is important to promote sustainability. A lot depends on involving the right people.

Different segments of the population will have varying interests in the analysis. **Community of interest** is the population or community group expected to receive health benefits from the project. **Stakeholders** are the people or organizations in the community who have something to gain by improving the health of the community of interest. **Collaborators** are members of the community of interest and stakeholders who become part of the team and make decisions related to the project. Designated advisors are the faculty instructor and organizational advisor(s) who share responsibility for the project and advise the team throughout the project. The Appendix to this chapter describes different levels of collaboration and provides examples of interest groups in the community.

Some collaborators self-identify; others have to be recruited. While it is ideal for the team to have a consistent group of collaborators, people frequently come and go. Community members are often more involved at one phase of the project than at others. In the longer term, the expectation is that the team and community collaborators will develop a responsive relationship and learn from each other.

The development of a collaborative relationship is dependent on the different parties making complementary contributions. The main contribution of the team is to provide leadership with the assistance of advisors, gather information, and foster a process that supports involvement and collaborative decision making. The contribution of the collaborators is to provide advice and information and eventually engage in the decision making to identify the issues for action that will be relevant to the community of interest. The involvement of collaborators is crucial in determining a feasible direction and providing support for the sustainability of the project.

The team needs to present the preliminary results of the analysis to collaborators in a way that is meaningful for them. The collaborators first need the background to the project and a description of how the team collected the data to obtain the community perspective. Even if they have been working with the team, they are unlikely to know everything. The topics that follow provide an outline for presenting the information to the collaborators:

1. Background on why the concern is important
2. What data was collected and how it was collected
3. Summary of the major concerns found in the qualitative and quantitative data
4. Summary of the strengths found in the qualitative and quantitative data
5. Comparison of the concerns and strengths with different groups who participated, with background statistics, and with the agency mandate
6. Preliminary conclusions on the present and preferred health situation, and gap analysis to identify the issues for action

Once the collaborators understand the process that was followed to collect and analyze information on the community, they will be in a much better situation to comment on whether it fits with their knowledge of the community.

The way the meeting is structured depends on factors such as the number of people present, how well you know them, and how well they know the project. When providing background information, keep the message simple and use clear language. People should not feel overwhelmed by the information. When giving the results, consider providing tentative conclusions or a couple of possible interpretations to stimulate discussion. It is important to avoid giving the impression that you have already decided what is important. This is a consultative process, and community members need to feel comfortable asking questions and expressing their true feelings. For example, when describing the barriers to health, the team could say "We found that most people we talked to mention a difficulty in getting good food. We did not know if this was because of the cost of food, transportation to grocery stores, knowing what food was good, or some other reason."

This approach suggests that the team has done the best it could in the situation to collect and analyze the data but may have inadvertently missed some things. The approach also acknowledges that the people in the community and the stakeholders have a more intimate knowledge of the situation than the team does and can add to the interpretation. As an example, I once led a research team involved in a survey with teenage girls about various health and social behaviors. The results indicated that a high percentage of the girls brushed their teeth regularly. The researchers were impressed until two teachers reported that the girls brushed their teeth to remove the cigarette smell from their breath!

---

**SCENARIO: Validating the Data with the Women and Defining the Issues for Action**

At the validation session, the team explains the results, comparing the items that interested most of the women who came to the lobby with those that received the most responses in the questionnaire. Two team members act as observers and feel that the women's nods and comments to each other indicate that most understand the process.

The team wants to further engage the women in the lobby to confirm their interests and validate the questionnaire data. They ask the women to stand beside one of four cards held by the team members. The first card shows pictures of healthy foods for women. The second shows healthy foods for babies, and the third, a shopping cart with a dollar symbol. The fourth has a question mark for people to offer other suggestions. Five of the 16 women present quickly move to the card showing healthy foods for women; five go the card with healthy foods for babies; and three women want to learn about healthy, low-cost food. Two women, who want to learn how to prepare different food, stand by the card with the question mark. The team feels that the women enjoyed demonstrating their choice and viewing the choices of others.

After the session, the team meets with the two collaborators to decide on the issues for action. The team and collaborators identify the three items from the present situation that received support throughout the assessment: (1) information on food for mothers (from progressive inquiry, questionnaire, validation); (2) information on food for babies (from progressive inquiry, questionnaire, validation); and (3) where to buy healthy, low-cost food (progressive inquiry, validation). With the preferred health situation being access to healthy, low-cost food for mothers and babies, the issues for action are providing information and support on obtaining healthy and low-cost food for mothers and babies. They had previously identified that the strengths are the interest shown by the women in learning about healthy foods and the support from collaborators and public health. They realize now that they will use the strengths when addressing the issues for action.

**Discussion Topics and Questions**

7. What aspects of the validation session make it easier for the women to provide their responses?

8. Why was it important to have observers watch the women's responses to the presentation?

## Develop Action Statements (Step 5c)

Once the team has defined the issues for action (concerns or strengths), the next step is to identify potential actions to reinforce the strength or to correct the deficit to achieve the preferred health status of the community. The development of action statements is an intermediary phase in the decision-making process with the community. The **action statement** is a summary of the assessment that identifies the community of interest and a concern or strength, and suggests feasible options to correct or reduce the concern and maintain or enhance the strengths.

Action statements are similar to a nursing diagnosis. A community or nursing diagnosis relevant to community health nursing practice is expressed through a four-part statement that identifies the following (Anderson & McFarlane, 2014; Ervin, 2002; Helvie, 1998; Neufeld & Harrison, 2000):

- Name or description of group
- Situation or response (concern or strength)
- Related-to factors
- Evidence

We focus on the first three parts, similar to the three-part community-oriented nursing diagnosis (Shuster & Goeppinger, 2003), and include the fourth part, evidence, as a following statement. Table 5.2 outlines the three parts of action statements.

### Community of Interest

The community of interest, or the people who are expected to receive health benefits, is often refined throughout the project, depending on factors such as the availability of resources and access to the community group. For example, a project to improve bicycle safety for children in grades 3 and 4 could start with all schools in a city, be reduced to an area or neighborhood, and finally, to one school.

### Concern or Strength

The concerns and strengths are determined during the interpretation and validation of data. The summation of concerns and strengths provides the focus for a project. Avoid the tendency to concentrate on health concerns; the strengths may be less obvious but they provide a building block for change. The next section discusses how to formulate statements for action that will guide interventions to address a concern or boost a strength.

**Table 5.2: Three-Part Action Statements**

| Part 1 | Part 2 | Part 3 |
|---|---|---|
| Community of Interest | Concern or Strength | Related-to Clause |
| Specific description of community of interest | State in terms of concern or strength from analysis and validation of assessment data | Factors related to preferred state that nursing in collaboration with others can change |

A properly constructed action statement to address a concern identifies a specific community group, a potential or actual concern, and the reason for this deficiency, which is potentially modifiable. For example, the following is a properly constructed action statement: "Women with young children living in low-income apartment buildings have difficulty obtaining healthy food for themselves and their children related to a lack of understandable and available information on healthy nutrition." In this example, both the status and related-to clause refer to a concern or risk. Detailing what is lacking in the provision of services, rather than using a broad term such as "lack of knowledge by the community members," provides more direction for action. As well, lack of knowledge infers that the women are deficient in something, whereas "lack of understandable and available information on healthy nutrition" places the onus on the health care system.

The action statements referring to strengths are formulated as "have potential for" followed by an improved health status. A properly constructed strength action statement identifies a specific community group with an actual or potential for strength, grounded in evidence of a demonstrated characteristic of the group. For example, the following is a properly constructed strength action statement: "Women living in low-income apartment buildings have potential for improving family nutrition related to their interest in learning about healthy food choices." In the example, note that both the status and the related-to clause are positive. In order to make this statement, the strength, that is, the level of interest in learning, would be based on evidence determined from positive responses to a specific question on the topic or other expressions of their interests. In contrast, a low score on a topic should not be interpreted as an indication of interest.

The health concerns, strengths, and preferred health situation are determined from primary data elicited from community members and stakeholders. When circumstances dictate that secondary data is the only available source of information, the elements would need to be checked, at least with stakeholders, and used cautiously.

### Related-to Clause

The **related-to clause** identifies the potentially modifiable factors that contribute to the concern or strength that community health nursing in collaboration with others can address. Four types of factors should be considered when action statements are developed:

1. Factors that can be changed
2. Factors that promote collaboration
3. Factors that define a nursing role
4. Factors that are manageable within a short-term project

Box 5.3 includes the description of these four factors.

At this point, most short-term projects usually have a total of two to five action statements, consisting of both concern and strength statements. In Chapter 6, you will determine the final or priority action statement.

## BOX 5.3
**Four Factors of the Related-to Clause in a Short-Term Project**

### 1. Factors That Can Be Changed

Relate the concern to factors that are potentially modifiable and strengths to factors than can be supported. For example, a community may feel that teenage drinking at school activities is unacceptable. Although age and developmental stage are not unrelated to this concern, they are not modifiable. Focus on relevant factors that can be changed, such as parents having limited skill with behavioral management strategies, community attitudes toward underage drinking, or the lack of alternative community activities for teens.

### 2. Factors That Promote Collaboration

To promote collaboration and engage the interest and support of community members, the terms in the related-to clause need to be understandable, relevant to the situation, and nonjudgmental.

Tips:
- Use terms familiar to the community, rather than medical terms such as "maternal attachment"
- Select actions that are likely to be strongly supported
- Specify why little has occurred thus far using nonjudgmental language. For example, attributing a low level of participation in exercise by new immigrants to "lack of interest/knowledge" suggests a total lack of interest, knowledge, or understanding in the population. This is rarely the case. Furthermore, it fails to consider social and environmental determinants, such as culture and language, and blames the victim. Low participation may be beyond the control of group members if health information is inaccessible, that is, unavailable in plain language or in the language spoken by members of the group.

### 3. Factors That Define a Nursing Role

Although community health nurses must consider all the social determinants of health (Commission on Social Determinants of Health, 2008), they do not necessarily have the expertise or resources to change them or provide all needed services directly. For example, community nurses in a management role are likely to be involved in intersectoral action at different levels of the health system to address broad issues such as unemployment, poverty, and poor housing. Community health nurses at the neighborhood level need to identify the factors they have the expertise and resources to address, either on their own or in collaboration with others. As well, it is important to describe what you are going to do in precise terms. For example, rather than proposing to "address language barriers," a more realistic role would be to "work with language teachers to provide useful health information that people can understand." In addition to being vague, "addressing language barriers" could be interpreted as teaching language skills, which is outside the nursing scope of practice.

### 4. Factors That Are Manageable within a Short-Term Project

Broad determinants of health, such as poverty, have to be broken down into manageable steps for short-term projects. Possible actions to deal with poverty are increasing communication among community members or service providers, identifying a location or structure to bring people together, or providing accessible information on community resources. It would be feasible for community health nurses to initiate these actions alone, or in collaboration with others, within a short time period with a view to these actions being continued by the community.

As the students start to consider their action statements, they remember that they initially thought their community group would be pregnant women and women with young babies because they were working with the public health prenatal and postnatal health program. However, they found that most of the women they met had children between one and five, and only one was pregnant. The students struggle at first to try to fit this population into prenatal and postnatal health. Their public health nurse advisor explains that since the apartment building is a small community, any teaching about healthy foods to a group has the potential for improving prenatal and postnatal health and family nutrition throughout the building.

The next consideration is whether to frame the item as a concern or strength. Several different sources of information (observations on the lack of inexpensive grocery stores in the area, specific comments from women and key informants, secondary data) place a lot more emphasis on the concern about obtaining good food rather than on the strengths. The strengths indicate the resources that can help to address the concerns. They lay out the information in the three-part table (Table 5.3) to help them clarify the communities of interest. By using Table 5.3, they can also check that Parts 2 and 3 are both negative for a concern or both positive for a strength, check that Part 3 is modifiable, and compare inclusiveness.

**Discussion Topics and Questions**

9. Why was "limited money for food" not included in the list of concerns?
10. Discuss the pros and cons of the following two statements: "Women have a lack of knowledge about healthy eating" and "Women lack access to appropriate resources for healthy eating."

**Table 5.3: Action Statements Showing Three-Part Format**

| Part 1: Community of Interest | Part 2: Concern or Strength | Part 3: Related-to Clause |
| --- | --- | --- |
| Pregnant women and those with babies living in the apartment building | experience difficulties in obtaining healthy food for themselves and their babies | [related to] lack of access to clear information on healthy, low-cost food. |
| Pregnant women and those with young children living in the apartment building | experience difficulties in obtaining healthy food for themselves and their families | [related to] lack of access to clear information on healthy, low-cost food. |
| Pregnant women and those with young children living in the apartment building | have potential for obtaining healthy food for themselves and their families | [related to] their interest in learning about healthy food, and support from collaborators and public health. |

## Summarize Assessment (Step 5d)

Once you have identified the action statements, you complete the assessment by summarizing and documenting the process and results in a report form shown in Appendix A.3.3 at the end of the text. The report provides a succinct record of what your team has accomplished and a ready reference to the main finding as the project develops. In addition to providing current data on the community that will inform action, others might also use the report to inform future projects by the organization.

The assessment report form, shown in Table 5.4, lists the sections of the assessment report and provides an example of the content that might be included. Use the information from your working documents to fill in the form. The suggested length of the

**Table 5.4: Completing the Assessment Report**

| Items | Directions |
|---|---|
| Key health issues of the population | Summarize national, provincial, and local statistics, and literature review with references (Step 2 in work plan). |
| Community of interest | Define present community of interest. |
| Assessment methods | Summarize the assessment methods, process, and sources of information. Include timelines and number and description of participants who provided primary data relevant to the topic of interest. Avoid giving identifying data, such as age, sex, SES, and place of residence, that might identify individuals. |
| Validated key results/ findings | Describe how the data was analyzed and validated with collaborators and the key findings:<br>– Present health situation, including concerns about health and strengths (assets, previous initiatives, amount of interest, resources) with supporting evidence<br>– Preferred health situation with evidence<br>– Issues for action |
| Action statements | List the action statements addressing concerns and strengths developed in consultation with the community that will guide the project. |
| Limitations | List any limitations to the assessment process identified during analysis and consultation. |
| Sustainability | Indicate ways to build on what has been done, for example, to develop a relationship with the community group, or to address an important health concern. |
| Recommendations | Identify possible future directions or opportunities for action with the community group. |
| Relevance for community health nursing | Identify the public/community health nursing standards or competencies exemplified in the assessment and proposed action. |
| Attachments | Data collection resources (e.g., questionnaires, focused discussion questions), community map, tables of data, excerpts of comments (with revealing information removed), reference list, and so on |

assessment report is two to four single-spaced pages, not including attachments. Appendix A.3.3 provides a blank form.

The first five items in the report (Table 5.4) provide a synopsis of the process used to determine the action statements. They constitute the first part of the project report (see Appendix A.3.3), which will be discussed in more detail in Chapter 8. The "Limitations" section identifies any factors that may have unduly restricted the data collection or interfered with the assessment process; for example, insufficient time and resources, or factors such as weather, that have limited progress but are beyond the control of the team. "Sustainability" refers to factors that influence the continuation of the project or of work with the community group. For example, the project may have brought together community members and helped them work together, thereby increasing community capacity, which in turn may sustain community action. The "Recommendations" section identifies what action the team and the community collaborators feel would help to direct the work of the project in the future.

Halfway through the project, the team is asked to give a verbal report of the assessment to the clinical instructor, advisor, and the advisor's manager in public health. They follow the same outline they used to present findings to the community (see "Validation and Definition of Issues for Action," above), updating it with information from the draft assessment report (see below). The presentation goes smoothly and the audience compliments them on how well they involved the community group.

### Draft Assessment Report

North American University, School of Nursing

Community Health Nursing Project in Collaboration with
    Old York Public Health Department

Promoting Healthy Women and Babies

October 15, 2015

Students: Ashley Blais, Tyler Jamison, Alexis Loreto, Lai-
    Ying Yeung

Agency Advisor: Andrea Ho

Clinical Instructor: Jessica Galica

Manager: Hannah Riley

#### Key Health Issues of the Population

Poor perinatal outcomes, such as low birth weight and death, are associated with many factors including smoking, drinking, low education level, and both young and older aged mothers (Public Health Agency of Canada, 2008; Maternal and Child Health Bureau, 2011), and poverty (Larson, 2007; Maternal and Child Health Bureau, 2011). Only 10 percent of non-English-speaking people in Old York attended prenatal classes in 2010 and 2011 compared to 20–50 percent for other population groups in the city ([fictional] Old York, 2011). The multilanguage building houses those on a low income, and just over 30 percent of the residents are single mothers or families with a child under two.

#### Community of Interest

Women with young children living in a low-income, multilanguage building

#### Assessment Methods

**Table 5.5: Method, Timelines, and Participants**

| Method | Timelines | Number of Participants | Description |
|---|---|---|---|
| Collection and review of secondary data | Sept. 10–Oct. 1 | N/A | |
| Mapping neighborhood | Sept. 10–Oct. 1 | N/A | Included food stores, laundry, bus stops, schools, post office, and so on |
| Key informant interviews | Sept. 17–24 | 4 | 2 volunteers from building, city support worker, manager of multicultural organization |
| Progressive inquiry | Sept. 24–Oct. 15 | 12 | Women from apartment building meeting in lobby |
| Questionnaire | Oct. 8–Oct. 22 | 20 | Women from apartment building not meeting in lobby |

*Validated Key Results/Findings*

Present health situation:

- Concerns: lack of access to (1) information on food for mothers (from progressive inquiry, questionnaire, validation); (2) information on food for children (from progressive inquiry, questionnaire, validation); and (3) resources for buying healthy, low-cost food (progressive inquiry, validation)
- Strengths: interest shown by the women in providing family with a healthy diet and learning about healthy foods; support from collaborators and public health (progressive inquiry, key informant interviews, validation)

Preferred health: Having access to healthy, low-cost food for mothers and families

*Issues for action*

Lack of access to information and support on healthy and low-cost food for mothers and families

*Action Statements*

- Pregnant women and those with babies living in the apartment building experience difficulties in obtaining healthy food for themselves and their babies related to lack of access to clear information on healthy, low-cost food.
- Women with young children living in the apartment building experience difficulties in obtaining healthy food for themselves and their children related to lack of access to clear information on healthy, low-cost food.
- Women with young children living in the apartment building have potential for obtaining healthy food for themselves and their families related to both their interest in learning about healthy food and support from collaborators and public health.

*Items not included*

Limitations, Sustainability, Recommendations, Relevance for Community Health Nursing, and Attachments

**Discussion Topics and Questions**

11. What is the benefit of documenting the assessment as it is occurring?
12. Why would collaborators want to know about the methods and number and type of participants before they consider the findings?

## Teamwork during Analysis

Moving into analysis signifies considerable progress by the team. The team has had to make plans to assess the community and follow through with the plans to collect assessment data. The progress will be manifested in team productivity, relationships, and increased comfort and knowledge of the community. Not least, this will bring a clearer understanding of the scope of the project. The team challenges while completing the substeps of Step 5 involve keeping the team organized and the morale high.

## Team Organization

The challenges of team organization are time management and coordinating tasks. You will probably feel that you have been doing a juggling act, learning about your community and communicating with more and more people. The data analysis requires working together more closely as a team to draw together the assessment data, interpret results, and define the issues for action.

### Time

As a rule, a team will be able to complete the analysis of data for a short project in one to two weeks. Keeping to this time frame requires a concentrated group effort. You may decide to work on tasks individually or in pairs and then come together to check each other's work. You need to get consensus before moving on to the next step. When you work methodically, keep track of your process, and summarize and double-check your actions and findings in the work plan and timeline, you are using your time efficiently. The assessment report provides a record of your approach; it is a major accomplishment and conveys to your advisors that you have followed a thorough process and analysis.

### Coordination

As the assessment phase draws to an end, it is particularly important that team activities are well coordinated. The start of data analysis, validation of findings with the community, and documentation is a lockstep process. By this stage of the project, the team has probably learned to delegate and report results when they meet each week; however, new skills will be called into play during analysis. The team needs to keep to timelines and can miss important details unless the team leader and recorder pay close attention to coordination and communication. Without adequate coordination, the time for action and evaluation can be shortchanged.

## Team Morale

During the final stages of assessment, team members will be spending considerable time working together. This is when you are likely to see that the team has reached the performing stage of team functioning and is beginning to see the benefits of its hard work. This is a good point to reflect on progress. The following questions can guide the discussion: "Are we learning what we wanted to learn? Are we learning what we expected to learn? What have I learned about working in a group? What have I enjoyed the most/the least? What individual and group skills can I now add to my résumé or CV?"

As well, if this is the end of your project, take some time to enjoy yourselves. In the future, you will probably have fond memories of being part of a team that was doing something worthwhile. Also, take some time to show appreciation for the people who have worked with you. In your presentation, name people who have been especially helpful. You may also want to give people a thank-you card or a letter that they can put in their personal file. Plan a party or some form of celebration to commemorate the work you have done and the friends you have made. Chapter 8 has more ideas for ending well.

## Summary

Analysis of the data, preparation of action statements, and documentation of results requires concentrated effort and draws on different skills than those used in data collection. The process of analysis is a worthwhile skill to learn because it applies to most situations where data is collected and indicates to the community that you are seriously considering their contribution.

Analysis of data also provides the opportunity to involve more community members and to consider the different categories of involvement. The involvement of collaborators, interested people from the community of interest, and stakeholders is particularly important while validating conclusions. Validation is important to ensure that the direction of the project is relevant for the community. The summary of the assessment can be carried forward by the team into the planning stage and used by the organization in future projects.

Teamwork during analysis shifts to working together to complete the analysis. Organization involving a consideration of the time remaining and coordination of activities is a priority, as well as maintaining morale.

## Classroom and Seminar Exercises

1. Using your community clinical situation, identify what decisions need to be made and who would be the decision makers in the following two phases of analysis:
   a. Classification of data into background, issues, and strengths
   b. Validation and definition of issues for action
2. Using at least two sources of data that you have available from your community clinical situation, explain how you would structure the presentation to obtain feedback on:
   a. the assessment data
   b. the present health situation
   c. the preferred health situation
   d. the issues for action
3. You are working on a team with a charity organization concerned with preventing heart attacks and strokes in your community. As part of your assessment of adults working/living in _____, you decide to identify the groups and organizations that could be involved in the project according to the following categories (see examples in the Appendix to Chapter 5):
   a. Community of interest
   b. Stakeholders
   c. Collaborators
   d. Designated advisors
4. Using the four points in Box 5.3 above, rewrite the related-to clause in the following action statement and discuss why the current clause is inappropriate: "Older adults attending Petoria Seniors Center have difficulty exercising related to their age, arthritis of the hips and knees, and myopia."

# References

Anderson, E., & McFarlane, J. (2014). *Community as partner* (7th ed.). Philadelphia, PA: Lippincott Williams & Wilkins.

Commission on Social Determinants of Health. (2008). *Closing the gap in a generation: Health equity through action on the social determinants of health.* Final Report of the Commission on Social Determinants of Health. Geneva: World Health Organization. Retrieved from http://whqlibdoc.who.int/publications/2008/9789241563703_eng.pdf

Ervin, N. (2002). *Advanced community health nursing practice: Population-focused care.* Upper Saddle River, NJ: Prentice Hall.

Helvie, C. (1998). *Advanced practice nursing in the community.* Thousand Oaks, CA: Sage.

Larson, C. (2007). Poverty during pregnancy: Its effects on child health outcomes. *Pediatric and Child Health, 12*(8), 673–677. Retrieved from www.ncbi.nlm.nih.gov/pmc/articles/PMC2528810/

Maternal and Child Health Bureau, US Department of Health and Human Services, Health Resources and Services Administration. (2011). *Child health USA 2011.* Retrieved from http://mchb.hrsa.gov/chusa11/

McKenzie, J., Neiger, B., & Thackeray, R. (2013). *Planning, implementing and evaluating health promotion programs: A primer* (6th ed.). Needham Heights, MA: Allyn and Bacon.

Neufeld, A., & Harrison, M. (2000). Nursing diagnosis for aggregates and groups. In M. Stewart (Ed.), *Community nursing: Promoting Canadians' health* (2nd ed., pp. 370–385). Toronto, ON: Saunders.

Public Health Agency of Canada. (2008). *Canadian Perinatal Report 2008.* Retrieved from http://phac-aspc.gc.ca/publicat/2008/cphr-rspc/index-eng.php

Shuster, G., & Goeppinger, J. (2003). Community as client: Assessment and analysis. In M. Stanhope & J. Lancaster (Eds.), *Community and public health nursing* (6th ed., pp. 342–373). St. Louis, MO: Mosby.

## Website Resources

International (NANDA-I): www.nanda.org

The NANDA-I website explains the process of developing nursing diagnoses and provides links to obtaining reference material.

# Appendix to Chapter 5

**Descriptions, Characteristics, and Examples of Interest Groups in the Community**

**Examples of Interest Groups in the Community**

| Category | Characteristics | Examples |
|---|---|---|
| Community of interest | Defined community group expected to receive health benefits from project | – Older adults attending a mall walking program<br>– Breast-feeding mothers in the city, area, or neighborhood<br>– Children in grades 5 and 6 in X school<br>– Women living on farms in County X |
| Stakeholders | People or organizations who can contribute to the health benefits of the community of interest | – Friends and families of the community of interest (e.g., adult children of elderly persons, families of breast-feeding women, parents of school-age children, or farm families in a county)<br>– Service providers in health care organizations, (e.g., public health departments, community health centers, clinics, and hospitals)<br>– Other health professionals (e.g., family doctors, parish nurses, pharmacists)<br>– Other sectors with an interest in the health topic (e.g., education, police, businesses, municipal and regional governments)<br>– Not-for-profit associations with a health interest (e.g., Heart and Stroke Foundation, Diabetes Associations, Mothers Against Drunk Driving [MADD], Shriners)<br>– Local support organizations (e.g., church outreach, afterschool programs, neighborhood groups, or older adults' associations) |
| Collaborators from the community | Volunteers who work closely with the core team at times but are not part of it. They can be members of the community of interest and/or stakeholders. | – In the Multilanguage Project, the two women working in the lobby of the building<br>– People from different agencies or organizations who are ready to provide assistance as needed |
| Designated advisors | People assigned to work with the team | – Faculty instructor and preceptor or advisor from the placement organization who advise the team throughout |

# Chapter 6

# Planning for Action—Step 6

Planning for action brings together the assessment and analysis from earlier chapters to prepare for action and evaluation. Theories provide a framework for planning and to guide learning, and in the process, demonstrate the benefits of using theories and models in practice. Planning for action guides you through building a foundation of knowledge and skills essential to community health nursing practice.

Planning begins with selecting a priority from among the action statements, then moves to determining a project goal. Identifying a strategy and evidence-based intervention comes next and requires critical thinking on different levels to consider evidence from theories and research, clinical practice, and the availability of resources. The final step in planning, developing measurable objectives, is a crucial skill needed to provide direction for the intervention. The homeless project featured in the scenarios demonstrates ways to work through these decisions and use planning tools, such as a work plan to document work and a timeline to sequence the activities and tasks.

Keeping the team on track during planning develops skills in effective decision making, documentation, and communication. As well, team evaluation helps to strengthen the team in preparation for action.

## Learning Objectives

After reading this chapter and answering the questions throughout the chapter, you should be able to:

1. Plan the action of a community nursing project using a theory-based approach.
2. Determine a priority action statement and goal with collaborators.

### Key Terms and Concepts

action • best practices: emerging, promising, best • Cochrane databases • Gantt chart • Generalized Model for Program Planning in Health Promotion • health impact assessment (HIA) • health goal • health literacy • health promotion strategies: community capacity building and organization, environmental and organizational change, health education, health policy/enforcement, (mass) health communication strategies • impact objectives: learning (awareness, knowledge, appreciation), ability, accomplishment, environmental • intervention • planning • Population Health Promotion Model • priority action statement • process objectives • SMART • theories • train-the-trainer • Transtheoretical Stages of Change Model

**SCENARIO: Improvement of Services for the Homeless**

A four-member student team is continuing a community project started by another team. The assignment is to plan and carry out a short-term intervention to improve an aspect of services for the chronically homeless. Several agencies providing services for the homeless in South Hampton are providing input to the project, which is part of a large program involving all levels of government to reduce homelessness and the effects of homelessness in the region. In preparation for the assignment, they review Steps 1 to 5 of the community health nursing process in previous chapters. At orientation, the team reviews the final assessment report and attachments (see Appendix to this chapter) from the previous community project and finds out that the community advisor who worked with the previous team will be working with them as well.

**Discussion Topics and Questions**

1. Identify two or three priorities for the team in the scenario above and discuss how you might address them in the first few weeks of the project.
2. Community health nurses must frequently work with data that has been collected by others. Discuss the benefits and challenges of planning action based on data that others have collected.

For suggested responses, please see the Answer Key at the back of the book.

3. Identify a health promotion strategy and evidence-based intervention to achieve the project goal by reviewing evidence from theory and research, clinical practice, community preferences, and available resources.
4. Develop measurable impact and process objectives.
5. Document and communicate plans.

## Overview of Chapters 6 and 7

Chapters 6 and 7 represent a change of focus from assessment to planning and taking action (implementation). This step in the community health nursing project builds on the health information, strengths, and concerns of the community gained during assessment, and in turn lays the groundwork for evaluation. Generally, the goal of community health nursing action is to promote health, build capacity, and increase access to the determinants of health while working collaboratively with others in the community. The process of planning and taking action is complex and intertwined, so we recommend that you read chapters 6 and 7 together.

The **Population Health Promotion Model** (Hamilton & Bhatti, 1996) provides an overview of the health promotion strategies identified in the *Ottawa Charter for Health Promotion* (World Health Organization, 1986) and a framework for understanding how health promotion strategies are applied. The "cube," illustrated in Figure 6.1, lists five broad approaches to promoting community health: strengthen community action, build healthy public policy, create supportive environments, develop personal skills, and reorient the health services. Underpinning these strategies are the values and assumptions of community health nursing practice, as detailed in Chapter 1, together with a strong and evolving knowledge base founded on research, experiential learning, and evaluation. The model shows that planners apply these strategies at different levels of the system, from the individual to society as a whole, to increase access to one or more of the social determinants of health listed on the front of the cube.

**Figure 6.1: Population Health Promotion Model (The Cube)**

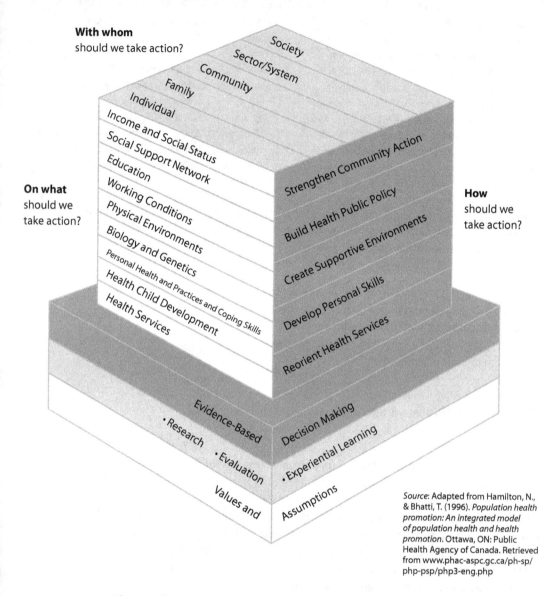

*Source:* Adapted from Hamilton, N., & Bhatti, T. (1996). *Population health promotion: An integrated model of population health and health promotion.* Ottawa, ON: Public Health Agency of Canada. Retrieved from www.phac-aspc.gc.ca/ph-sp/php-psp/php3-eng.php

The Population Health Promotion Model is a framework for understanding health promotion interventions that, although not research-based, is an informed synthesis of factors important for planning. The cube provides a simple illustration of three types of factors: population, issue, and an overview of types of health promotion interventions. The three-dimensional aspect of the cube (Figure 6.1) can be illustrated by considering a health concern, for example, bicycle safety in an inner-city neighborhood. The assessment data indicates that many children are riding rusty old bikes and do not use bicycle helmets. Several determinants of health are implicated, such as unsafe physical environments and lack of access to healthy child development, as well as low income. From the action side of the cube, we might consider using strategies to develop the personal skills of the children or try to strengthen community action to repair the bicycles, depending on the strengths and resources and preferences of the community.

Community health nursing practice requires an understanding of the fundamental strategic approaches in the cube and of the most common evidence-based approaches, termed interventions, which make up each strategy. The evidence, derived from theory or models, tested by research or by application in practice, describes the conditions required for the implementation approach to work. The stronger the evidence, the more likely an intervention will achieve the desired goal when the circumstances are similar and when the approach can be applied as intended. Planning evidence-based approaches to address community concerns and support community strengths, in collaboration with a community group, is the focus of this chapter.

## Plan Action (Step 6)

The purpose of planning is to determine priorities for action, translate these into specific goals and objectives, and identify evidence-based action to meet the goals. **Planning** is a decision-making process that identifies priorities from assessment, lays out expected goals and objectives, and specifies the strategies and interventions needed to achieve the goals and objectives. **Action** is implementing planned activities to improve health. The **intervention** is the actions or experiences to which the priority population will be exposed between the beginning and end of a program (McKenzie, Neiger, & Thackeray, 2013).

Box 6.1 expands Step 6 within the context of the community project. Although the substeps are presented in sequence, the process is more a dance of "two steps forward, one step back" rather than "step-by-step.".

It will come as no surprise that planning the care of a community group is more complex than that of an individual and that, to be effective, planning community care requires meaningful collaboration with community members and stakeholders. Consider the example in Box 6.2.

Planning a project with a community group is one of the most challenging aspects of community work. The mall walking example emphasizes the importance of involving those affected by a concern in determining the solution, taking time to talk to people, consulting with colleagues, and not jumping to conclusions. While it may seem faster to make decisions alone, this runs the risk of not considering the range of factors that affect the health of people

BOX 6.1

**Step 6 in Completing the Community Health Nursing Project**

ASSESS
1. Orient to community project
2. Assess secondary data
3. Assess physical and social environment
4. Assess primary data
5. Analyze assessment data

PLAN
6. **Plan action**
   a. **Select priority**
   b. **Identify goal**
   c. **Identify strategy and evidence-based intervention**
   d. **Develop impact and process objectives**

ACT
7. Take action

EVALUATE
8. Evaluate results and complete project
9. Evaluate teamwork

BOX 6.2

**Developing a Mall Walking Program**

A community health nurse has started to work with some older adults who manage a walking program in a shopping mall. At the first meeting, she learns the program is becoming more popular, especially among those who use walkers or wheelchairs. Now, some walkers are complaining that because of the slower pace of the group, they can no longer walk as fast as they would like. The nurse agrees to lead a working group to deal with the concern. At the first meeting, she presents the group with a plan that places people into walking periods according to their mobility: fast walkers, unassisted slow walkers, and those using wheelchairs, walkers, or canes, with each group walking at a different time. Her plan is met with stunned silence. She had not considered that people might want to walk with their friends.

living in the community. Avoiding costly mistakes justifies the time and effort required for collaboration in planning.

Taking action to promote community health depends on a variety of factors and requires input from people in different organizations. The planning process provides an opportunity to bring together people with different views to work out feasible, relevant outcomes. In the process, the community members become collaborators in the project, forging a relationship that is important for the success of the project. Community members do not become collaborators by chance. People get involved because they have an interest in the project, and you have fanned that interest by including them in meetings and consulting them on decisions. For example, the nurse in the mall walking example could have asked for ideas from the walkers and provided them with options to consider. Once community members have collaborated on a plan, they are likely to stay on track with its implementation and see it through the many delays and difficulties that are a natural part of living and working in the community.

At the community level, planning is based on knowledge of the broad community and an in-depth knowledge of the community group. Planning involves the team, collaborators from the community, and stakeholders working together. This broad collaboration helps to ensure that the plan is thorough and feasible. Creativity, critical thinking, negotiation, teamwork, and clear written and verbal communication are some of the necessary skills for planning. The following sections guide you through the community health nursing planning process.

## Select Priority (Step 6a)

The purpose of priority setting is to determine which concern to address from a range of alternatives (Chapter 5). The selected statement becomes the priority action statement. The **priority action statement** is the action statement that meets defined criteria to represent the most prominent and amenable concern or strength of the community group. A thorough analysis of assessment data identifies the priority action statement that nursing action, in collaboration with the community, could address.

Planners (team members, community collaborators, and stakeholders) must consider many factors when deciding on a priority. A key aspect of priority setting is to identify who will be involved in making the decision and what type of process will be used to determine the priority.

Setting a priority is not a value-free process, and those who may be involved in determining priorities bring many different perspectives. The example in Box 6.3 identifies some of the different perspectives that people in the community might hold on a particular topic.

As discussed in Chapter 5, there are different categories of people who may be involved in a project and in making decisions. The core planners usually make day-to-day decisions; however, selecting priorities is one point where it is vital to involve people with different perspectives to ensure that health action will be relevant to the community as a whole and will be sustainable.

On a practical level, the team needs to branch out from its core group and seek representation from the different community groups who may be affected. In this way, people can give input and the process becomes more transparent. For example, in Box 6.3, if potential communities of interest (people with young children, older people, golfers) or stakeholders (community health practitioners and business leaders) are not involved in the decision making, they may quickly make their dissatisfaction known and possibly withdraw support for the project. The town council could also lose credibility. Although most can appreciate that it is not possible to meet every need, people still need to feel that decisions are fair, and that their issues and concerns have been heard and might be addressed in the future. That feeling of fairness will encourage support for a final decision based on broad input and will help pave the way for a successful outcome.

The actual process used to select a priority is the next consideration. A clear framework helps to make the selection of a priority as objective and transparent as possible. An important element of this framework is the health impact of actions. A **health impact assessment (HIA)** aims to enhance the positive aspects and minimize the aspects of a program or project that may have negative effects on the health of different groups in the population (McKenzie et al., 2013). The following framework for selecting priorities is based on five priority-setting questions (McKenzie et al., 2013, p. 99) augmented by considerations about health impact assessment:

1. What is the most pressing need? What issue is of most concern to the community? Is this a concern for groups with inequitable access to the social determinants of health and low capacity to take action? How many people are affected by the concern and how severe is the threat to health (mortality and morbidity; poor health status; unsafe environment)?

2. Are there resources adequate to deal with the problem? That is, are there sufficient people, supplies, and funds to act?

3. Can the problem best be solved by a health promotion intervention, or could it be better handled through other means? Is there potential to build capacity in the community?

4. Are effective intervention strategies available to address the problem? Are there equitable and evidence-based strategies, theories, or promising practices that could address the problem? Does action on this concern fit with the mandate of the community organization? Would another organization or government office be better suited to deal with the concern?

5. Can the problem be solved in a reasonable amount of time?

The process used to select priorities can be informal or formal. An informal approach is appropriate with smaller groups, especially groups that are familiar with the concerns.

> **BOX 6.3**
> **Different Perspectives Involved in Selecting a Community Priority**
>
> The town council of a small community has funding for a project to increase physical activity and social interactions, which in the long term could have an impact on morbidity and mortality. Community residents identify three possible options in a community consultation: build a playground, make sidewalks more accessible for wheelchairs and strollers, or expand the municipal golf course. In deciding what to do, decision makers might have different criteria in mind.
>
> For example, a community health nurse, thinking about the social determinants of health, might want to modify the physical environment to increase access to activity for the less mobile. A business leader might favor options with the potential to attract business and tourism. If the council wanted to increase the town image as a retirement community, it might be interested in promoting safety and recreation for retired people. The final decision would be influenced by the criteria selected, the persuasiveness of the arguments, and the ability to reach a compromise that would provide some satisfaction for everyone.

For example, planners can explain the various options at a community meeting and use the five questions listed above to get input. Other options may come up during the discussion. For example, it might be possible to combine options, by taking action that "kills two birds with one stone," as the saying goes. Another option might be to phase in action, dealing with one concern at a time.

The more formal approach of ranking options using the criteria above is appropriate when more people are involved. For example, in the situation described in Box 6.3, the town council could invite representatives of community groups and other stakeholders to rank the three options: build a playground, improve the sidewalks, or expand the golf course. The meeting would likely start with a short presentation on the funding requirements (to increase physical activity and social interactions) and information on each option identified during the community consultation. To facilitate the process, participants could use a scoring sheet to rank each option on a scale of 1 to 10 according to the five-question framework described above. A tally of responses indicates the community's favored option.

In some projects, it may be necessary or convenient to combine the final steps of assessment—the validation of findings and development of action statements—with the priority-setting exercise. There are pros and cons to this. Two community meetings provide the opportunity to build relationship with community members more gradually, but this must be weighed against the time and resources required to organize two meetings instead of one.

The end result of selecting a priority, the priority action statement, provides direction and substantiation for the plan. As depicted in Table 6.1, each part of the priority action statement is linked to a component of the plan (Vollman, Anderson, & McFarlane, 2008). These components are discussed in the following sections.

## Identify the Goal (Step 6b)

Once the priority action statement is selected, the next step for planners is to translate this into a goal for action. A **health goal** provides direction toward improving the health of a particular population. For example, a health goal identifies the focus of the action—individuals and families, the community, or larger aggregates—and specifies a clear endpoint/outcome, thereby setting boundaries on what is to be accomplished. In turn, this informs the choice of strategies to promote health, build capacity, or increase access to the social determinants of health, as shown in the cube in Figure 6.1 (Hamilton & Bhatti, 1996).

**Table 6.1: Relationship of the Priority Action Statement to Components of the Plan**

| Part of Action Statement | Relationship | Component of Plan |
|---|---|---|
| Parts 1 and 2: Name of group and concern or strength | links to | Goal and objectives |
| Part 3: Related-to clause | links to | Strategy and intervention for action, described in objectives |
| Evidence | links to | Evaluation measures |

At their first meeting, team members get to know each other and orient themselves to their community health project. They review the final assessment project report (see Appendix to this chapter), which includes the following three action statements:

- The homeless are at risk for hypothermia and frostbite related to limited daytime activities and spaces, warm clothing, and information on how to protect themselves from the cold.
- The homeless are at risk for poor nutrition related to lack of nutritious food.
- The homeless have a mutual support system related to consistently helping others to find food, shelter, and social events.

Before proceeding, team members take time to acquaint themselves with the community and introduce themselves to the key informants. In addition to making contact, they need to confirm that the situation has not changed and to learn more about effective ways to work with the homeless. The Homeless Coalition will meet in one week to set priorities, so they want to be prepared for that meeting.

At the shelters, they find there is still a high interest in learning about protection from frostbite and hypothermia. When a couple of men start telling them how a friend experienced severe frostbite last year, more join in with their own experiences.

While talking to shelter staff and the homeless men and women, team members pick up useful information about how to work with the group. Staff have told them about how one person came in to give a presentation and then showed a series of slides about the importance of healthy foods without giving any chance for discussion. In contrast, another presenter provided information in simple language and pictures, based on the food available in the shelter, and asked questions. The second person stimulated a good discussion. Team members realize that an interactive approach will be most appropriate at the shelters.

The planning session with the Homeless Coalition opens with a brief discussion to bring the group up to date. At first, everyone seems quite overwhelmed at the prospect of finding sufficient daytime spaces, healthy food, and adequate clothing, and the need to increase daytime drop-ins. Then the project leader says, "Well, we can't do everything at the same time. We need to decide on priorities and work from there." Her statement lessens the tension in the room.

Since they know the priority is shelter and clothing, the student team works with the Coalition leader to take the group through the questions that will help them select a priority action: Are there resources adequate to deal with the problem? Can the problem best be solved by a health promotion intervention, or could it be better handled through other means? Are effective intervention strategies available to address the problem? Can the problem be solved in a reasonable amount of time? (McKenzie et al., 2013, p. 99).

The participants admit that providing daytime space will be challenging without extra funds. However, the Coalition reports that they have sufficient funds to provide drop-ins at two shelters this winter; they will open for two hours, during the morning and afternoon. The Coalition asks the team to build on the interest shown by some shelter residents and work with them to inform people about the new arrangements. As well, they invite the team to take the lead in developing and providing some sessions on how to keep warm when on the street. The team agrees with their request. The final priority action statement is: "The chronic homeless residents in two shelters are at risk of hypothermia and frostbite related to limited access to daytime drop-ins and to information on ways to stay warm and protect themselves from the cold."

**Discussion Topics and Questions**

3. After referring to the final assessment report in the Appendix to this chapter, identify why poor nutrition was considered a lower priority than the risk of hypothermia and frostbite.
4. What elements of the health impact assessment (HIA) were included in the priority-setting process?

In terms of the planning process, the project goal is derived from the priority action statement and informed by the supporting evidence (see Table 6.1, above). It is the positive expression of the group's concern or barrier to health, or it addresses how the strengths of the group might be maintained. Comprised of two parts, the goal describes, simply and concisely, who will be affected and what will change (McKenzie et al., 2013). It answers the question "How will this project provide future benefit for the population?" For example, if the priority action statement is "School-age children are at risk of smoking," the goal would be "School-age children are at reduced risk of smoking." When the priority action statement identifies strengths, the goal will be to maintain that strength.

Identifying the goal is a considerable step forward; however, the endpoint is still broad. Further definition of the goal is achieved by determining which evidence-based health promotion strategy and intervention are the most relevant and by defining the specific objectives that will guide each step of the action. Box 6.4 explains the relationship among the three components.

There is a hierarchy to the goal and objectives (McKenzie et al., 2013), in that the goal sets the criteria for the objectives and strategy. From another perspective, both must be directly relevant to achieving the goal. This process of specifying objectives to guide the most appropriate course of action is based on knowledge of evidence-based health promotion strategies.

## Identify a Strategy and Evidence-Based Intervention (Step 6c)

Determining a strategy and evidence-based intervention occurs in phases. First, assessment data provides a context for deciding which strategy would be most appropriate. The general category of health promotion strategies includes a range of approaches. Box 6.6, below, identifies the most common ones. Next, consider which evidence-based interventions, appropriate for the strategy, you might use, alone or combined with others. In this critical part of the project, carefully consider the available sources of evidence from theory, research, and practice.

### Health Promotion Strategies

**Health promotion strategies** are "any planned combination of educational, political, environmental, regulatory, or organizational mechanisms that support actions and conditions of living conducive to the health of individuals, groups and communities" (Joint Committee on Health Education and Promotion Terminology, 2012). Health promotion strategies promote community health through action on the social determinants of health.

In large health promotion programs based on ecological models of health, community researchers select strategies that will interact across multiple levels of the system

**Health Promotion Strategies**

**Health education** is "any combination of planned learning experiences based on sound theories that provide individuals, groups, and communities the opportunity to acquire knowledge and the skills needed to make quality health decisions" (Joint Committee on Terminology, 2012).

**(Mass) health communication strategies** involve informing and influencing individual and community decisions to enhance health using forms such as mass media, media advocacy, risk communication, public relations, entertainment education, print materials, or electronic communication (McKenzie et al., 2013).

**Community capacity building and organization** includes "an orientation to community that is strength based rather than need based and stresses the identification, nurturing, and celebration of community assets" (Minkler & Wallerstein, 2005, p. 4). It is also the "process by which community groups are helped to identify common problems or goals, mobilize resources, and in other ways develop and implement strategies for reaching the goals they have collectively set" (Minkler, Wallerstein, & Wilson, 2008, p. 288).

**Environmental and organizational change** strategies include modifying the physical, economic, service, cultural, psychological, and political environments surrounding people (McKenzie et al., 2013) to create a health-supporting environment.

**Health policy/enforcement** strategies are mandated or regulated, and include executive orders, laws, ordinances, policies, regulations, rules, and position statements (McKenzie et al., 2013) to achieve specific health goals in a society.

(individual/family, small group, community, society) to promote the health of specific populations (Sallis, Owen, & Fisher, 2008). The community health nursing projects in this text tend to focus on the use of strategies at the group and community level that complement strategies aimed at the broader system.

There is not a common classification of the health promotion strategies; both the number and names for the strategies vary. For example, the Population Health Promotion Cube in Figure 6.1 identifies five strategies. McKenzie and colleagues (2013) identify six broad categories and four "other" types, and the Public Health Nursing Section (2001) of the Minnesota Department of Health identifies 17 types of public health interventions. Box 6.5 lists and defines the five broad strategies discussed in this text.

The naming of the health promotion strategies in Box 6.5 is somewhat arbitrary but provides an entry point to understanding the different approaches. While there is considerable overlap in the definition and application of strategies in practice, they do represent distinct approaches to changing behavior and/or creating environments that support health. Furthermore, it is widely recognized that the strategies work in synergy and that using multiple strategies at different levels of the system has greater impact than the use of a single strategy.

Each strategy uses a range of associated methods and approaches, called interventions, to expose the priority population to planned actions or experiences. For example, suppose you want to promote the health of employees in Company A and decide to start small by encouraging more frequent use of the stairs. Interventions might include distributing health information on the fitness benefits of using the stairs in pamphlets or posters, offering a workshop presentation, or instituting a policy that elevators are to be used only by people with a disability. The pamphlets, posters, and presentation are interventions associated with a health education strategy; the restricted use of the elevators is associated with both organizational and policy change strategies. Since interventions are easier to understand than the broader health promotion strategies, determining an evidence-based intervention with your community group is a very important step in planning; it helps to focus the action for everyone.

Since health education is perhaps the most frequently used group strategy, we discuss it in detail to explore what to consider when selecting a strategy and associated interventions. Subsequent chapters will examine other strategies. Chapters 10 and 11 address the strategy of community capacity building and organization, and Chapter 12 discusses health policy/enforcement. Examples of environmental and organization change and mass communication strategies occur throughout the remaining chapters.

Health education aims to provide individuals and collectives with the opportunity to learn knowledge and skills to make healthy decisions (McKenzie et al., 2013). In a review of health promotion concepts, the World Health Organization (Regional Office for the Eastern Mediterranean, 2012) concluded that effective health education increases health literacy. **Health literacy** is the capacity to access and use health information to make appropriate health decisions and maintain basic health. The potential to increase the health literacy of the audience is a crucial consideration in developing learning materials. Chapter 7 discusses health literacy in detail.

Once your team has decided to use a health education strategy, the next decision is deciding on one or more interventions. Building on the example to increase stair use described above, you would consult the research literature to determine which educational approaches had worked in similar circumstances. Usually you find that it is better to use more than one method. Before intervening, you would collect baseline, or pretest, data on the current use of the stairs. Repeating the data collection at the end of the intervention, that is, gathering posttest data, would allow you to evaluate the success of the intervention.

Health education strategies are applicable to individual or group settings. For example, in counseling or tutoring, a professional provides individualized help and support to develop knowledge and skills and foster changes in behavior. Even if the counseling occurs in a group setting, the purpose is individual behavior change, that is, each person in the group will reduce smoking or adopt a healthier lifestyle. One type of counseling is behavior modification, based on the stimulus response theory (McKenzie et al., 2013).

Health education acknowledges the influence of environment on health behavior and on learning and includes actions to modify the environment to support learning. This can range from providing a quiet place for people to work in groups to providing bus passes or child care so people can access a health education intervention. Another example is identifying when and where a person smokes and counseling individuals on ways to change that environment (McKenzie et al., 2013).

**Train-the-trainer** is a particular type of health education used to extend the reach of health providers and build community capacity. Train-the-trainer means that lay workers are taught to deliver services in their own community. Ideally, the approach builds on existing skills in the community, for example, drawing on experienced mothers to support new mothers with breast-feeding or infant care. Another example is that of grandmothers in Africa who are working to support each other in caring for children who have lost both parents to HIV (Grandmothers to Grandmothers Campaign, n.d.). Child-to-child is a specific form of train-the-trainer that involves children in the assessment and planning process to improve their health and the health of the family or the community (Child-to-Child Trust, 2013).

## Evidence-Based Interventions

Since bringing about change in the community is costly in terms of time and effort, it is especially important that the strategies and interventions used with groups and populations are effective. As mentioned in Chapter 1, the evidence for practice comes from theory, research, clinical experience, community preferences, and available resources. Models and frameworks draw on a number of theories and research findings to help understand problems in a particular situation (Glanz, Rimer, & Viswanath, 2008).

Clinical expertise is based on practice experience combined with reflection and evaluation. You can learn about practice by consulting with your faculty clinical instructors and community advisors, as well as reviewing case studies and examples of community initiatives in similar situations. Community preferences have been determined during assessment, analysis, and priority setting. You determine the availability of health care resources for an intervention through discussion with your advisors. The following section will focus first on the evidence base derived from theories and models, and then from research and practice.

Theories and models can guide strategies and interventions by providing a lens through which to view a problem and explain how to address it. **Theories** prevent us from reinventing the wheel and allow us to improve it by testing and altering the wheel for different situations (Budgen, Cameron, & Bartfay, 2010).

When reviewing theories and models, consider how they could help you to accomplish the project goals. For example, the Population Health Promotion Cube (Figure 6.1, above) can be used to situate your project in terms of the population group and relevant determinants of health, and to identify potential strategies, one of which is health education. When considering health education strategies, more than one theory may be pertinent. Theories that explain how knowledge is taken in, processed, and stored are particularly pertinent. The learning theories include Knowles's assumptions about adult learners and social learning, and cognitive, humanistic, behavioral, and developmental learning theories (as cited in Allender, Rector, & Warner, 2010). For example, a research study aimed at reducing adolescent risk-taking behavior would likely be informed by theories of adolescent development. It is important to note that although researchers usually situate their initial studies within a theoretical framework, later published reports might not identify those theories.

The three models frequently used to guide health education interventions use the concepts of phases or staging: the Generalized Model for Program Planning in Health Promotion (McKenzie et al., 2013), the Transtheoretical Stages of Change Model (Prochaska, Redding, & Evers, 2008), and the Health Communication Program Cycle found in the National Cancer Institute's (2008) Pink Book. The first two are described below; the Cycle is discussed in Chapter 7.

The **Generalized Model for Program Planning in Health Promotion** identifies five stages of learning that lead to behavior change: awareness, knowledge, appreciation, ability, and accomplishment, augmented by environmental supports (McKenzie et al., 2013). The first three stages reflect a change in understanding; the last two reflect a change in behavior. These stages were determined from an analysis of the educational and ecological assessment of the PRECEDE-PROCEED program planning model (McKenzie et al., 2013). Simply put, movement from one stage to another is facilitated by stage-specific interventions that increase learning and/or change the environment. The environmental interventions are designed to support changes in learning and/or behavior by modifying

**Table 6.2: Stages in the Generalized Model for Health Planning in Health Promotion**

| Learning | Awareness means being conscious of a health concern at a basic level. Being aware of a potential risk to health or the possibility of taking action provides an incentive to learn how to maintain or improve health. |
| | Knowledge refers to the level of understanding required to comprehend the implications of a health concern in order to take action. |
| | Appreciation means having developed a positive attitude toward the need to do something about a health concern that enables a person to deal with it and moves them to take action. This entails thinking that action is possible and will be worthwhile. |
| | Ability means possessing the necessary skills or ability to engage in health-enhancing behavior. The amount of effort required to acquire a skill and ability can vary, as anyone learning to give an injection or to ski realizes. With technical skills, it helps to observe others and have the opportunity to practice. |
| Behavior Change | Accomplishment means demonstrating the behaviors or actions that will resolve the problem and, in the longer term, progress to health improvement. This is more than a demonstration of ability; it requires that the behavior becomes habitual and incorporated into daily life. Some examples: following an exercise regime, meditating daily to deal better with stress, or consistently using chronic disease self-management approaches to prevent complications. |

Environmental Change underpins learning and behavior change by reducing barriers or strengthening resources to support healthy behavior.

*Source*: Adapted from McKenzie, Neiger, & Thackeray, 2013.

the nonbehavioral causes of a health problem present in the social, physical, and/or psychological service environment (McKenzie et al., 2013). The final stage, accomplishment, identifies the behavioral change expected to lead to health improvement. Table 6.2 summarizes the stages of the model.

A theory-based model that is frequently used to explain behavior change is the Transtheoretical Stages of Change Model. The **Transtheoretical Stages of Change Model** explains how individuals progress over time through predictable stages of change when adopting and maintaining health behavior change (McKenzie et al., 2013). This model, which integrates processes and principles from major theories of health behavior intervention, has been applied to a wide variety of individual problem behaviors, such as smoking cessation, exercise, mammography screening, and stress management (Prochaska, Redding, & Evers, 2008). While the model applies mainly to individual behavior change, it has applications to groups and collectives. For example, applications at the broader community level have addressed smoking and multiple-behavior change programs (Prochaska et al., 2008).

One of the many important messages from research on the Transtheoretical Stages of Change Model is that "[t]he majority of at-risk populations are not prepared to act and will not be served effectively by traditional action-oriented behavior change programs" (Prochaska et al., 2008, p. 103). This conclusion is based on findings from studies that show approximately 40 percent of smokers in the United States are in precontemplation (not thinking of changing) and 40 percent are in contemplation (thinking of changing possibly in six months). That leaves only 20 percent of the smoking population ready to change their risk behavior.

The model is very useful in that it encourages us to think about behavior change as a relatively slow process. It reminds us that the individual must actively engage in modifying problem behaviors to achieve lasting change. It is important to note that significantly greater effect sizes are found when all of the four main/key constructs of the model (stages of change, processes of change, decisional balance, and self-efficacy) are applied (Noar, Benac, & Harris, 2007). In other words, merely determining the stage of change is not enough; it is necessary to support efforts to work through the processes of change, make decisions, and increase self-efficacy. The model is important because it explains the complex and long-term process of behavior change. (See "Website Resources" at the end of this chapter for a link to the model.)

As well as theories and concepts developed from research and practice, systematic reviews of research on a particular topic or best practice guidelines provide a rich source of evidence that can be used to guide interventions. Keep in mind, though, that the amount of research available on a particular community health topic varies greatly according to the number of people at risk, the severity of the risk, the availability of research funding, and other factors. For example, researchers have appropriately focused on decreasing smoking levels for decades, but research on the use of sunscreen preparations, water safety, or vitamin D is just beginning. Even less research may be available for specific population groups, such as isolated rural older adults or recent immigrants whose first language is not English.

Possibly the best known resource for locating trustworthy and credible information to inform practice is the Cochrane databases. The **Cochrane databases** bring together health practitioners, researchers, patient advocates, and others in a global network to conduct rigorous systematic reviews of primary research on specified health care interventions using a defined process and explicit criteria. Two valuable resources pertinent to community and population health are the *Guide to Community Preventive Services* (Community Preventive Services Task Force, 2015) in the US and the *Canadian Best Practices Portal* (Public Health Agency of Canada, 2013). Both are described in the "Website Resources" along with other links.

Furthermore, numerous organizations assemble practice guidelines and provide Web-based resources and education to promote evidence-informed decision making by health professionals. For example, the Registered Nurses' Association of Ontario (2014) has best practice guidelines that summarize the best available evidence on topics relevant to community health nurses, such as facilitating client-centered learning, embracing cultural diversity, enhancing healthy adolescent development, and supporting and strengthening families.

Experienced practitioners are another source of information on best practice, particularly when there is consensus. One group, the Association of Maternal Child Health Programs (AMCHP, 2014), seeks to improve practice by disseminating public health interventions that have a base of support but have not been rigorously evaluated. The **best practices** program is a continuum of three levels of practice, **emerging** practices, **promising** practices, and **best** practices, that reinforces the importance of sharing information from well-conducted, thorough evaluations of new and innovative practice to determine what works and what does not (AMCHP, 2014). The cumulative efforts contribute to the knowledge base of community health nursing practice. The systematic process and evaluation included in the short-term projects in this text would contribute to the emerging practice area. Box 6.6 describes the criteria for each level of the best practices program.

BOX 6.6

**Definition of Emerging, Promising, and Best Practices Included in the AMCHP (2014) Best Practices Program**

**Emerging Practice:**
- Incorporates the philosophy, values, characteristics, and indicators of other positive/effective public health interventions
- Is based on guidelines, protocols, standards, or preferred practice patterns that have been proven to lead to effective public health outcomes
- Incorporates a process of continual quality improvement that accumulates and applies knowledge about what is working and not working in different situations and contexts
- Incorporates lessons learned, feedback, and analysis to lead toward improvement or positive outcomes
- Has an evaluation plan in place to measure program outcomes, but does not yet have evaluation data available to demonstrate effectiveness or positive outcomes

**Promising Practice:**
- Fills the criteria for emerging practice and has been or is being evaluated
- Has strong quantitative and qualitative data showing positive outcomes, but does not yet have enough research or replication to support positive public health outcomes that can be generalized

**Best Practice:**
- Has been reviewed and substantiated by experts in the public health field according to predetermined standards of empirical research
- Is replicable and produces desirable results in a variety of settings
- Clearly links positive effects to the program/practice being evaluated and not to other external factors

Even though many sources of evidence are available, the process of finding the best evidence to guide an intervention is not always straightforward. There are different ways to do it depending on time and experience. Experienced researchers and program planners have sufficient resources and time to conduct an extensive literature review to identify evidence-based strategies/interventions that have been proven effective in addressing similar situations. An alternative, and quicker, approach is to check websites that document "best practices." We provide a list of websites for evidence-based interventions searchable by age, population, and concern at the end of the chapter.

To give an example of what you might expect to find on a website, assume you want to identify an evidence-based health education intervention to prevent or reduce smoking in school-age children or youth. To start, you would search a best practices website for public/community health, such as Community Preventive Services Task Force, US (2013), and/or Public Health Agency of Canada (2013). The search reveals several well-documented interventions meeting consistent measures of success. Box 6.7 describes one of these, the Tar Wars program.

### Identifying the Evidence-Based Intervention

The theories, models, and sources for evidence-based interventions, described in the section above, help you to determine the applicability of an intervention to your situation and provide guidance on how to use it. Your priority setting has identified community preferences. The remaining evidence-based considerations are clinical expertise and available resources. Critical thinking and discussions with your advisors and collaborators, along with your knowledge of the community, will help you to decide which intervention(s) is the most likely to succeed.

Resist the temptation to jump into action too quickly. For example, if you decide on a health education strategy, do not automatically leap to preparing a pamphlet or

BOX 6.7
**Example of an Evidence-Based Intervention to Reduce Tobacco Use in Children, the Tar Wars Program**

The Tar Wars program has provided a "tobacco-free" education program to 9 million fourth- and fifth-grade students in the US and worldwide over the past 25 years. The Tar Wars program includes a classroom presentation about the short-term health effects and consequences of tobacco use, better uses for the money usually spent on tobacco, the influence of the tobacco industry, and the skills needed to make positive health decisions and take personal responsibility for well-being. The second component invites students to enter a poster or video into a well-publicized school, state, or national contest.

The program documents incorporate concepts of self-efficacy, observational learning, and incentive motivation found in Bandura's theory of social cognitive learning (see Glanz, Rimer, & Viswanath, 2008, p. 171). As well, the program is consistent with evidence-based US guidelines for programs to prevent tobacco use and addiction in school health (National Center for Chronic Disease Prevention and Health Promotion, 1994) and recent reviews of effective practice (Peters, Kok, Ten Dam, Buijs, & Paulussen, 2009; Thomas, Micucci, Ciliska, & Mirza, 2005).

A review of the results by your team could provide further information, for instance, on the settings, students, and presenters, to make decisions about whether or not the approach is appropriate for your situation. The approach could be applied as part of a short-term project and would assist planners to think more broadly about evidence-based interventions.

*Source*: Adapted from American Academy of Family Physicians, 2013.

giving a presentation without considering what other possible intervention options would best achieve your goal.

Once you have decided on your intervention, you usually have some ideas on how you will carry it out. At this point in planning, it is helpful to give your intervention a title that conveys the broad approach you will take. The title of the intervention helps to focus thinking and explain the project to others. You could call it your "working title." For example, the working title for an intervention to increase the use of stairs in Company A could be "A Presentation to Provide Information on the Health Benefits of Using the Stairs." If you later find out that this approach does not fit with the way the organization functions and need to change the intervention, you can always preface the new title with "Working Title 2."

## Develop Impact and Process Objectives (Step 6d)

As discussed earlier, the goal of an intervention provides focus and sets a boundary on the action, and the objectives provide specific direction. Using the Generalized Model for Program Planning in Health Promotion, McKenzie and colleagues (2013) describe the health behavior change likely to result in improved health as movement through sequential levels of learning and behavior change objectives within a supportive environment. The stepwise progression highlights the importance of allowing time to complement and build on earlier learning rather than skipping a step or expecting the process to occur all at once.

The three commonly used types of objectives that lead to behavior change are: outcome, impact, and process. Outcome objectives are the observable and measureable broad changes in health in the priority group, such as reduced levels of smoking in immigrant men. Since the projects in this text occur over a relatively short time, we focus

The team converts the priority action statement into the goal: "The homeless residents in two shelters are at decreased risk of hypothermia and frostbite." Thinking about possible interventions, they anticipate that offering daytime drop-ins will help to decrease the risk of hypothermia and frostbite due to the lack of shelter but will not fully address the problem.

The students determine that access to daytime shelter is dependent on the homeless residents knowing when the shelters are open and taking advantage of the opportunity to gain respite from the cold. They reason that the challenges will be to get the information out on opening hours and to draw people in. Shelter announcements and posted schedules might not be enough. It seems obvious that one should get in out of the cold whenever possible, but the shelter workers say some people are forgetful; they tend to get distracted and need constant reminders. As well, team members have noticed that shelter residents do not pay much attention to written material, possibly because they have difficulty reading or need glasses. They decide that word-of-mouth is the best communication method to use.

The team worries that the goal leaves out a lot until the instructor reminds them to look at the assessment data. Considering the first related-to clause, "limited daytime activities and spaces, warm clothing, and information on how to protect themselves from the cold" from the second scenario in this chapter, above, the team is aware that many homeless men and women do not have adequate winter clothing—they especially lack warm socks, hats, and mitts. From staff, they learn there are donations of warm clothing available. Perhaps this could be distributed with tips on how to stay warm. As well, the team wants to build on the strengths they have identified.

Considering the challenges—promoting the drop-ins, and providing information and resources for dealing with the cold—the team identifies that the best strategy to meet their needs is health education. They start considering what would be the most effective way to communicate information on protection from the cold weather. Should they provide information on posters and handouts, in a presentation, or provide demonstrations in a workshop, or would a combination of methods work best? Turning to the literature, they do not find anything about protecting the homeless, or anyone else, from the cold in the research databases available through their organization.

A search of the Internet, however, produces practical information on health care for the homeless and ways to deal with the cold on US military websites. All these sites mention using the buddy system to reduce cold injuries in others. This means encouraging friends to check each other for red or white skin on the face or ears. From their assessment, which documents that several residents talked about helping each other out, the team members feel that this might be something that would work. As well, they plan to use Knowles's principles of adult learning, social influence theory, and the Health Communication Program Cycle (National Cancer Institute, 2008; see Chapter 7 in this text) in designing the intervention. They plan to work collaboratively with the homeless residents to distribute the information about the daytime drop-ins and about dealing with the cold.

After discussing their limited findings from the literature and what they have learned from the staff and homeless residents, they report to the Homeless Coalition. They propose that the main intervention will be interactive, small-group workshops prepared in collaboration with the residents. The workshops will include reminders about the shelter hours and information on seeking shelter, dressing for the cold, and possibly other ways to protect themselves from the cold. The Coalition agrees that the proposal is feasible and relevant.

**Discussion Topics and Questions**

5. Discuss how to formulate a possible goal from the priority action statement: "The homeless residents have a mutual support system related to helping others find food, shelter, and social events."

6. How does the related-to clause contribute to the relevance of an intervention?

on the objectives with shorter timelines, that is, impact and process objectives. **Impact objectives** specify the measurable changes in learning, behavior, and the environment that need to occur in the priority community and environment to achieve the health goal (McKenzie et al., 2013). Impact objectives are an intermediate point on the path to the ultimate goal. Impact objectives include learning objectives, action or behavioral objectives, and environmental objectives.

Learning objectives are the educational tools needed to achieve the desired behavior change, and include a hierarchy that begins with the least complex and builds to the most complex (McKenzie et al., 2013). Complexity includes time, effort, and resources required to accomplish the objective. **Awareness objectives** are the least complex and indicate that the community will have some preliminary idea of the presence of the health concern. **Knowledge objectives** build on awareness to expand the information the community has about the health concern. **Appreciation objectives** build on the awareness and knowledge to attain and maintain an attitude that enables or motivates the community to deal with the health concern. Learning objectives contain elements of awareness, knowledge, and appreciation to prepare or motivate the community to obtain the ability to change health behavior.

**Ability objectives** build on awareness, knowledge, and appreciation for the community to develop the necessary skills to demonstrate the desired healthy behavior. **Accomplishment objectives** define the ongoing behavior change that is needed to resolve the health concern because the behavior is incorporated into the everyday lives of the community group.

**Environmental objectives** indicate changes that are needed to reduce the social, physical, psychological, service, and/or political factors related to the health concern (McKenzie et al., 2013). Environmental objectives may be as immediate as providing warm clothing or sanding icy sidewalks, or as broad as using social media to change attitudes about single-sex couples or advocating changes in social assistance payments.

The application of impact objectives is illustrated by the example of seeking to increase home safety for toddlers by parents attending a well-child drop-in provided by a Parents' Resource Center. Starting with the learning objectives, the parents need to be aware that certain situations in the home can be unsafe for toddlers. This awareness may seem obvious, but some people may not even consider injuries in the home while being very concerned about injuries in the yard or street. Second, the parents need to know what type of situations in the home could be unsafe. Third, the parents need to appreciate the need to take action to improve home safety. If the first three objectives are combined into a learning objective, the objective could be "The parents are ready to learn more about home safety." Fourth, the parents need to have the ability to improve home safety. To experience a change in behavior, the parents need to accomplish the task of addressing home safety on a regular basis. Throughout or at some point during learning and behavioral changes, the environment needs to be modified to support change. The environment objective could involve providing bus passes to attend an educational event on home safety.

Figure 6.2 illustrates the hierarchy of changes, or stages of learning, leading to behavior change provided earlier in Table 6.2. For simplicity, we combine the first three objectives of increasing/developing awareness, knowledge, and appreciation into the learning objective. Be aware, however, that in some situations, especially with large populations, the focus could be on raising awareness or increasing knowledge.

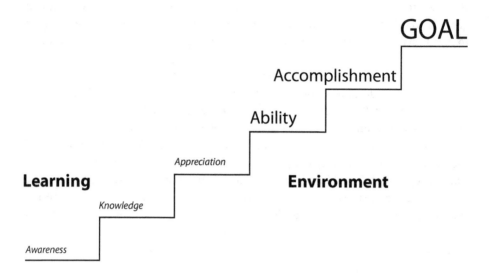

The first consideration when developing impact objectives for the health education model is to determine what level of learning or behavior change is feasible for the intervention you are planning in relation to the intended outcome of the project. This will depend on your situation. If you have been conducting an assessment with a community group for a few weeks, you have some understanding of where they are on the continuum. Based on the assessment process, you may have determined that the group are aware and have some knowledge and motivation to take action on the health concern identified in the priority action statement. In that case, you would appropriately focus on developing participants' ability. If you have taken over an assessment completed by others, or your community group has changed, you will need to conduct a quick reassessment to determine the concerns and interests of the community group at the present time.

When developing learning and behavioral objectives for interventions, you need to keep in mind whose behavior is expected to change. The Generalized Model (McKenzie et al., 2013) describes a continuum of change. In other words, the "who" in the learning and behavioral objectives needs to refer to the same group. For example, if the "who" of the learning objective is "parents of toddlers attending the Resource Center," the "who" of the ability objective would be the same.

In some projects, you could have two potential communities of interest, a community group and a provider for the community group. For example, in the project with parents of toddlers, referred to above, you might also consider the staff of the Resource Center. We do not recommend having two communities of interest for small-scale projects (especially for teams of two to four) because it means doubling the number of objectives and work. An alternative approach would be to include the staff in the environmental objective. We suggest favoring involvement with community members over staff to increase your skill in dealing with more varied opinions.

As discussed earlier, the environmental objective is concerned with changing the social

**Table 6.3: Draft of Process and Impact Objectives**

| Process Objectives (needed to attain impact objectives) | Impact Objectives (to support behavior change) |
| --- | --- |
| Develop and distribute information on unsafe home situations and options to improve safety. | *Learning*: Parents express interest in learning how to improve home safety for toddlers. |
| Book room and equipment. Develop, test, and deliver interactive workshop. | *Ability*: Parents identify unsafe situations and how to make them safe. |
| Offer follow-up discussions about home safety at drop-in. | *Accomplishment*: Parents report checking regularly for unsafe home situations. |
| Arrange for bus passes and monitor use. | *Environment*: Parents receive bus passes to attend workshop. |

or physical environment to support learning. The responsibility for doing this usually resides with the team or with someone other than the community group. Collaborating with Center staff, as described above, provides a supportive environment for change.

**Process objectives** specify the actions taken by the team that will lead to achievement of the impact objectives and, ultimately, the goal. Another term for process objectives is program activities (Anderson & McFarlane, 2014). They break the intervention down into manageable steps and answer the question "What actions should the team take to bring about each of the impact objectives?"

Careful planning is necessary to make the process objectives comprehensive and help you to avoid being overwhelmed. Before considering the process objectives on their own, a useful exercise is to map out some of the process objectives in relation to the impact objectives. Table 6.3 presents the draft for objectives for an interactive workshop for parents on home safety.

Table 6.3 helps you become more aware of the sequence and timing of actions. Three aspects are important. The first is the staging of the impact objectives to allow time for the progression from learning to behavior change to occur, as discussed in the previous section. The second factor is the obvious need to complete the action described in the process objective in order to achieve the expected changes described in the impact objective. Less obvious in this table is the third factor, the sequencing and monitoring of the tasks required to carry out each process objective.

Process objectives address three types of interrelated team activities:

1. Develop, test, and deliver the intervention.
2. Make the arrangements for delivering the intervention, such as securing the required equipment, finding a place for educational activities, and advertising events.
3. Evaluate or monitor that the intervention is being carried out as planned, including seeking feedback from all involved and making adjustments as necessary.

Although identified separately, the three actions are interrelated. For example, prior to providing a workshop, you need to develop and test the content and delivery of the information session, organize the workshop location, and make sure the required resources and equipment are available. Not least is taking steps to ensure you have the

**Table 6.4: Example of Three Tasks Associated with One Process Objective**

| Process Objective (needed to attain impact objective) | Impact Objective (to support behavior change) |
|---|---|
| Develop and distribute information on unsafe home situations and options to improve safety.<br><br>Tasks:<br>• Develop and test a poster on unsafe home situations and options to improve safety with at least two staff and two parents.<br>• Arrange for team member to put up posters in prominent locations in Resource Center.<br>• Check with team and staff about the reaction of people to the posters (e.g., Did many read the posters? Did they ask questions? Did they seem interested?). Clarify any misunderstandings if necessary (formative evaluation). | *Learning*: Parents express interest in learning how to improve home safety for toddlers. |

required audience. Some of these actions, such as finding a location and promoting attendance, need to occur as soon as possible, while others can be left until later.

Table 6.4 provides an example of the three types of tasks associated with the process objective "Develop and distribute information on unsafe home situations and options to improve safety."

Program planning uses the term "formative evaluation" (McKenzie et al., 2013) for the testing and seeking feedback that is an inherent part of nursing practice. This might include obtaining feedback on a draft poster with questions such as "What did you like? What didn't you like?" and "What would you keep? What would you change?" or asking specific questions about other aspects of an intervention. For example, during a rehearsal of some aspect of the intervention, participants may be asked to evaluate a speaker's delivery style or to give feedback on practical arrangements: "Was the room suitable? Could you hear what was being said?" These questions help you adjust the content and delivery of an intervention so that they are relevant to the project and to the needs of the community group.

The timeline (also called a Gantt chart), first presented in Chapter 4, assists in scheduling the tasks in sequence (Ewles & Simnett, 1999). A **Gantt chart** is a table with activities listed in the left-hand column and dates across the top and is used to plan the timing of activities (see Table 6.5 in the scenario below). Learning how to use a timeline or Gantt chart is a necessary skill for teamwork and community health nursing practice.

### Guidelines for Defining Impact and Process Objectives

This section describes how to write impact and process objectives to give clear direction for action and, most importantly, provide a framework for evaluation. Bear in mind that both types of objectives can be broken down to give more detailed direction.

A well-written objective answers four questions (McKenzie et al., 2013):

1. *Who* is expected to respond or change?
2. *What* response or change is desired?

3. *When* will the response or change occur?

4. *How much* change will occur?

In an impact objective, "who is expected to change" refers to the community of interest. For example, "who" might be defined by a geographical location, age, gender, or relationship to others, such as "parents of toddlers attending a Parents' Resource Center." Process objects are usually written as imperative statements directing the unstated "you" to complete the action. The unstated "you" refers to the team. For example, the team members will complete the process objective "Develop draft resources materials and processes for testing with community group."

It is important to use explicit verbs to specify the desired change or action. For example, verbs such as "identify," "state," "list," or "compare and contrast" are more specific and easier to measure than vaguer terms such as "understand" and "realize" (Ervin, 2002; Vollman et al., 2008). Process objectives specify actions such as "develop" or "make arrangements." Both impact and process objectives should specify a time deadline.

**SMART** is an acronym used to describe the criteria for writing objectives, that is, they should be Specific, Measurable, Appropriate, Reasonable, and Timed. Box 6.8 explains the SMART criteria.

Most people can determine whether or not an objective is written using terms that are specific and measurable. It will identify explicitly who or what is expected to change, in what way, and by how much, and give the time frame for the change to occur. However, the SMART criteria include two important requirements—that the changes are appropriate and reasonable. Only people familiar with the actual situation can determine if these criteria are met in the objective.

For example, consider an event to increase students' awareness of the six ways that the tobacco industry influences smoking by youth (National Center for Chronic Disease Prevention and Health Promotion (US) Office on Smoking and Health, 2012). The following objective has been prepared: "By January 30, 20 percent of the youth attending South Bend School will identify three of the possible six approaches that the tobacco industry uses to increase smoking by youth." The objective has the required parts, is specific, and appears measurable; however, it would be inappropriate and unreasonable if the school did not have the equipment needed to show images of industry influences from websites and movies, or if there was insufficient time allowed for it to occur.

Impact objectives require that the nature and amount of expected change be clearly stated to make them measurable. The example given above specifies both the percentage of students who must change and by how much (identify three of six methods used by tobacco industry). Sometimes the change might be moving from one group to another, for example, from a smoker to a nonsmoker, which is not as easy to determine and requires further definition, such as "Has not smoked a cigarette in the past three months."

Determining the degree of change specified in impact objectives is not an exact science. Sometimes there is data to establish a baseline for continuing assessment. While it may not be completely reliable, it supports an informed estimate, or a realistic goal to aim for. A more likely situation is that the numbers are based on population estimates and can vary considerably in small sample sizes. Usually the change represents reasonable

The team is figuring out how the chosen intervention will bring about the behavior change before they start to write the objectives. They start by asking, and answering, several questions:

Question: "Who will be doing the learning and making the behavior change?"

Answer: "The homeless residents of the two shelters."

Question: "What behavior change do we expect from our intervention?"

Answer: "The homeless residents will use the shelters when they are available and take other steps to protect themselves from the cold."

Focusing on taking protection from the cold, they ask, "What do the homeless residents need to learn?" With the Generalized Model (McKenzie et al., 2013) in mind, they provide a possible answer: "Appreciate the importance of getting out of the cold and learning other ways to protect themselves from the cold." They then ask, "How will we know they are able to do this?" Possible answers are "The homeless residents will attend the shelters, dress warmly, and possibly seek out tips for protecting themselves from the cold." Then they ask, "What will we need to do to get that to happen?" At this point they start brainstorming various ideas as to what the team will do and what they will encourage the shelter staff and residents to do. Ideas include working with shelter staff and residents to spread the word about the opening hours, make the shelters welcoming, and distribute warm clothing.

The students decide to work in pairs, one at each shelter, so the staff and residents will get to know them. Since the drop-in times are different at each place, the whole team will be available to deliver both workshops. Before starting on the workshops, they realize that they need to encourage the shelter residents to attend the drop-ins during the daytime so that they come to know and appreciate the importance of (a) getting out of the cold and (b) obtaining warm clothing and other information about protection from the cold. They feel that the sooner they get the message out, the more likely the residents will attend.

In planning the workshops, they agree to use an interactive approach to encourage the residents at each shelter to give feedback about the drop-ins, the hours and activities, what they like and what they do not like, and to share ideas about ways of keeping warm when outside. They ask for ideas on a name for the workshop, and one resident suggests "Beating the Cold." Others quickly rally around the name and the team realizes that it would bring people together.

The team decides that the lead pairs might adapt the approach in each setting, based on what they have found effective in their preliminary interactions. For example, they have noticed in one shelter that residents talk in small groups, with a few hanging around within earshot; in the other, they all gather in small groups. They might also provide additional information, such as using the buddy system to identify signs of frostbite or hypothermia, if participants show interest. After numerous changes based on feedback, they draft the following list of impact and process objectives, which they have arranged to review with the shelter staff, community group, and coalition members. In particular, they want advice on how they might evaluate the impact objectives.

### Learning
By March 4, at least half the people using the overnight accommodation in the two shelters will have attended the daytime drop-in once in two weeks.

Process objective for learning: Put up posters and collaborate with staff to spread the word to the residents at each shelter about the hours for the daytime drop-ins, January 28 to March 4.

### Ability
By March 18, half the participants attending a workshop on protection from the cold will demonstrate ability to dress warmly.

Process objective for ability: Prepare, deliver, monitor, and seek feedback on interactive workshops on dressing warmly, March 11 and 18.

### Environment
By March 18, staff and a group of residents in both shelters have spread the word about the drop-ins.

**Table 6.5: Gantt Chart for *Beating the Cold* Workshops—Revised February 14, 2015**

| Process Objectives[1] | Name | January 21 | January 28 | February 4 | February 11 | February 18 | February 25 | March 4 | March 11 | March 18 | March 25 |
|---|---|---|---|---|---|---|---|---|---|---|---|
| *Learning*: Increase readiness for workshops.<br>– Put up posters.<br>– Engage participants in discussion on the value of seeking shelter and protection from cold. | Angie & Cheryl | X | X | X | X | X | X | X | | | |
| – Identify a name for the workshops. | Elsa & Greg | X | X | X | X | X | X | X | | | |
| *Ability*: Deliver workshops. | All | | | | | | | | X | X | |
| – Search for evidence-based interventions in the literature, theory, and from shelter staff and Coalition members. | Elsa & Greg | X | X | X | | | | | | | |
| – Draft workshop agenda and review with shelter staff. | Elsa & Greg | | | | X | X | | | | | |
| – Locate or develop relevant educational resources. | Elsa & Greg | | | | X | X | X | | | | |
| – Test and adjust resources and processes. | All | | | | | X | X | X | | | |
| *Environment*: Engage with shelter staff and residents to spread the word about drop-ins and workshop. | All | | | | X | X | X | X | X | X | |
| Make arrangements. | | | | | | | | | | | |
| – Arrange for space to deliver workshops in shelters. | Angie & Cheryl | X | X | | | | | | | | |
| – Organize equipment (VCR) and snacks. | Angie & Cheryl | | | X | X | | | | | | |
| – Arrange seating prior to workshop and clean up after. | All | | | | | | | | X | X | |

*Note*: 1. Monitoring and seeking feedback on action is part of every process objective.

*continued on the following page*

continued from the previous page

**Process Objective for Environment**

Work with shelter staff to identify and coach three key residents to spread the word about the drop-ins, February 11 to March 18.

The team prepares a Gantt chart to help them keep on track and delegate tasks fairly. Table 6.5 details the process objectives by tasks and time.

As they develop the objectives and Gantt chart, the team members revise the earlier objectives and tasks until they flow smoothly. They find this makes the plan more workable. There are still some areas of uncertainty; for instance, they know some of the changes they have anticipated (such as "half the residents" in the shelter for the learning objective, or "half the workshop participants" for the ability objective) are just an educated guess because they are not sure how easy it will be to get the homeless residents to participate. Now

that they have the Gantt chart drafted, they bring their work plan up to date. The beginning sections of their work plan are provided in the Appendix to this chapter.

At times, they feel frustrated with the process. They really just want to get started! On a more positive note, however, when they finish the draft of the Gantt chart, they realize that the actions in the early objectives are laying the groundwork and will help to create a buzz. When they get the timelines down, they feel quite proud of themselves and like hearing others comment on how well they have laid out their plan.

**Discussion Topics and Questions**

7. Discuss the pros and cons of determining objectives by asking questions, as in the scenario.
8. How does the environmental objective in the scenario contribute to learning and behavior change?

expectations based on experience and discussion with the advisors and collaborators, and is a "best guess." Similarly, the more explicit the process objectives are, the easier they are to measure. For example, specifying the Web-based materials and written resources, and providing the outline for an "interactive discussion," in the workshop, provide measures of quality for the process objectives.

## Teamwork during Planning

By the planning stage of the project, the team usually knows how to work together and with the community, and should have a clearer understanding of the project. The team dynamics may come under pressure during planning. At this time, you must make decisions in a relatively short period based on a minimal amount of information about different factors. Another difficulty is maintaining timely communication. A team evaluation during the transition to planning is particularly valuable to keep the team on track before taking action.

### Decision Making

During planning, the team makes decisions about the nature and scope of an intervention, maps out the impact and process objectives, determines timelines, and identifies those responsible for completing the activities. This is not a straightforward, step-by-step procedure. Putting the plan in writing helps the team see what is expected to happen. Two forms are available to document the tasks and monitor progress: Part 2 of the work plan (see Appendix A.3.1b) and a timeline (Gantt chart) relevant to the implementation of the project (see Appendix A.3.2a). The work plan provides an overview of the key steps in planning, carrying out, and evaluating the project and provides space to enter the anticipated results and the expected completion date. This helps you to envisage the flow of the project and understand how each step will contribute to the result. As shown in Table 6.5, the timeline/Gantt chart expands a section of the work plan, laying out when tasks begin and end. The Appendix to Chapter 6 provides an example of a beginning work plan for the scenario in this chapter.

One approach to developing process objectives is to delegate the two aspects to different team members. For example, half the team could take the lead in developing the intervention and resources and the other half could make the practical arrangements. Each subteam can record the results in a common timeline/work plan, report on progress, and obtain feedback at team meetings. In addition to coordinating efforts, this provides opportunity for everyone to be involved in the overall process and maximizes learning. Using the work plan or timeline/Gantt chart to inform the meeting agenda also helps to keep it current.

During planning, teams will often feel that they are being pushed to make decisions before they are ready. For example, advisors may recommend scheduling activities, such as booking a room for an anticipated presentation, before the team has fully thought through what they will be doing. They do not know if they are they planning a workshop or a health fair. However, they do realize that they need a room no matter what they decide on. From experience, advisors know it is easier to cancel a booking than to find a room in the community at short notice. Similarly, the team may be advised to schedule time on a meeting agenda of a community group that only meets once a month. The team may not initially appreciate these timing deadlines, and so it is wise to follow the advice of people who have done this before.

Another reason for pushing the team to make planning decisions as quickly as possible is simply to move the project along and allow sufficient time to take action. Although planning is important, it can consume a considerable amount of time. Keep in mind that plans can be changed. Sometimes inconsistencies or conflicts become apparent only after you have made decisions. For example, a bus strike, a hurricane, an outbreak, such as a measles or virus (H1N1), or even cuts in funding are just some reasons for having to change plans at the last minute. A very beneficial side effect of creating a plan with others is that you have all agreed on the purpose of the plan and can make adjustments to keep going in the right direction.

Follow advice and the suggested timetable shown in Chapter 2, Table 2.1, to determine a reasonable amount of time to devote to planning based on your course schedule. Be prepared to review the plan and make adjustments as needed.

## Communication

Planning is a time of intense activity, and at times teams have to make decisions based on a limited amount of information. You may feel uncomfortable distributing tentative ("half-baked") ideas, but it is important to share your thinking so that your advisors and collaborators can provide feedback or alert you to possible conflicts or opportunities. There are several ways to do this. You can use your weekly summary (Chapter 2) to pose questions and request feedback from the people on your distribution list. For example, attach a draft work plan and/or Gantt chart to the summary as early as the second or third day of working on the plan. Be certain to note the revision date at the top of the work plan and suggest a deadline for feedback.

Expect to deal with most feedback on the plan at the weekly team meeting and document changes in a revised work plan/timeline/Gantt chart or weekly report. Back and forth communication between clinical times often leads to confusion, since all team members may not be included or have time to check their email. If necessary, designate one team member to deal with unexpected issues. A good communication system helps to keep everyone up to date and is particularly important when things are changing rapidly.

## Evaluation

An evaluation of the roles and responsibilities of team members and team functioning should occur at least halfway through the collaborative action project, or sooner if designated in your team agreement. You will note that the team in the homeless project scenario evaluated the teamwork every second week (see Appendix to this chapter). By this point in the project, team members should be sharing the workload, contributing ideas and listening to each other, and bringing up differences rather than avoiding confrontation. As well as being essential for carrying out the project, working well together is necessary for developing a good relationship with people in the community.

Teamwork does not always go smoothly. Chapter 2 explains the storming process and gives examples of how to deal with upsets. It is important to address differences, as this frees up energy for the project. Otherwise, the team and the project will only limp along. Teams that have unresolved issues also have a tendency to blame other people for their problems. A steady litany of complaints can be a clue for the need to go through conflict resolution, as described in Chapter 2. The results of a team evaluation are included in the fifth item of the weekly report (Appendix A.2.3).

## Summary

Planning is not optional when working in the community; it is a necessity. As Benjamin Franklin said, by failing to prepare, you are preparing to fail. Planning with others, setting objectives, and deciding on a course of action lays the groundwork not only for what you will do over the coming weeks or months but also for how you relate to other members of your team. The process of planning provides both direction and flexibility to deal with unforeseen barriers and to capitalize on unexpected opportunities. Most important of all is the fact that planning provides the team with a shared vision to achieve the desired outcomes during action and evaluation.

Chapters 6 and 7 fit together. Chapter 6 focuses on the process of planning an evidence-based intervention; it refers to evaluation but does not go into detail. The objectives developed in Chapter 6 makes the plan concrete and measurable. Determining how to evaluate the objectives and the success of an intervention is discussed in Chapter 7. In addition, Chapter 7 examines the specific tasks related to the development of materials and making arrangements in more depth. A quick review of both chapters will assist you to keep on track as you plan, implement, and evaluate an intervention.

Teamwork during planning can be stressful because of the decisions that need to be made in a fairly short period of time with limited information. However, when the team realizes that the plans are not set in stone and can be revised as the circumstances require, they can progress in completing the plans and communicating with each other and collaborators, and benefit by conducting a team evaluation before they launch into action.

## Classroom and Seminar Exercises

1. Discuss why having knowledge about something does not necessarily mean that you have the ability to use the knowledge.
2. Discuss how environmental supports, which could improve attendance at a well-baby drop-in, relate to the principles of primary health care.
3. Based on the information in Box 6.3, which of the three options, playground, accessible sidewalks, or expanded golf course, would best meet the funding requirements (increase physical activity and social interaction) and priority-setting questions? Explain your answer.
4. Using action statements that you have developed from a community assessment or from the draft Assessment Report in Chapter 5, determine and document the following in a work plan:
   a. A priority action statement with the community group
   b. The project goal
   c. An evidence-based intervention
   d. The impact objectives
5. Using your clinical situation (or the Chapter 5 scenario), identify how the four aspects of evidence-based interventions, (a) theory, models, research; (b) clinical expertise; (c) community preferences; and (d) available resources, were, or could be, used in the selection of an appropriate intervention.

## References

Allender, J., Rector, C., & Warner, K. (2010). *Community health nursing: Promoting and protecting the public's health* (7th ed.). Philadelphia, PA: Lippincott Williams & Wilkins.

American Academy of Family Physicians. (2013). *Tar Wars*. Retrieved from www.aafp.org/about/initiatives/tar-wars.html

Anderson, E., & McFarlane, J. (2014). *Community as partner: Theory and practice in nursing* (7th ed.). Philadelphia, PA: Wolters Kluwer Health/Lippincott Williams & Wilkins.

Association of Maternal Child Health Programs (AMCHP). (2014). *Best practices program*. Retrieved from www.amchp.org/programsandtopics/BestPractices/Pages/BestPracticeTerms.aspx

Budgen, C., Cameron, G., & Bartfay, W. (2010). Program planning, implementation, and evaluation. In J. Hitchcock, P. Shubert, S. Thomas, & W. Bartfay (Eds.), *Community health nursing: Caring in action* (1st Can. ed., pp. 284–324). Toronto, ON: Nelson Education.

Burns, N., & Grove, S. (2011). *Understanding nursing research: Building an evidence-based practice* (5th ed.). Maryland Heights, MO: Elsevier Saunders.

Child-to-Child Trust. (2013). The child-to-child approach. Retrieved from www.child-to-child.org/about/index.html

Ciliska, D., & Ganann, R. (2011). Research. In L. Stamler & L. Liu (Eds.), *Community health nursing: A Canadian perspective* (3rd ed., pp. 155–170). Toronto, ON: Pearson.

Community Preventive Services Task Force, US. (2013). *Guide to community preventive services* (the Community Guide). Retrieved from www.thecommunityguide.org

Ervin, N. (2002). *Advanced community health nursing practice.* Upper Saddle River, NJ: Prentice Hall.

Ewles, L., & Simnett, I. (1999). *Promoting health: A practical guide.* London, UK: Bailliere Tindall.

Glanz, K., Rimer, B., & Viswanath, K. (2008). Theory, research, and practice in health behavior and health education. In K. Glanz, B. Rimer, & K. Viswanath (Eds.), *Health behavior and health education: Theory, research, and practice* (4th ed., pp. 287–312). San Francisco, CA: Jossey-Bass.

Grandmothers to Grandmothers Campaign. (n.d.). *About us.* An Initiative of the Steven Lewis Foundation. Retrieved from www.grandmotherscampaign.org/

Hamilton, N., & Bhatti, T. (1996). *Population health promotion model.* Retrieved from www.phac-aspc.gc.ca/ph-sp/php-psp/php3-eng.php#Developing

Joint Committee on Health Education and Promotion Terminology. (2012). Report of the 2011 Joint Committee on Health Education and Promotion Terminology. *American Journal of Health Education, 43*(2).

McKenzie, J., Neiger, B., & Thackeray, R. (2013). *Planning, implementing and evaluating health promotion programs: A primer* (6th ed.). Needham Heights, MA: Allyn and Bacon.

Minkler, M., & Wallerstein, N. (2005). Improving health through community organizations and community building: A health education perspective. In M. Minkler (Ed.), *Community organizing and community building for health* (2nd ed., pp. 26–50). New Brunswick, NJ: Rutgers University Press.

Minkler, M., Wallerstein, N., & Wilson, N. (2008). Improving health through community organizing and community building. In K. Glanz, B. Rimer, & K. Viswanath (Eds.), *Health behavior and health education: Theory, research, and practice* (4th ed., pp. 287–312). San Francisco, CA: Jossey-Bass.

National Alliance to End Homelessness. (2013). *Chronic homelessness.* Retrieved from www.endhomelessness.org/pages/chronic_homelessness

National Cancer Institute. (2008). *Pink book: Making health communication programs work.* Retrieved from www.cancer.gov/cancertopics/cancerlibrary/pinkbook/page4

National Center for Chronic Disease Prevention and Health Promotion. (1994). Guidelines for school health programs to prevent tobacco use and addiction. *Morbidity & Mortality Weekly Report, 43*(RR-2), 1–18.

National Center for Chronic Disease Prevention and Health Promotion (US) Office on Smoking and Health. (2012). *Preventing tobacco use among youth and young adults: A report of the Surgeon General* (Chapter 5). Retrieved from www.ncbi.nlm.nih.gov/books/NBK99238

Noar, S., Benac, C., & Harris, M. (2007). Does tailoring matter? Meta-analytic review of tailored print health behavior change interventions. *Psychological Bulletin, 133,* 673–693.

Peters, L., Kok, G., Ten Dam, G., Buijs, G., & Paulussen, T. (2009). Effective elements of school health promotion across behavioral domains: A systematic review of reviews. *BioMedCentral Public Health, 9*(182). Retrieved from www.biomedcentral.com/1471-2458/9/182

Prochaska, J., Redding, C., & Evers, K. (2008). The transtheoretical model and stages of change. In K. Glanz, B. Rimer, & K. Viswanath (Eds.), *Health behavior and health education theory, research, and practice* (4th ed., pp. 97–165). San Francisco: Jossey-Bass.

Public Health Agency of Canada. (2013). *Canadian best practices portal*. Retrieved from http://cbpp-pcpe.phac-aspc.gc.ca/?s=+&post_type=interventions

Public Health Nursing Section. (2001). *Public health interventions: Applications for public health nursing practice*. St. Paul, MN: Minnesota Department of Health.

Registered Nurses' Association of Ontario. (2014). *Nursing best practice guidelines*. Retrieved from http://rnao.ca/bpg

Sallis, J., Owen, N., & Fisher, E. (2008). Ecological models of health behavior. In K. Glanz, B. Rimer, & K. Viswanath (Eds.), *Health behavior and health education theory, research, and practice* (4th ed., pp. 465–485). San Francisco, CA: Jossey-Bass.

Thomas, H., Micucci, S., Ciliska, D., & Mirza, M. (2005). Effectiveness of school-based interventions in reducing adolescent risk behaviours: A systematic review of reviews. Hamilton, ON: City of Hamilton, Public Health Services. Retrieved from www.ephpp.ca/PDF/2005_Reduce%20Adolescent%20Risk%20Behav.pdf

US Department of Housing and Urban Development. (2012). *2012 Annual Homeless Assessment Report* (Vol. 1). Retrieved from www.onecpd.info/resources/documents/2012AHAR_PITestimates.pdf

Vollman, A., Anderson, E., & McFarlane, J. (2008). *Canadian community as partner* (2nd ed.). Philadelphia, PA: Lippincott Williams & Wilkins.

World Health Organization (WHO). (1986). *The Ottawa Charter for Health Promotion*. Retrieved from www.who.int/healthpromotion/conferences/previous/ottawa/en/index1.html

World Health Organization (WHO), Regional Office for the Eastern Mediterranean. (2012). *Health education: Theoretical concepts, effective strategies and core competencies*. Retrieved from http://applications.emro.who.int/dsaf/EMRPUB_2012_EN_1362.pdf

## Website Resources

### Planning

Child-to-Child Trust: www.child-to-child.org

This site provides a description of the child-to-child approach and includes lessons that are appropriate for children of different ages.

KU Work Group on Health Promotion and Community Development, *A Model for Getting Started*: http://ctb.ku.edu/en/get-started

The KU web page on getting started is organized according to the planning process and provides links to different sections of the Tool Box. The "how-to tools" use simple, friendly language to explain how to perform the different tasks necessary for community health and development.

Public Health Ontario, *Online Health Program Planner*: www.publichealthontario.ca/en/ServicesAndTools/ohpp/Pages/default.aspx

The OHPP website states that it is an online, interactive planning tool, designed to help you make evidence-informed programming decisions through a series of interactive worksheets.

**Systematic Reviews and Best Practices**

Cochrane Collaboration: www.cochrane.org

The website identifies the different groups and fields within the Cochrane Collaboration. Groups include the Tobacco Addiction Group. The most relevant field is Health Promotion and Public Health. Each group and field provides a list of reviews relevant to its area. A full search of Cochrane databases is available through institutional libraries.

Community Preventive Services Task Force, US, *Guide to Community Preventive Services (the Community Guide)*: www.thecommunityguide.org

The Community Guide is based on a scientific systematic review process and answers questions critical to almost everyone interested in community health and well-being.

Evidence for Policy and Practice Information and Co-ordinating Centre (EPPI-Centre): http://eppi.ioe.ac.uk/

The UK EPPI-Centre website states that it is committed to informing policy and professional practice with sound evidence. It is involved in two main areas of work: (1) systematic reviews that include developing methods for systematic reviews and research syntheses, conducting reviews, supporting others to undertake reviews, and providing guidance and training in this area; and (2) research use that includes studying the use/non-use of research evidence in personal, practice, and political decision making, supporting those who wish to find and use research to help solve problems.

Health Nexus, *Your Health Promotion Specialist*: http://en.healthnexus.ca/

This Ontario health promotion service website states that it supports individuals, organizations, and communities to strengthen their capacity to promote health in Ontario and beyond. Their work is grounded in the *Ottawa Charter for Health Promotion* and they view health broadly. The four aspects of what they do are: (1) build capacity, (2) connect communities with resources, (3) form partnerships, (4) advocate for change, and (5) provide services in both English and French.

KU Work Group on Health Promotion and Community Development, *Databases of Best Practices*: http://ctb.ku.edu/en/databases-best-practices

This web page provides a list of comprehensive Web-based resources and links to categorical websites on specific issues, including adolescent pregnancy and chronic diseases.

National Collaborating Centres for Public (NCCPH) Health: www.nccph.ca/en/home.aspx

NCCPH states that the six National Collaborating Centres (NCCs) for Public Health promote and improve the use of scientific research and other knowledge to strengthen public health practices and policies in Canada. They identify knowledge gaps, foster networks, and translate existing knowledge to produce and exchange relevant, accessible, and evidence-informed products with practitioners, policy makers, and researchers. The centres are: Aboriginal Health (NCCAH), Determinants of Health (NCCDH), Environmental Health (NCCEH), Healthy Public Policy (NCCHPP), Infectious Diseases (NCCID), and Methods and Tools (NCCMT).

Public Health Agency of Canada, *Canadian Best Practices Portal*: http://cbpp-pcpe.phac-aspc. gc.ca/?s=&post_type=interventions&st=all

This website provides the opportunity to search for best practice interventions using a broad range of icons representing aspects such as health risk (tobacco, obesity, alcohol), age, location, country (Canadian, International, US), and determinants of health.

Registered Nurses' Association of Ontario, *Nursing Best Practice Guidelines*: http://rnao.ca/bpg

This site offers best practices guidelines prepared by and for nurses working in institutions and the community, on subjects ranging from "Prevention of Falls and Fall Injuries in Older Adults" to "Primary Prevention of Childhood Obesity."

## Theories

Cancer Prevention Research Center, *Transtheoretical Model*: www.uri.edu/research/cprc/transtheoretical.htm

This site provides a detailed discussion and overview of the Transtheoretical Model.

National Cancer Institute, *Pink Book–Making Health Communication Programs Work*: http://cancer.gov/pinkbook

The Pink Book provides a framework for the development of health communications and includes a variety of resources, including a method to calculate literacy level.

The Transtheoretical Model and Stages of Change: www.sfu.ca/uploads/page/18/GERO820_2012_Transtheortical_Mode.pdf

This presentation visually illustrates the model and its constructs, and provides examples for use with older people. Limitations of the model are discussed.

World Health Organization (WHO), Regional Office for the Eastern Mediterranean, *Health Education: Theoretical Concepts, Effective Strategies and Core Competencies*: http://applications.emro.who.int/dsaf/EMRPUB_2012_EN_1362.pdf

This report from the WHO summarizes theoretical concepts, effective strategies, and core competencies in health education, and provides a foundation document to guide capacity.

# Appendix to Chapter 6

**Final Assessment Project Report**

Eastern University College, School of Nursing
Community Health Nursing Project in Collaboration
with the Homeless Coalition of South Hampton
Improvement of Services for the Chronically Homeless
December 5, 2014
Students: Greg Dupuis, Angie Greely, Cheryl Mukherjee,
Elsa Sarraf
Agency Advisor: Michael George
Clinical Instructor: Sarah Reid-Lafontaine
Manager: Allison Renee

**Key Health Concerns of the Population**

Chronic homelessness is defined as individuals who
have been homeless for a year or longer, or who
have had four episodes of being homeless in the last
three years and have a disability (US Department of
Housing and Urban Development, 2012). According
to the National Alliance to End Homelessness (2013),
members of this group tend to have high rates of
behavioral health problems including severe mental
illness and substance abuse disorders, conditions
that may be exacerbated by physical illness, injury, or
trauma. Therefore, the homeless are frequent users of
emergency services, crisis response, and public safety
systems. The Alliance states that the most effective
intervention is providing permanent housing and
support. In 2012, around 100,000 individuals accounted
for 16 percent of all homelessness on a given night (US
Department of Housing and Urban Development, 2012).
In South Hampton, the Homeless Coalition identified
that approximately 850 people had been homeless in
2013. Of those, 18 percent (150 people) were chronically
homeless, and 90 percent were men; all were between
25 and 75 years old.

Community of Interest: 150 chronically homeless in
South Hampton

**Assessment Methods and Timelines**

**Assessment Methods**

| Method | Timelines | Number of Participants | Description |
|---|---|---|---|
| Collection and review of secondary data | Sept. 10–Oct. 1 | N/A | Obtained statistics from government and association websites related to homelessness. |
| Mapping downtown | Sept. 10–24 | N/A | Identified organizations and services provided to the homeless. |
| Key informant interviews | Sept. 17–24 | 15 | Interviewed one staff member from each homeless shelter. |
| Meetings with Homeless Coalition | Sept. 24, Oct. 29, Nov. 26 | 8–12 | Met with representatives from homeless shelters and other services. |
| Survey using questionnaire | Oct. 29–Nov. 19 | 3–5 in 15 shelters, 60 total | Staff gave out the invitation to participate to chronically homeless individuals. Invitation included informed consent, which was checked by team before offering questionnaire. |

## Validated Key Results/Findings

The table below indicates the issues for action and associated evidence. The team developed these concerns and strengths after consulting with Coalition members individually.

The Coalition organized a referral system with staff and the homeless residents the following week, so issues related to running out of food were not included.

### Issues for Action

| Issue | Evidence |
|---|---|
| Finding sufficient food[1] | 90 percent of homeless had difficulties obtaining sufficient quantities of food. 12 of 15 agencies talked about often having too much or too little food each day. |
| Lack of shelter | 70 percent of homeless had a concern about finding shelter from the cold, getting warm clothing, having no warm place to gather during the day, lack of activities during the day, not knowing how to prevent frostbite, and not knowing about activities. |
| | Three people almost died from hypothermia the previous winter and there were 20 incidents of severe frostbite (reports from staff). |
| Quality of food | 55 percent of homeless stated boredom with food choices. 14 of 15 staff identified that most of the food was donated bread, potatoes, doughnuts, and other sweet goods. The nutritional value of the food available most days was substandard compared with national standards. |
| Support system | 45 percent of homeless stated that they gained satisfaction from passing on information or taking someone to get help. |

*Note:* 1. This problem, identified by shelter staff, was reported and acted upon.

### Action Statements

- The homeless residents are at risk for hypothermia and frostbite related to limited daytime activities and spaces, warm clothing, and information on how to protect themselves from the cold.
- The homeless residents are at risk for poor nutrition related to lack of nutritious food.
- The homeless residents have a mutual support system related to consistently helping others to find food, shelter, and social events.

### Limitations

In some cases, participants invited to complete the questionnaire did not understand what was involved even after several explanations. That meant that approximately two of five approached could not be included.

### Sustainability

The Homeless Coalition has funding to continue the project for the next six months. Some of the shelter staff and residents have shown interest in acting on the issues.

### Recommendations

Continue to work on coordinating services among agencies for the homeless.

Involve chronically homeless individuals in planning and carrying out further action.

Initiate action with government that will lead to permanent supportive housing for the chronically homeless.

### Relevance for Community Health Nursing

Working to improve services for the chronically homeless addresses equity and social justice, a basic tenet of community health nursing that underlies the public and community health nursing standards and competencies.

### Attachments (*not attached in this example*)

- Mapping of homeless resources in downtown area
- Key informant questions and responses (identifying information removed)
- Procedure for recruiting chronically homeless for survey
- Questionnaire for chronically homeless
- Data from questionnaire
- Process used to analyze data

# Plan, Action, Evaluation Work Plan for Improvement of Services for the Homeless

Plan, Action, Evaluation Work Plan for Improvement of Services for the Homeless—
Revised February 14, 2015 (5th week of project)[1]

| Steps (time period) | Results Summary, with Completion/Revision Date |
|---|---|
| **PLAN** | |
| 6. Plan action (Jan. 7–Feb. 14) | |
| a. Set priority (Jan. 7–21) | Jan. 7. Orientation to project. Jan. 14. Met with staff and some residents to discuss concerns and possible interventions. Concern about cold among homeless residents remains high. Jan. 21. Met with 7 members of Homeless Coalition and used questions to set priority. Priority action statement: "The chronic homeless residents in two shelters are at risk of hypothermia and frostbite related to limited access to daytime drop-ins and information on ways to stay warm and protect themselves from the cold." |
| b. Identify goal (Jan. 21) | Jan. 21. The homeless residents in two shelters are at decreased risk of hypothermia and frostbite. |
| c. Identify strategy and evidence-based intervention (Jan. 21–Feb. 1) | Feb. 1. Health education strategy using intervention of interactive small group workshops on protection from the cold that includes information about seeking shelter, dressing for the cold, and possibly other ways to protect themselves. Intervention approved by Coalition. |
| d. Develop impact and process objectives (Feb. 1–14) | Feb. 14. *Learning*: By March 4, at least half the people using the overnight accommodation in the two shelters will have attended the daytime drop-in once in two weeks. Process objective for learning: Put up posters and spread the word to staff and participants in both shelters about the hours for the daytime drop-ins, Jan. 28 to March 4. *Ability*: By March 18, half of the participants attending a workshop on protection from the cold demonstrate how to dress warmly. Process objective for ability: Deliver, monitor, and seek feedback on workshops on dressing warmly, March 11 and 18. *Environmental*: By March 18, staff and a group of residents in both shelters spread the word about the drop-ins. Process objective for environment: Work with shelter staff to identify and coach three key residents to spread the word about the drop-ins, Feb. 11 to March 18. |
| **ACT** | |
| 7. Take action (Feb. 7–March 7) | |
| 9. Evaluate teamwork (Feb. 14, March 28) | Feb. 14. Reviewed team agreement and compared it to present functioning. Team found planning stressful but quieter ones learned to speak up so they are heard. Feel we are now in performing stage! |

Note: 1. Steps 7 and 8 are not yet completed and are therefore not included in the table. See Appendix A.3.1b.

# Chapter 7

# Taking Action—Step 7

· · · · · ·· ··· ···· ·· ·· · ··· ·· ·· ·· ·· ·· ·· ·· ·· · ·· ·· ·· ·· · ·· ·· ·· ·· · ·· ·· ·· ·· ·· ··◀

This chapter is where your plans will come to fruition through the implementation of an intervention adjusted to meet the needs of the community group. As well, you will learn to develop and use evaluation measures to collect data on the project objectives. Although many things will be happening at the same time, such as developing the intervention and making arrangements, your plan will assist you and your collaborators in keeping on track.

You will find the tailoring process, which involves drafting some material, trying it out with collaborators, making adjustments, and repeating the process, enlightening. The use of a pilot test can assist you in tailoring the intervention to your situation and increase your confidence. Consideration of the culture and literacy level of participants during the tailoring process is brought out in the scenario of a team working in a supermarket to improve back health.

Implementing and evaluating the intervention is a rewarding experience. It is exciting to be part of a team and community effort, and it produces valuable resources and community learning that will continue to develop.

## Learning Objectives

After reading this chapter and answering the questions throughout the chapter, you should be able to:

1. Tailor and test an intervention based on a plan, evidence-based resources, and feedback from community members and stakeholders.
2. Incorporate health literacy and cultural safety in the intervention design.
3. Develop and incorporate evaluation measures based on a plan.
4. Make arrangements to deliver tailored intervention.
5. Implement the intervention with the assistance of community members and stakeholders.
6. Document and communicate action.

> ### Key Terms and Concepts
>
> communication channel · cultural safety · engaging people · evaluation measures · Health Communication Program Cycle · impact evaluation · interaction · marketing · message · message concepts · message content · pilot test · plain language · process evaluation · social support · tailored intervention · tailoring

Four community health nursing students are assigned to an injury prevention project at a large supermarket. The Health and Safety Committee of the supermarket has requested the project because of figures indicating a high number of work-related back injuries. The store manager supported the request. The chair of the Committee, an Occupational Health Nurse, is the students' agency advisor.

The team has 12 weeks to complete the project. During the first two weeks, they meet with their faculty instructor and the agency advisor, and then the Health and Safety Committee. They are taken on a tour of the premises, spend time becoming familiar with the layout and functioning of the supermarket, and review the statistics on injuries and lost days of work provided by their advisor. They conduct a search of the research literature on preventing back injuries and find a few possible evidence-based interventions on reducing back injuries in the workplace using a workshop format.

The team determines that the "stockers," the employees who move the cases of food and stock shelves, have the highest number of lost days of work due to back pain. The stockers work the night shift and are from diverse backgrounds and cultures. The team uses progressive inquiry (see Chapter 4) with the stockers during one weekday and one weekend night shift to determine their thoughts about back injuries. They find out,

sometimes with the help of stockers who can interpret various languages, that most stockers are concerned about back injuries and like the idea that the store is planning education sessions for them.

In the third week, the team meets with the Committee to review preliminary ideas and put forward a proposal to develop and test a workshop on back health. The Committee accepts the proposal and surprises the team by suggesting that a committee member, Letecia, work with them and learn to conduct the workshop. With Letecia's involvement, they find that detailing the plan is much easier. For example, she advises them to meet with the managers early to gain their support and to determine where and when to conduct the workshops. They update their work plan as follows:

### Priority action statement

Stockers have the potential for improved back health related to their expressed interest in avoiding injury and to the commitment of the Health and Safety Committee to introduce effective measures to reduce back injuries. Evidence: (1) Injury statistics for previous three years show back pain is the most common cause for lost days of work, (2) stockers are the employees having the most lost days of work due to back pain, (3) there is no training to prevent back injury for staff, and (4) the Health and Safety Committees is interested in providing training and support to reduce back injuries.

## Take Action (Step 7)

The exciting part of community projects is working directly with community members, organizations, and service providers to implement an intervention to bring about change. Developing, testing, and using the intervention is the reward you receive from planning well. When you are taking action, you may find situations that you did not consider or encounter events beyond your control, all of which have to be accommodated. Taking action is the "acid test" for your plan.

Taking action involves adjusting, or tailoring, the plan to the community and time-lines and then carrying out planned activities. Taking action on a planned intervention is the seventh step in the application of the community health nursing process in a community project. Box 7.1 displays the step and substeps. Step 7 is where you actually work out the details of the plan and carry it out.

**Project goal**

Stockers have improved back health.

**Intervention strategy and related theory, models, and research**

Health education intervention involving an interactive workshop and materials on preventing back injury, and training Health and Safety Committee members to provide the workshop. Models: Generalized Model for health education program planning (McKenzie, Neiger, & Thackery, 2013) and Health Communication Program Cycle (National Cancer Institute, 2008). Expand Internet search on back injury prevention to Cochrane databases and best practice websites.

**Impact objectives**

(*Note*: Learning objectives—awareness, knowledge, and appreciation—are not included because stockers are already interested and motivated.)

**Ability objective**

By November 10, 60 percent of participants in back injury prevention workshops for stockers demonstrate safe lifting techniques.

**Accomplishment objective**

By November 17, 40 percent of trained stockers demonstrate safe lifting techniques at work.

**Environmental objective**

By November 14, 75 percent of Health and Safety Committee members are trained to provide back injury prevention workshops to all shifts on a regular basis.

**Process objectives**

The team drafts the process objectives to meet the goal and objectives in a Gantt chart. The September 30 version of the Gantt chart is provided in Appendix 7.1.

**Discussion Topics and Questions**

1. What assessment methods did the team use?
2. What aspects of the team's situation helped them to prepare a plan using a health education strategy in a relatively short period of time?

For suggested responses, please see the Answer Key at the back of the book.

Although the first three action steps are presented in a certain order, in reality they are done concurrently (as illustrated in the Gantt chart in Appendix 7.1) so that everything comes together when you implement the tailored intervention.

## Tailor the Intervention (Step 7a)

Once you have identified an appropriate evidence-based intervention, you must tailor the intervention to the community group and situation. **Tailoring** means adapting the content and delivery of an intervention to reach a specific group based on assessed needs and interests, taking into consideration the local culture. A **tailored intervention** is an intervention that has been tested and successfully adapted through feedback from the community group.

Three factors increase your understanding of the community as you prepare to tailor the intervention: culture, health literacy, and collaboration. The cultural makeup of the community group influences how receptive they might be to health information. Health literacy affects what they will be able to understand and use. Collaboration, now more than ever during the project, can greatly assist you in understanding and addressing issues related to culture, literacy, and the particular community situation.

## Culture

Culture is an important influence on society, a determinant of health, and, therefore, a necessary aspect to consider while tailoring the intervention. Entwined in the fabric of our lives, culture includes the values, norms, symbols, ways of living, traditions, history, and institutions shared by a group of people.

Culture has two important dimensions: (1) primary cultural factors, linked to race, ethnicity, language, nationality, and religion; and (2) secondary cultural factors, linked to age, gender, sexual orientation, educational level, occupation, income level, and acculturation to mainstream (Center for Substance Abuse Prevention, 1994). For example, teenagers are influenced by their individual family culture as well as the norms, values, and symbols that comprise teen culture in their locale. In relation to health care, culture is the attitudes and beliefs from a person's background (upbringing and environment) that become integrated into health behaviors and attitudes, and affect responses to health messages and materials (National Cancer Institute, 2008).

Orientation to the cultural makeup of your community begins with a review of the sociodemographic data and continues with observations of community life and interactions with community members. Learning how people act, respond, and engage in health and health care requires an understanding of the concept of cultural safety.

The concept of cultural safety in the delivery of health care arose from experiences of working with Maori in New Zealand (Papps & Ramsden, 1996). It refers to a proactive social justice approach to providing health care that does not compromise a person's real or perceived ability to receive effective care. **Cultural safety** exposes and manages unequal power relations (Aboriginal Nurses Association of Canada, 2009) and "enables safe service to be defined by those who receive the service" (Papps, 2005, p. 23).

According to the Aboriginal Nurses Association of Canada (2009), cultural safety goes beyond a mechanical acknowledgement and respect of differences, or practitioners having the skills, knowledge, and attitudes to apply concepts such as cultural awareness, cultural sensitivity, and cultural competence. Action-oriented cultural safety requires an appreciation of the complexity of "culture" and is in alignment with the advocacy role of nurses and the nursing profession (Aboriginal Nurses Association of Canada, 2009). This means that we must consider our own attitudes and beliefs, and policies and practices, to provide services that are truly accessible to people who differ from us either in primary or secondary cultural aspects. Cultural safety means developing respectful relationships and consistently checking with intended audiences to find out if the messages and services are relevant to them.

For example, think about the images portrayed in health messages: the symbols and metaphors; visual cues, including clothing, jewelry, hairstyles, and the actors; and language and music that convey culture (National Cancer Institute, 2008). A good approach is to

The main concern when preparing health information is that people value and be able to act on the information. As a rule, people who have been at school more than 12 years can read and use the information in a written text. They can fill out forms, use math, and problem solve. This ability goes down if they are worried or anxious about their health. Many people, however, have fewer years at school, are unable to see, hear, or speak well, or come from different cultures and perhaps do not speak English well. This means they are unable to read quickly and act on written text, especially if it includes filling in forms, math, or problem solving. When sick or worried, such tasks would be impossible. Yet, if a person wants to join a program to quit smoking, she or he would need to do these four tasks. The person would need to (1) read about options and programs to quit smoking, (2) use a map and fill out a form to apply to a program, (3) use figures to arrive at a cost for the program or for travel, and (4) problem solve in setting a goal for the program.

In the paragraph above, we purposely tried to use shorter sentences and words with less than three syllables. After rewriting and testing it many times on an online readability site (ReadabilityFormulas.com, 2013), we obtained the following result: "Readability Consensus Based on 8 readability formulas, we have scored your text: Grade Level: 5, Reading Level: easy to read. Reader's Age: 8–9 yrs. old (Fourth and Fifth graders)." Although that level of readability is good for the general public, it would still be too challenging for people with low literacy who are trying to make health decisions, especially when they are stressed.

consistently try out messages with people from the intended audience. Being respectful and open to the perspective and ideas of people from different cultures in your intended audience will help to make the health messages meaningful to them.

**Health Literacy**
Health literacy is closely related to culture and must also be included in tailoring the intervention. As discussed in Chapter 1, the values of equity and social justice underpin community health nursing. A major contributor to health inequity is that many people are unable to act on health information because they do not understand it. Therefore, when you prepare health messages, you must consider the health literacy of your intended audience.

People with low literacy suffer more from negative health outcomes, lower incomes, and less community engagement, all associated with poorer health and quality of life (Rootman & Gordon-El-Bihbety, 2008). In international studies of adult literacy and life skills (ALL), four aspects of literacy are used: (a) prose, (b) document, (c) numeracy, and (d) problem solving (OECD and Statistics Canada, 2011). Health literacy is more complex than general literacy because it requires mastering the four aspects, often simultaneously (Rootman & Gordon-El-Bihbety, 2008). Box 7.2 explains how literacy influences health action.

Health literacy is a fundamental issue of fairness and basic human rights, and a requirement for achieving of health. The *National Action Plan to Improve Health Literacy* (US Department of Health and Social Services, 2010) states that "Improving health literacy—that is, the degree to which individuals have the capacity to obtain, process, and understand basic health information and services needed to make appropriate health decisions—is critical to achieving the objectives set forth in Healthy People 2020 and, more broadly, key to the success of our national health agenda" (p. iii). In Canada, the discussion paper *Intersectoral Approach for Improving Health Literacy for Canadians* (Public Health Association of BC, 2012) states that health literacy is critical to the capacity of Canadians to manage their health and is recognized as a determinant of health—one that is closely related to other social determinants of health such as literacy, education, income, and culture. Health literacy requires the involvement of individuals as well as health-related systems and health care providers.

In both Canada and the US, the people most likely to have low literacy and low health literacy are those over 65, recent immigrants, minority groups, and people with low income (Canadian Council of Learning, 2008; National Network of Libraries of Medicine, 2014). First results from the survey of adult skills by the Organization for Economic Co-operation and Development (2013) rate countries on proficiency in three areas: literacy, numeracy, and problem solving in technology-rich environments. The scores from each country are rated "above average," "average," and "below average." The countries of Finland, the Netherlands, Norway, and Sweden rate above average on all three. Canada and the US are below average on numeracy. Canada is average on literacy, and above average on problem solving, while the US is below average on both (Organization for Economic Co-operation and Development, 2013).

People with low literacy and low health literacy are less likely to take preventive measures such as mammograms, Pap smears, and flu shots. Furthermore, when compared to those with adequate health literacy, studies show that patients with limited health literacy enter the health care system when they are sicker (National Network of Libraries of Medicine, 2014). Therefore, community health professionals must be prepared to make programs accessible to people in all sectors of the population. This includes taking responsibility for helping people to understand and use health information so they can choose a healthy lifestyle, know how to seek medical care, and take advantage of preventive measures (National Network of Libraries of Medicine, 2014).

When health materials and processes are written and explained in plain language, they provide health access to a greater number of people. Throughout the text, we have identified effective approaches to addressing low health literacy in preparing health information and provided examples. For example, Chapter 4 includes an example of an assessment questionnaire written in plain language for people with a low literacy level. Appendix 7.2 provides more information on, and approaches to, health literacy.

### Collaboration

At this time collaboration with the community group and organization becomes increasingly meaningful. Reaching out early to other people and organizations allows you to take advantage of different strengths and encourages their continued involvement.

Table 5.4 in Chapter 5 lays out the categories of people that community health nurses may encounter. In a project involving school children, for example, you would want the stakeholders, such as teachers and parents, to work with you and therefore become collaborators. If the project focused on bicycle safety, you might involve the police and businesses that sell bikes. If the project goal was to improve heart health, you could approach a public health nutritionist and the local chapter of the American Heart Association or the Heart and Stroke Association (Canada).

You can promote collaboration with community members and organizational staff by establishing a regular meeting time and place for the project, if you have not already done so. Depending on your setting, the place could be an empty office, classroom, boardroom, or a corner in the cafeteria, as long as it has chairs, a table, and some measure of privacy. You want to create a climate where people are comfortable sharing ideas. Regular meetings provide an opportunity to get input on your preliminary ideas, or drafts, before making any decisions about whether they are useful or not. While meeting, actively seek input and provide frequent opportunities for giving feedback. Ask "What worked well?" and "What did not?" Community workers and organizers are frequently able to draw on past experience in the community and give examples of key insights, such as how different approaches failed until they figured out how the group wanted to learn.

Although the project team should request advice and help from others, it is responsible for maintaining movement toward the project goal. This means treating community feedback as only one source of information among others. Consider feedback together with the information you gather from theory, research, and community nursing practice before deciding what action to take. Look for the trends, rather than trying to respond to every single comment. Be aware that if you make too many changes, you will be forever testing, rather than making the content more relevant. Usually, when team members are prepared to listen and work with the community, they will produce something that is beneficial. Although projects are time-limited, collaboration promotes long-term sustainability.

Sustainability is the degree to which a program (or project) instituting change is continued after the initial resources are expended (Oldenburg & Glanz, 2008). Sustainability involves both developing resources that are relevant to the community of interest and stakeholders, and recruiting people willing and able to continue using the resources. Usually continued use of project resources depends on the commitment of stakeholders associated with the organization supporting the project. You can prepare stakeholders to take over by drawing them into the team and team-building activities so that you learn the necessary knowledge and skills together.

## Tailoring a Health Education Intervention

The strategy of health education and the Health Communication Program Cycle (National Cancer Institute, 2008) will be used to illustrate the approach to tailoring an intervention. The Health Communication Program Cycle has appeared in texts and been used for over 25 years by many organizations to design successful health communication programs. The **Health Communication Program Cycle**, from the *Pink Book—Making Health Communication Programs Work*, has four stages that guide the development and delivery of relevant health messages to a heterogeneous audience (National Cancer Institute, 2008). The four stages are shown in Figure 7.1. The first two stages of the Program Cycle are concerned with planning and development; the last two stages are concerned with implementation and evaluation. As you probably realize, these stages are similar to the community health nursing process.

### Planning Health Education Communication
A useful starting point when planning to develop health education messages is to ask "Who is my intended audience? What health message do I want to convey?" and "What is the best means (or channel) of communicating with this audience?" You likely have a good sense of the answer from working with the community and can check out your ideas with community members and advisors. Keep in mind that collaboration, culture, and health literacy are key considerations when communicating health education messages.

**Figure 7.1: Health Communication Program Cycle**

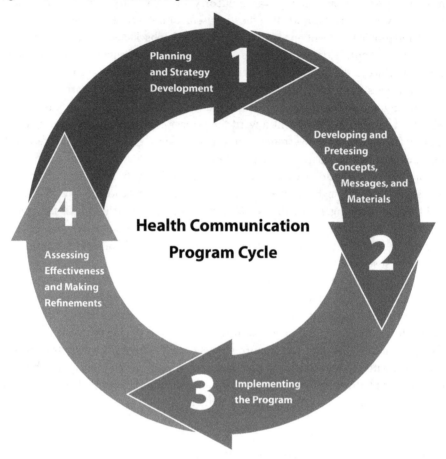

*Source*: Adapted from the National Cancer Institute. (2008). *Pink book—Making health communication programs work.* Retrieved from www.cancer.gov/cancertopics/cancerlibrary/pinkbook/page4

The channel of communication is an important concept used in the Health Communication Program Cycle. A **communication channel** is the way or ways that you convey information to your intended audience. Since every audience is different and each channel has pros and cons, you must consider both when selecting a channel. The basic channels of communication—nonverbal, oral, and written—can be augmented by technology: telephone, radio, TV, email, and Internet (Bowman, 2002). A channel permits different types of **interaction**: one-way communication (e.g., mass media), two-way communication, or both (National Cancer Institute, 2008). Two-way channels support discussion between individuals, groups, or larger audiences and are the most effective forms of communication.

Keep in mind that although a channel, such as a talk and slide presentation with handouts, combines the three principal channels of communication—oral, written, and nonverbal—and has the potential to be interactive, it is not interactive unless it provides an opportunity for back-and-forth discussion, for example, by including a question-and-answer session or group work.

The choice of channel will vary according to the information you want to convey. For example, if you want to tell someone about a meeting, you can talk in person, by phone, by email, or by posting a notice. If you want to counsel, convince, persuade, or

**Table 7.1: Ideas for Channels**

| Type of Channel (based on type of communication) | Examples and Considerations |
|---|---|
| Interactive (two-way) | Individual: A one-on-one discussion is the most effective way of providing health education tailored to the individual. This approach is also the most time-consuming and costly if it relies on delivery by a health professional. Some health messages can be passed on through friends, family members, hairdressers, counselors, clergy, or coaches. This can occur face-to-face, on the telephone, by email, or by interactive digital media such as Skype. |
| | Group: Brown bag lunches, classroom activities, Sunday school discussions, neighborhood gatherings, and club meetings provide opportunities for communication and interaction with groups. Digital media can also be used. Group discussions have the potential to bring out different opinions and perspectives and can be used to affirm health messages. |
| | Community or Organization: Meetings with larger bodies, face-to-face or by Internet, for example, town hall meetings or work events for all staff, are two-way when they provide the opportunity for discussion and clarification and can be used to enhance motivation and reinforce action. The involvement of community organizations can lend credibility. For example, not-for-profit organizations, such as those related to heart and stroke, diabetes, and cancer, have a strong advocacy role and can expand the reach of health messages. |
| Interactive digital media (one- and two-way) | Telephone, email, Internet websites, bulletin boards, newsgroups, chat rooms, CD-ROMs, and kiosks can be used to communicate one-on-one or with large numbers of people. Because these channels allow us to deliver highly tailored messages and receive feedback from the intended audience, they can be used for both interpersonal interaction and mass communication. Use of digital media can have cost and equipment implications, and requires careful consideration of potential ethical issues and security of information. If you choose to use interactive digital media to communicate health messages, you must ensure that your website is associated with a credible health care organization and has security features.<br><br>See the reference list on the National Cancer Institute website for a description of different types of Internet and digital media. |
| Mass media (one-way) | Print and digital media can be used to distribute health information to a large number of people through direct mail, billboards, newspapers and magazines, radio, and network and cable television. You can choose the medium most likely to reach an intended audience, but you cannot guarantee that the message will be received. Mass media, when used alone, is less likely than two-way channels to move people to action. |

Source: Adapted from the National Cancer Institute, 2008.

inform someone about eating a healthy diet, you will need more structure, such as a counseling session or a speech supported by a slideshow and demonstration, or through a booklet with "how-to" instructions. Table 7.1 provides ideas on the different channels that you could use.

On a final note, remember that you can combine different channels to reinforce what you want to say. For example, mass media can encourage people to seek or accept

**Developing Messages on Mammograms That Are Meaningful across Cultures and Ages**

The National Cancer Institute's (2008) Office of Communications conducted separate focus groups with women in different ethnic groups and older women to find messages about mammography that were appealing and important to them. The participants first indicated, individually, which of 10 motivational messages they found the most and least appealing. The moderator then led an in-depth discussion about the participants' knowledge, attitudes, and behaviors concerning breast cancer and mammography. Across focus groups, the following message elements were viewed most positively:

- Breast cancer can develop at any time.
- All women are at risk—even those age 65 and older, or those without a family history.

- Mammograms can detect breast cancer early.
- Early detection can save lives.

Messages indicating fear, older age, and sometimes gender were turnoffs—participants stated that cancer is a risk for all people; people of a certain age (e.g., 40 or 50) should not be singled out. The notion of a mammogram being able to "save lives" was persuasive not only because it was positive but also because it did not distinguish between age groups. In general, messages that seemed to tell women what to think were considered offensive, while messages that were phrased as an explanation or encouragement were deemed more effective.

personal health counseling. As well, information delivered by poster, website, or through lunchtime discussions, all possible in an organizational setting, can work in synergy, which means that the combined effort is more than the sum of each component.

### Developing and Pretesting Concepts, Messages, and Methods

The second stage of the Program Cycle (National Cancer Institute, 2008) guides the development and testing of communication messages and methods. The **message** in health communication is a concise statement that you want people to understand and remember. The process includes the following actions: reviewing existing materials, developing and testing message concepts, and developing and testing message content and delivery methods. Each element is addressed in detail below.

The review of existing materials involves seeking, through collaborators and the Internet, any possible content that you could use or adapt. Consider messages and approaches that best fit your purpose. For example, if you wanted to develop messages about increasing the number of people getting the flu shot, you might initially ask people about their experiences, search the Internet, and watch what is being said in newspapers, on the radio, on TV, or on social media. Potential resource material might be videos, fact sheets, pamphlets, computer programs, games, or electronic material. You need to review these "found" materials critically to determine if they meet your criteria and are appropriate for your situation. You will find a beginning list of credible websites for health information in "Website Resources" at the end of this chapter.

**Message concepts** are the different ways that information about an issue can be formulated (National Cancer Institute, 2008). To continue with the flu shot example, possible message concepts are: "The flu shot can improve your health," "The flu shot can protect you from getting sick," and "The flu shot can reduce the spread of the flu to others." Since some message concepts and the way they are expressed will be more relevant for some and less relevant for others, you need to write the different viewpoints in sentence or point form and try them out. One way to do this is to hold a focus group (see Chapter 4) with a community group to identify which statements are the most

After learning about the various channels, the team feels that they made the right decision to develop an interactive workshop to discuss back health safety with their multicultural participants. The workshop format also provides the opportunity to observe, discuss, and obtain feedback on the meaningfulness of the materials and approach for the participants, especially those with lower literacy skills.

A search of US government websites (www. thecommunityguide.org) for existing resources related to workplace health yielded a comprehensive resource on safety training for grocery store employees (Occupational Safety and Health Administration, 2004) that they passed on to the Committee. However, the prize find was a 2007 booklet entitled *Ergonomic Guidelines for Manual Material Handling*, published by the Research and Education Unit (Cal/ OSHA Consultation Service), Division of Occupational Safety and Health, California Department of Industrial Relations (2007). The booklet provided explanations and illustrations for all types of lifting situations and advice for changing the environment to improve safe lifting. The training section had the following introduction:

Training is most effective when it is interactive and fully involves workers. Below are some suggestions for training based on adult learning principles:

1. Provide hands-on practice when new tools, equipment, or procedures are introduced to the workforce.
2. Use several types of visual aids (e.g., pictures, charts, videos) of actual tasks in your workplace.
3. Hold small-group discussions and problem-solving sessions.
4. Give workers many opportunities for questions. (p. 10)

The team decides to include the four principles in the workshop and asks Letecia to review the material to help them consider how to make it accessible to people from a variety of cultures and with challenges in understanding English. The team has learned that Letecia started working at the grocery store when she first came to the US and could only speak a few words in English. After looking at the material, she says that what helped her most was a person who spoke fairly slowly and showed her what they wanted. Then she remembers that she did not ask questions because she was afraid of not knowing the right words. The team starts to think about how to use her information when planning the workshop.

Based on the Health Communication Program Cycle (National Cancer Institute, 2008) research, the team delegates two members to search for a video that demonstrates the safe lifting techniques included in the booklet. They find a 25-minute video with all the right elements and have sufficient funds in their budget to order a copy.

Team members brainstorm what message concepts they might convey about back safety at the workshop. They come up with three message concepts: "Safe lifting prevents back injuries," "Training to lift correctly means less sick time," and "Learning to lift safely makes you stronger at home and work." They feel that the stockers in the pilot tests might have better ideas.

**Discussion Topics and Questions**

3. Discuss how the team is using the Health Communication Program Cycle and the *Manual Material Handling* booklet to develop the intervention.
4. Based on the difficulties Letecia identified related to low literacy, what changes might the team consider for the workshop?

meaningful and which reflect the words of the participants. This testing will also help to determine if the messages are culturally appropriate and written in plain language. Box 7.3 describes an approach for developing appealing messages about mammograms.

### Developing and Testing Message Content and Delivery Methods

Once you have identified the most relevant message concept, the next step is to develop the content that will support the message. **Message content** is written material that provides positive and specific information about the message. For example, content about the flu shot could include statistics identifying the reduction in people getting the flu after a flu shot, testimonials from people who got the flu shot, and where and when to easily find a place to get a flu shot.

You then consider the best channel to deliver the message to your intended audience. For example, Mike Evans (2011), a physician working in preventive medicine, determined that the message "23 and 1/2 hours: What is the single best thing we can do for our health?" was effective. The catch phrase of "23 1/2 hours" and the presentation of evidence before he even mentions exercise help to capture people's interest, possibly because it makes them figure out that his message is "Spending half an hour a day being active is the single best thing we can do for our health." He also decided to produce a 9-minute video and post it on YouTube to get his message out to as many young adults as possible. The video shows a cartoonist's hand illustrating the author's verbal message, and the evidence to support it, on a white board. The message, delivery, and content are appropriate for quickly reaching a large number of young adults. The 2011 version has "gone viral."

You may be reluctant to start developing the materials because you have not done sufficient research to develop content or to test what you have. For some topics, such as smoking cessation, you could prepare for a year and never find all the information that could be relevant. The best approach is to start early with a few ideas and then expand and test until most agree with the message and direction.

When you are crafting your message and developing the content and delivery method, you need to test as you go to make sure the different elements are effective; that is, that they engage the intended audience. **Engaging people** involves interacting with them in a way that interests them and holds their attention. Engagement improves when messages are "sticky" or, in other words, when the message is important to them and they remember it.

Observing how participants respond, asking questions, and listening to feedback provides qualitative data that allows you to monitor engagement during the development and testing of intervention messages and methods. In Chapter 6 an example was introduced that dealt with seeking to increase home safety for toddlers by parents attending a well-child drop-in provided by a Parents' Resource Center. Using this example, you ask the parents to provide you with individual feedback on pictures depicting different home situations, and observe that the parents are reluctant to respond. Obviously responding individually is not working and when you ask what would work, they say they would like to talk it over with others. Since this seems reasonable and increases engagement, make the change. If, at the next testing session, you observe that the approach is working and members of the group are discussing their ideas with each other, you can then move forward.

Before completing your intervention, ensure that you try out, or pilot test, all or part of your content and methods with the intended audience. A **pilot test** is a structured testing method to provide feedback on draft content and methods including timing and audience reactions and suggestions. This rehearsal of sequenced content and delivery is more formal than the requests for feedback on specific content that you have been doing up to this point. The information you receive from the pilot test is invaluable in ensuring a successful intervention.

Based on experience, we recommend one or two pilot tests, especially when you have limited contact with your intended audience. In the early development of student projects, one team was developing public health resources for winter recreation safety. The team collected assessment data from grades 4 to 6 in four schools but had no access to

After Letecia informs the team that the manager is not likely to agree to more than an hour and a half for the workshop, the team starts figuring out how to fit everything into that time frame. They have to include a 25-minute video, a demonstration on lifting techniques, and a posttest. Based on theory, the booklet, and access for people with low literacy, they also need time for participants to share their experiences with back pain before the video and to give feedback during the workshop.

The two team members who observed lifting techniques on the job prepare and conduct the demonstration, and develop a checklist to monitor the return demonstration. Since the other two will lead the workshop, they develop the schedule and script. The following box provides their outline for the pilot with three half-hour blocks.

They plan a rehearsal and conduct two pilot workshops, each with at least four participants. At the rehearsal they present their parts following the outline and using a stopwatch. The demonstration takes 15 minutes rather than 10, so they reduce the number of techniques based on observations of what is most relevant to the stockers. Going into the first pilot workshop, everyone feels quite

confident about performing his or her part. Immediately after the pilot they debrief and share initial impressions. Overall, they feel satisfied but have some concerns. Each team member then reflects on his or her own performance—what went well and what they would like to improve next time. The leader says she learned that there was too much content on statistics; she will talk with Letecia about how to reduce it. She feels good about how the discussions went but notes that only two people did the talking, although others showed interest. Another member agrees to put together suggestions for changing the demonstrations because participants were reluctant to repeat the lifting techniques in front of everyone. At the end of the pilot, one stocker suggested the slogan "Watch my back!" and demonstrated what that meant. The rest seemed to agree, and the team decides to try out the slogan in the second pilot.

They make changes for the second pilot test: they replace the presentation on back injury statistics in the workplace with a short fact sheet using plain language, and have the participants identify correct and incorrect techniques modeled by the Safety Committee as a posttest rather than a return demonstration. They draft a new ability objective:

*Ability objective*

By November 10, 60 percent of participants in back injury prevention workshops for stockers will identify safe lifting techniques.

When they present the suggested changes to their instructor and the Health and Safety Committee, the changes are accepted. Everyone agrees that the team has made the changes based on good evidence without losing the essential elements of the workshop.

**Discussion Topics and Questions**
5. What were the benefits of holding a team rehearsal and the first pilot test?
6. What would make it easier or more difficult to speak up during the team debriefing session?

---

**Outline for Pilot Workshop for Back Injury with Timelines**

23:30–24:00
Introduction (5 minutes)
Introduction of participants (5 minutes)
Presentation on the effects and causes of back pain from work injury (10 minutes)
Discussion about personal experiences of back pain (10 minutes)
24:00–00:30
Show video on lifting techniques (25 minutes)
00:30–01:00
Demonstrate lifting techniques (10 minutes)
Volunteers perform techniques as posttest (10 minutes)
Feedback session (5 minutes)
Summary (5 minutes)

students while developing the intervention. They booked six "back-to-back" sessions to deliver a presentation on the safe use of sleds and toboggans at the end of project. At the first school, the team quickly realized that students were bored. They worked late that night to liven up their delivery and were able to rescue the remaining presentations, but they were stressed. The usual practice when repeating a presentation several times is to consider the first presentation, and possibly the second, as a pilot, and allow time to make some changes.

## Make Practical Arrangements for the Delivery of the Intervention (Step 7b)

In tandem with developing and testing a health intervention, it is essential to complete the practical arrangements for delivering the tailored intervention in a timely fashion. The arrangements include fixing the date, time, and location for planned activities; obtaining necessary supplies; and ensuring the participation of the intended audience. As well as securing the date and location for delivering the intervention, the immediate requirement is to organize what is needed to facilitate the initial part of the development of the intervention. Later on, the focus will change to organizing and obtaining resources for the testing and adaptation of the intervention.

Think about where, when, and with whom you will deliver your tailored intervention. Some factors might already be in place, but it is important to check that dates and the location fit your availability and the availability of your intended audience. For example, planning for a healthy eating workshop for older adults involves contacting the people working with the older adults to determine when the older adults could be available, and when and where you could meet with them. For planning purposes, include the arrangements in process objectives once they are confirmed. For example: "Deliver an interactive workshop on five fruits and vegetables a day to older adults at the Sunnyside Community Center on a Wednesday between Nov. 1 and Nov. 14."

Once you have a clear picture about what form your intervention will take (e.g., workshop, poster campaign, and so on), you will have an idea of what supplies and equipment you will need. You may need equipment to deliver a slide presentation, for example, or access to a computer, paper, and a printer to produce fact sheets, pamphlets, and displays. Determine potential sources and the availability of these items, and have them ready when needed. Another practical consideration is funding. The sponsoring agency might provide a budget for a community project, or you may need to request funding for resources or special services such as translation or equipment rental. If no funding is available, organizers will need to scale back the project.

It is never too early to think about how you will reach the intended audience of your intervention. For small community projects, this audience will likely be the community group with whom you are working. Nevertheless, you want to reach as many of the potential audience as possible.

Approaches used in the marketplace can assist in attracting participants to the planned activities. **Marketing** has four components: the product, or what is being offered (or, in other words, the message); the price or costs in terms of time or money; the place in terms of location and accessibility; and the promotion or communication strategy used to let people know about the product, how to get it, and the benefits they will receive

**Activities to Recruit People for the Action**

### Advertising

Advertising involves preparing and distributing a notice about the event or opportunity. Depending on what population group you want to reach, the distribution can involve the following: a newspaper, website, email, social media, poster, and handouts or pamphlets. Staff and key people can aid in the distribution of the notice.

### Social Opportunities

Social activities, gatherings, and social networks provide opportunity for people to interact with each other. They may include food, music, or other forms of entertainment. Some social activities, such as parties or sharing a meal, allow more freedom to interact and form friendships. Although social activities are a form of incentive, they are likely to attract different people than those wanting a prize.

Social activities offering support may encourage some to participate in a health intervention. **Social support** is the perception and actuality that one is cared for through one or more of the four types of supportive behaviors: emotional support, instrumental support, informational support, and appraisal support (Heaney

& Israel, 2008). As well, people can be drawn to an activity for mutual support, also called self-help or peer support, because they have a concern that they want to share and seek to learn from others who have the same concern.

### Incentives

People can be encouraged to participate in activities through financial or nonfinancial offers, such as the opportunity to receive a token gift or to win a donated door prize. To be effective, the incentive should be available to anyone who attends, be meaningful to the participants as determined during assessment, and should not conflict with health promotion goals (McKenzie et al., 2013).

### Competition

Some people are drawn to participate in an activity if it involves a contest between different groups. The rules for the contest and the prizes need to be clear and fair and appropriate for the age group of the intended audience.

---

(McKenzie et al., 2013). Marketing strategy, or the way of attracting people to participate, includes using social activities, advertising, incentives, and/or competition (McKenzie et al., 2013). These activities are described more fully in Box 7.4. The social dimension is particularly important; providing an opportunity to interact with others individually, in a group, or in a community setting is a key drawing feature. Knowledge of the community and discussions with collaborators will assist with the selection of appropriate marketing activities. Marketing strategies may also be useful when designing interventions for taking action, as described in Chapter 6.

As you move closer to delivering the tailored intervention, most of the practical arrangements should be in place, other than last-minute organizational details. Even so, it is necessary to monitor plans and be ready to respond to unexpected changes. For example, a school principal might ask you to expand a health fair to include additional classrooms.

By this time you will have some idea of the level of community interest in the planned activities but marketing will continue to be important to ensure participation. This is another opportunity to involve community members in spreading the word by invitation or word-of-mouth. Paying attention to the details may seem mundane but helps to ensure successful delivery of the intervention.

On a final note, in some projects, training others to carry out or continue a health education intervention is an important focus from the outset. The most practical approach

Based on the Gantt chart in their plan, two team members know they have to organize a location for the workshop with the store manager but find it difficult to arrange a meeting. Eventually, they meet and, with Letecia's help, negotiate the use of the staff room for the hour-and-a-half workshop, and receive permission for a Committee member to bring in a TV and video player. While thinking about how to market the workshop, the team decides to emphasize the opportunity to get information, learn with others, and provide mutual support to prevent back injuries. They feel that the prospect of mutual support will encourage the stockers to participate and keep using the safe lifting techniques after the workshop. They advertise these ideas in colorful one-page posters, which they post around the work and lunch areas. Members of the Health and Safety Committee add their voice by "talking up" the statistics and workshop with the stockers.

The team meets to scope out the details of the plan, including who will do what and when, and update the Gantt chart. Table 7.2 shows the details added under the item "Advertise workshop: Poster, staff announcements."

**Discussion Topics and Questions**

7. Discuss how the advertising and marketing of the workshops could influence the impact.

8. What methods would the team use to keep track of what each member was doing each day?

**Table 7.2: Expansion of One Item in Gantt Chart for Supermarket Back Health—Revised October 6, 2014**

| Process Objectives | Name | September 22 | 29 | October 6 | 13 | 20 | 27 | November 3 | 10 | 17 | 24 |
|---|---|---|---|---|---|---|---|---|---|---|---|
| **Advertise workshop: poster, staff announcements** | | | | | | | | | | | |
| Determine message for posters and announcements, number of posters needed | Denny & Marie | | | X | | | | | | | |
| Draft and test posters with others, pass on announcement message | Denny & Marie | | | X | X | | | | | | |
| Print and post posters | Denny | | | | | X | | | | | |
| Observe and ask about usefulness of posters | Denny & Marie | | | | | X | X | X | | | |

for a short-term project is to have the potential trainees work along with the team in the final stages of preparation. This allows the trainees time to document the process for their own purposes and ask questions when they do not understand. The delivery of the intervention, followed by a debriefing session, can be used as a rehearsal for the trainees.

## Develop Evaluation Measures (Step 7c)

Evaluation is a cornerstone of all nursing practice and is particularly important in the community where it can be challenging to follow a systematic evaluation process. The documentation of community health interventions contributes to the identification of promising practices (Association of Maternal Child Health Program, 2014), and the consistent use of evaluation in all aspects of community health nursing practice contributes to the continual improvement of professional practice.

The evaluation of short-term projects usually focuses on measuring the process and the impact of an intervention in relation to the project goal and objectives. **Process evaluation** involves monitoring and recording what happened and when during the implementation of the tailored intervention (McKenzie et al., 2013). Sometimes termed "formative evaluation," process evaluation, as described in Chapter 6, informs and guides the development and delivery of an implementation to make sure it is consistent with goals and objectives and community needs. This type of evaluation allows you to answer the question "Was the intervention carried out as planned?" Process evaluation is based on the premise that if you can demonstrate that you carried out an evidence-based intervention, adjusted for your situation, then you should achieve the predicted results.

The broad aim is to document exactly what intervention was delivered, when, and to whom. This means monitoring the intervention as it really happened as opposed to what you planned to do. Monitoring involves checking to see if the intervention was implemented as planned according to the Gantt chart or logic model by (a) recording the number of events, presentations, products, and so forth; (b) documenting that there was sufficient participation by an adequate number of participants from the community of interest; and (c) keeping track of external factors, such as competing events, weather, illness, and so on (McKenzie et al., 2013).

The required information can be gathered through observation, using simple counting measures and checklists; by asking questions (progressive inquiry); and by using simple questionnaires. Similar approaches and tools are used to complete an assessment (Chapter 4). It also means being alert to contextual factors that might influence an intervention—factors that might reduce or increase participation in one setting, or cause an unexpected change of plan. As an example, when you implement a tailored intervention, you may find that not as many people show up at one session as expected because of a competing event, or the DVD player does not function and your backup overheads stimulate less discussion than the video would have. Your process evaluation can later draw on the attendance data and be informed by a note of the external factor of the nonfunctioning DVD player. That data will contribute to the analysis of the results. The aim is to have a complete factual account of the delivery of the intervention, including a record of the collaboration with community partners and the development and maintenance of collaborative relationships.

Similarly, monitoring the collaboration with community members and stakeholders involves keeping track of the progress of relationships and identifying what strategies do or do not work. The usual approach in practice would be to track key aspects of the collaboration in field notes or a diary. As an example, you might document efforts to engage community members in the project, such as providing regular meeting opportunities to discuss involvement, and reflect on how well each one works. Another option is to document significant events such as a disagreement with a collaborator and its impact on the project. You may also choose to use such incidents as part of reflective practice using the tool in Appendix A.2.5.

**Impact evaluation** is a summative evaluation that measures changes in learning and behavior in the community of interest (McKenzie et al., 2013) after using a health education strategy and intervention. The focus is on relatively short-term outcomes in contrast to the longer-term impacts on health that may take several years to manifest. This requires gathering data before and after the intervention to measure what changes, if any, occur. Such data may be gathered by using pretest and posttest questionnaires to assess changes in knowledge or skill, or by gathering qualitative data through interviews and focused discussions.

Similar to the collection of assessment data, the collection of evaluation data requires that you have informed consent, which includes informing people about who you are, the project you are working on, how the data will be used, and the fact that they have a right not to contribute. For verbal evaluation methods, provide the explanation at the beginning of the session; for example: "We are going to ask you some questions about how you feel about the activities you have been doing. You can respond or not to the questions. We will use the responses to evaluate the activities." For a written evaluation, provide an information letter explaining who you are, who you are working with, why you are collecting the information, and how the information will be used in planning or evaluating this or future projects or programs. You need to assure people that their names or specific information about them will not be asked. This is part of ethical practice.

### Developing Evaluation Measures

The first step in evaluation began by writing process and impact objectives using the SMART criteria, as described in Chapter 6. As you recall, one requirement is that the objectives are measureable. The next step occurs during the action phase, when the requirements for data collection are considered. The **evaluation measures** specify the data required to determine whether or not a process or impact objective has been achieved and define how the data will be collected. Often this means choosing from a range of methods. The evaluators need to decide which method(s) is the most reliable and feasible based on timing, availability of resources, and acceptance by the community group.

To determine appropriate impact evaluation measures, ask the question "What evidence (data) will tell me that the objective has been met, and how will I collect this evidence?" When developing the measures, consider how easy it will be to collect the data. If it is not possible to gather the required evidence, the measures or objective will need to be changed. Try to keep the type of evidence you need as simple as possible to improve consistency and analysis. For example, it is simpler and likely more reliable to ask questions such as "Do you exercise at least three times a week?" requiring a simple "yes/no" answer, rather than asking "Do you exercise 30 minutes on most days?" or "Do you exercise consistently?" The last two questions require the respondent to make subjective judgments about "most days" and "consistently." Also, when considering measures, remember that people are usually more willing to respond verbally than to fill out a lengthy questionnaire, but they may not be as truthful as they would be if the evaluation were anonymous (e.g., written).

Table 7.3 provides possible measures to evaluate the impact of a health education intervention with parents of toddlers to improve home safety. The evaluation measures indicate what data to collect, how it should be collected, and how it should be recorded. The dates for each objective provide the deadline for completing the collection of evaluation data.

Developing process and impact measures often involves preparing forms to gather the specified data in a consistent fashion. Once the requirements are established, draft a form and then try it out (formative evaluation) with a few people. Since process evaluation deals with monitoring, typically the forms are used to document the number of participants, check off actions, or record comments.

With impact evaluation, the forms may be designed for completion by team members

**Table 7.3: Examples of Objectives and Evaluation Measures for Improving Home Safety for Parents of Toddlers**

| Impact Objectives | Possible Evaluation Measures |
|---|---|
| Learning: By Feb. 14, 40 percent of parents at Resource Center express interest by signing up for workshop on how to improve home safety for toddlers. | Count the number present and the number signing the workshop sheet. Document results. |
| Ability: By Feb. 28, 30 percent of mothers in workshop identify and correct at least 3 of 4 unsafe situations in a picture. | Provide each woman a picture that includes 4 unsafe situations. Ask each woman to circle and number the unsafe situations and write below the picture (or draw on the picture) how to correct each numbered situation. Collect the completed pictures and collate the results on a checklist. |
| Accomplishment: By March 14, 20 percent of mothers from workshop include one new safety measure into their daily routine. | After the workshop, contact the women to determine whether they are using a new safety measure at home. Document the number reached, the number not available, and the number using at least one measure at home. |
| Environmental: By Feb. 28, the Parents' Resource Center will provide bus passes for the safety workshop. | Document whether the bus passes were available, how easy it was for the women to get the bus passes, and how many women picked up the bus passes. |

**Table 7.4: Example Form to Tally Evaluation Data: Identification of Appropriate Safety Measures**

| Participant Number (do not use names) | Cover Electrical Outlets | Use Safety Gate on Stairs | Remove Figurines | Place Cleaning Materials out of Reach |
|---|---|---|---|---|
| 1 | Missed | Yes | Yes | Yes |
| 2 | Missed | Yes | Yes | Missed |
| 3 | Yes | Yes | Yes | Missed |
| 4 | | | | |

or by participants. For example, consider the ability objective in Table 7.3 above: "By Feb. 28, 30 percent of mothers in workshop identify and correct at least 3 of 4 unsafe situations in a picture." This evaluation measure suggests preparing a checklist of the four items. Table 7.4 shows how such a checklist might be completed. The evaluator could question participants about their responses to gain insight into participants' reasoning. This feedback could be used to evaluate the effectiveness of the health safety information and possibly provide insight into how to adjust content and/or the clarity of the unsafe situations.

## Implement the Tailored Intervention and Conduct Evaluation (Step 7d)

This step, that of implementing an intervention that has been carefully tailored to the community group and evaluating the results, is when all the theory, plans, and arrangements come together. Whether the health promotion intervention is a workshop on healthy eating or advocacy on the proper use of child car seats, this is the most intensive period of a community project. It is also the exciting part! You may be a bit nervous but at the same time feel prepared because you have followed a logical process, honed community health nursing practice skills, and learned to collaborate with advisors and the community as you went along.

The collection of data occurs at different times during or following the intervention. For example, when you deliver the intervention to the intended participants, you will collect process evaluation data on how many attended, the components of the intervention, and what unexpected events might have occurred. The collection of data to evaluate impact objectives occurs according to the time specified in the objective.

As you deliver the intervention and collect evaluation data, you will be getting some sense of the response of the community group. Things may go smoothly or not exactly as planned; there may be some rough parts. The response you receive from participants could be quite different from your expectations and not what you anticipated. Many factors can influence reactions, such as the weather, or an upsetting news item, or a room that is too cold or hot. Be realistic and try not to set your expectations too high.

You may believe that the information and skills provided to participants is easy to learn, but you have been working with this type of information for a few years. Many participants have not had that opportunity. Participants may need time to reflect and appreciate the value of what they have learned. Theory supports that idea. The Transtheoretical Stages of Change Model (Prochaska, Redding, & Evers, 2008) emphasizes that behavior change takes time. Results that indicate that participants liked the intervention and learned something worthwhile is sufficient for short-term projects. Pay attention to first impressions and immediate feedback but, most importantly, learn from evaluation, the focus of the next section.

## Teamwork during Action and Evaluation

Leadership, decision making, and documentation are ongoing concerns at this stage of the project. As well, the team may face two new challenges: maintaining morale and expanding the team membership.

### Leadership and Decision Making

At this stage of the community project, the plan has been translated into concrete steps and must be carried out in accordance with timelines. The leader has overall responsibility for overseeing the implementation, and it can be challenging to coordinate activities, delegate effectively, make quick decisions, and maintain a collaborative approach. Team members are also allocated tasks on which the project depends, such as developing a checklist or conducting an evaluation. If they are unable to complete the work as requested, they need to alert the team in a timely fashion so that plans can be adjusted. All team members have to contribute effectively to maximize the team effort for successful implementation.

When the team first thought about evaluating the workshop, they considered administering a questionnaire before and after the workshop to measure change. They had already observed the stockers at work, so they would base the test on the most common methods of lifting and carrying. After becoming aware of the limited English capabilities of the participants, however, they decide a written questionnaire is not appropriate. Some of the stockers would find it difficult to explain what they do in English but would be able to physically demonstrate their activities. Therefore, the team decides it would be more appropriate to demonstrate safe lifting and carrying, and then observe and record practices while the stockers are working. The team reasons that by using the initial observations and then again observing after the workshop, they will have pre- and post-workshop performance measures. Letecia agrees with their plan and encourages them to observe in different areas of the store.

Team members construct a draft form to evaluate the lifting and carrying practices of the stockers based on their initial observations and the criteria given in their reference booklet. Three team members, working independently, use the form to document their observations at different periods and locations during the night shift. Staff is told to expect this. One person asks not to be observed, and they respect this request; the others are a little self-conscious initially but soon settle back to their usual practice.

After reviewing the results with the stockers, the observers change the form to include documentation of where incorrect lifts occur. They then repeat the observations. They feel satisfied that the form is easy to use and captures the essential features of proper lifting and carrying.

Before the second pilot test of the workshop, the team reviews the Health Communication Program Cycle (National Cancer Institute, 2008) and the results from the field notes on the first pilot test. They realize that identifying the number asking questions did not accurately capture the interest of participants who had limited language skills. Two team members had noted that all participants were listening and nodding most of the time, even if they didn't ask questions.

For the second pilot test, the team decides to evaluate the following aspects: (1) timing, (2) interest shown by participants, and (3) the rating of correct and incorrect lifting by Committee members, using thumbs-up for correct and thumbs-down for incorrect.

During the second pilot, the results are the same. Only half ask questions, and all show interest in what is being said and demonstrated. When the team discusses the observations with Letecia and the Committee, the Committee members explain that newer employees, especially those with limited English, tend to learn over time on the job. They emphasize the importance of the workshops in preparing the more experienced stockers who, in turn, will assist others with the new techniques.

Originally, the team planned to train three members of the Health and Safety Committee after the second pilot workshop. Now, they feel they might combine this training with the workshops to make the best use of time. The trainees agree; they will attend the first workshop as participants, attend the debriefing, and take on leadership roles in the second one.

The team is well prepared for the first official workshop; all know their parts and the evaluation measures are in place. After the workshop, they have evaluation data from the Committee member demonstrations and ratings from the follow-up evaluations, together with field notes from team members. They follow the same procedures for the second workshop except that Committee members take part in the delivery and evaluation along with team members.

Because the Health and Safety Committee is pleased with the work of the team, the team fills in the following statement in the results column in the work plan: "All members of the Health and Safety Committee have indicated, individually and collectively, that the workshops are working well." Appendix 7.1 provides the team's work plan completed up to November 3. After November 3, the team recorded the results directly in the project report.

Note: This scenario continues in Chapter 8.

### Discussion Topics and Questions

9.  What is the benefit of making observations of the lifting techniques before the workshops?
10. How reliable are the workshop numbers collected on the correct and incorrect demonstrations during the workshop?

## Documentation

As the project moves from planning to implementation, team members may find they are dealing with many forms of documentation. In addition to the ongoing weekly report, the planning tools—work plan and/or timeline/Gantt chart—become more detailed and have to be kept up to date. The team and instructor need to work out what combination of forms will best meet their respective needs. Some teams shorten the weekly report and communicate using the Gantt chart and work plan. Another option is to complete sections of the project report form as the work is completed (discussed in Chapter 8) and attach it to the weekly report beginning about halfway through the project. This early action will save the team some scrambling at the end.

## Collaboration

Up to this point, community members and stakeholders may have had limited involvement in making decisions. Although some may be quite comfortable with the formal planning approaches required in community health nursing practice, others may not. As an example, I was part of a team working with a group of women in a small town to put on a healthy living festival at their community center. Very few came to the team meetings, but the ones who came enjoyed planning with us. When we asked why so few attended, they said that some women preferred to get the information at the food store checkout or the post office as they went about their daily activity. They explained that these women did not have the patience for meetings but were more than willing to pitch in when given a task. Their communication system worked well, and the festival was a great success.

Most community members are likely to enjoy taking action. Ideally, this stage of the community project is the time to include community members more fully in what you are doing. Just as team members in the initial stage of development need a defined task to feel comfortable, the same is also true of community members who show an interest in joining the team. One approach is to give information on all available tasks and ask people to choose what they would like to work on. If a new member is taking on a complicated task, a team member can volunteer to work with them. Similarly, if new members are hesitant to take on a task, a team member can invite them to partner on a task. Everyone should have something to do. Community members bring expertise from living in the community and many other resources that you may not know about. By enlisting them in your action, your team will gain access to a greater wealth of resources and a much better chance for success.

## Maintaining Morale

Although the community project has taken shape and results are beginning to appear, there are still uncertainties to contend with. The pressure of developing resource materials can create shared anxiety: the workload is growing, time is limited, and things do not always run smoothly. When the response from the community is not very positive, or plans need adjusting, team members may feel demoralized and concerned about how the group is performing. Recognize this as a normal reaction, and encourage team members to take time to express their feelings.

People can feel anxious or worried for many reasons: one person may feel they are not performing as well as expected or fear they may have led the team astray; another may feel frustrated when participants do not seem to appreciate all the time and effort the team has put into the project. Such thoughts are not unlike those you might experience when you receive a low grade on a paper or exam. The difference here is that this situation is more public and there is shared responsibility. Sometimes people are unable to accept a poor result and start blaming others. When these thoughts are expressed, the team needs to acknowledge them in order to move on. If this does not work, the leader might suggest using conflict resolution or critical reflection (see Appendix A.2.5).

Another strategy would be for the team to focus on the lessons they have learned from, for example, trying to complete the project without community input. After recognizing that they are on the wrong track, team members can gain satisfaction from the knowledge that they have faced facts and taken action to save themselves from a continuing disaster. One necessary action that you must take when the evidence is mounting that the project is not going well is to seek assistance from your supervisor/instructor and from stakeholders and community members. No matter the reason, it is best to acknowledge the problem, explain the situation, and ask for assistance in working out a feasible solution. Being truthful about a problem and working with the community to resolve it is far more worthwhile in learning about community health nursing practice than producing a package of educational materials that might or might not be useful.


## Summary

Taking action builds on the plans made in Chapter 6 to prepare students and new practitioners to implement and evaluate a tailored intervention. Tailoring the intervention, developing evaluation measures, and making arrangements occur at the same time. During the development, teams learn to consider culture and literacy level, and use marketing strategies to recruit participants. The result of the action is an evidence-based intervention that is relevant to the community group.

Teamwork during action is particularly challenging, because team members are often working on different aspects of the intervention and have difficulty coming together to make decisions. However, collaborative decision making, coordination, and documentation of activities are particularly important to ensure that the intervention is completed and collaborators are involved. Morale may also be an issue at this busy time as team members may feel that they have not been able to overcome a change in circumstance to accomplish what they had planned. A focus on what has been accomplished and what is feasible in the remaining time can give a boost to their spirits.

## Classroom and Seminar Exercises

1. Document possible action and results in the taking action section of the collaborative work plan (see Appendix 7.1) for the Supermarket Back Health scenario.
2. Discuss the value of having an environmental objective in the Back Health scenario and in your clinical experiences.
3. Using an issue such as weight reduction, increasing exercise, or safe sexual practices, complete the following exercises:
   a. Define and use a relevant theory to guide a community project with high school students in a situation you specify.
   b. Locate databases or websites with systematic reviews of relevant research on your chosen topic.
   c. Suggest community groups or organizations that might have an interest in the issue.
   d. Explain how you would involve community members in addressing the issue.
4. Based on the findings on mammogram messages in Box 7.3, what might be an appealing message for increasing the number of women who get a mammogram?

## References

Aboriginal Nurses Association of Canada. (2009). *Cultural competence and cultural safety in nursing education: A framework for First Nations, Inuit and Métis nursing.* Retrieved from www.anac.on.ca/Documents/Making%20It%20Happen%20Curriculum%20Project/FINALFRAMEWORK.pdf

Association of Maternal Child Health Program. (2014). *Best practices program.* Retrieved from www.amchp.org/programsandtopics/BestPractices/Pages/BestPracticeTerms.aspx

Bowman, J. (2002). *Business communication: Managing information and relationships.* Retrieved from http://homepages.wmich.edu/~bowman/channels.html

Canadian Council of Learning. (2008). Healthy Literacy in Canada: A Healthy Understanding. Retrieved from http://www.ccl-cca.ca/CCL/Reports/HealthLiteracy/

Center for Substance Abuse Prevention. (1994). *Following specific guidelines will help you assess cultural competence in program design, application, and management* [Technical Assistance Bulletin].Washington, DC: US Government Printing Office.

Evans, M. (2011). *23 and 1/2 hours: What is the single best thing we can do for our health?* Available from www.youtube.com/watch?v=aUaInS6HIGo

Heaney, C., & Israel, B. (2008). Social networks and social support. In K. Glanz, B. Rimer, & K. Viswanath (Eds.), *Health behavior and health education: Theory, research, and practice* (4th ed., pp. 189–210). San Francisco, CA: Jossey-Bass.

McKenzie, J., Neiger, B., & Thackeray, R. (2013). *Planning, implementing and evaluating health promotion programs: A primer* (6th ed.). Needham Heights, MA: Allyn and Bacon.

National Cancer Institute. (2008). *Pink book—Making health communication programs work.* Retrieved from www.cancer.gov/cancertopics/cancerlibrary/pinkbook/page4

National Network of Libraries of Medicine. (2014). *Health literacy.* Retrieved from http://nnlm.gov/outreach/consumer/hlthlit.html

Occupational Safety and Health Administration. (2004). *Guidelines for retail grocery stores.*
Retrieved from www.osha.gov/ergonomics/guidelines/retailgrocery/retailgrocery.html

OECD (Organisation for Economic Co-operation and Development). (2013). *OECD Skills Outlook 2013: First Results from the Survey of Adult Skills.* Retrieved from www.oecd.org/site/piaac/Skills%20volume%201%20%28eng%29--full%20v12--eBook%20%2804%2011%202013%29.pdf

OECD (Organisation for Economic Co-operation and Development) and Statistics Canada. (2011). *Literacy for life: Further results from the Adult Literacy and Life Skills Survey.* Retrieved from www.statcan.gc.ca/pub/89-604-x/89-604-x2011001-eng.pdf

Oldenburg, B., & Glanz, K. (2008). Diffusion of innovations. In K. Glanz, B. Rimer, & K. Viswanath (Eds.), *Health behavior and health education: Theory, research, and practice* (4th ed., pp. 303–333). San Francisco, CA: Jossey-Bass.

Papps, E. (2005). Cultural safety: Daring to be different. In D. Wepa (Ed.), *Cultural safety in Aotearoa New Zealand* (Chapter 2). Auckland: Pearson Education New Zealand.

Papps, E., & Ramsden, I. (1996). Cultural safety in nursing: The New Zealand experience. *International Journal for Quality in Health Care, 8,* 491–496. Retrieved from http://intqhc.oxfordjournals.org/content/8/5/491.full.pdf

Prochaska, J., Redding, C., & Evers, K. (2008). The transtheoretical model and stages of change. In K. Glanz, B. Rimer, & K. Viswanath (Eds.), *Health behavior and health education: Theory, research, and practice* (4th ed., pp. 97–165). San Francisco, CA: Jossey-Bass.

ReadabilityFormulas.com. (2013). *Free text readability consensus calculator.* Retrieved from www.readabilityformulas.com/free-readability-formula-tests.php

Research and Education Unit (Cal/OSHA Consultation Service), Division of Occupational Safety and Health, California Department of Industrial Relations. (2007). *Ergonomic guidelines for manual material handling.* Retrieved from www.cdc.gov/niosh/docs/2007-131/pdfs/2007-131.pdf

Rootman, I., & Gordon-El-Bihbety, D. (2008). *A Vision for a Health Literate Canada. Report of the Expert Panel on Health Literacy.* Retrieved from http://www.cpha.ca/uploads/portals/h-l/report_e.pdf

US Department of Health and Human Services, Office of Disease Prevention and Health Promotion. (2010). *National Action Plan to Improve Health Literacy.* Washington, DC: Author.

## Website Resources

Agency for Healthcare Research and Quality (AHRQ): www.ahrq.gov
AHRQ's extensive website has health care information on priority populations and searchable health topics. Research tools and data include "State Snapshots," which compare a selected state to all others on a range of indicators.

American Cancer Society (ACS): www.cancer.org
The ACS web page tab "Stay Healthy" includes topics on how to stay healthy, tools and calculators, cancer screening, and cancer prevention news.

Centers for Disease Control and Prevention (CDC): www.cdc.gov
The CDC website has extensive lists of information on topics such as adolescent and school health, food safety, and healthy weights. The Healthy Communities Program includes a web page with links to the National Networks for Community Change.

Public Health Agency of Canada, *Health Promotion*: www.phac-aspc.gc.ca/hp-ps/index-eng.php

An extensive searchable website that includes such topics as seniors, pregnancy, mental health, and healthy living.

Office of Disease Prevention and Health Promotion, *healthfinder.gov*: www.healthfinder.gov

This website is very useful both as a resource for individuals and to prepare health education materials.

National Institutes of Health, *Health Information*: http://health.nih.gov/

This web page on health information provides access to an extensive database.

US Department of Health and Human Services: www.hhs.gov/

This site is a hub for government health information, including links to specific websites such as "stop bullying.gov," "Be Tobacco Free.gov," and "Let's Move!"

**Gantt Chart for Supermarket Back Health**

**Gantt Chart for Supermarket Back Health—Revised September 30, 2014**

| Process Objectives | Name | September | | October | | | | November | | | |
|---|---|---|---|---|---|---|---|---|---|---|---|
| | | 22 | 29 | 6 | 13 | 20 | 27 | 3 | 10 | 17 | 24 |
| **Develop workshop on back health.** | | | | | | | | | | | |
| Draft workshop agenda and presentation. | Denny & Marie | X | X | X | X | X | | | | | |
| Search for resources online with advisors, and locally. | Denny & Marie | X | X | X | | | | | | | |
| Test and revise pilot workshop (two groups of 4 to 5 stockers). | | | | | | X | X | | | | |
| Train employees to give workshop (3). | | | | | | X | X | | | | |
| Conduct two workshops (7 to 12 stockers each). | | | | | | | | X | X | | |
| Organize workshop. | | | | | | | | | | | |
| Meet with store manager to agree on workshop timing and attendance. | | | X | X | | | | | | | |
| Locate and book space for workshops and final presentation to Committee. | | | | X | | | | | | | |
| Advertise workshop: Poster, staff announcements. | | | | | | X | X | X | X | | |
| Prepare and clean up room for pilots and workshops. | | | | | | X | X | X | X | | |
| Evaluate change in lifting techniques. | | | | | | | | | | | |
| Develop pre- and post-evaluation measures. | Stephanie, Jose, & Letecia | | X | X | | | | | | | |
| Observe and document lifting behaviors. | Stephanie, Jose, & Letecia | X | X | X | | | | | | | |
| Conduct process (formative) evaluation. | All | X | X | X | X | X | | | | | |
| Evaluate workshops. | | | | | | | | X | X | | |
| Evaluate on-site lifting. | | | | | | | | | | X | X |

# Work Plan for Supermarket Back Health

**Plan, Action, and Evaluation Work Plan for Supermarket Back Health—Revised November 3, 2014**

| Steps & Activities[1] (number and time period) | Results Summary, with Completion Date |
|---|---|
| **PLAN** | |
| 6. Plan action (Sept. 8–29) | |
| a. Select priority | Stockers have the potential for improved back health related to their expressed interest in avoiding injury and to the commitment of the Health and Safety Committee to introduce effective measures to reduce back injuries. Evidence: (1) injury statistics for previous three years show back pain is the most common cause for lost days of work, (2) stockers are the employees having the most lost days of work due to back pain, (3) there is no training to prevent back injury for staff working nights, and (4) the Health and Safety Committee's interest in providing training and support to reduce back injuries. (Sept. 22) |
| b. Identify goal | Stockers have improved back health. (Sept. 22) |
| c. Identify strategy and evidence-based intervention | Provide health education workshop on back injury, train Health and Safety Committee members to provide workshop. Theory: Health Communication Program Cycle (National Cancer Institute, 2008). Identified 2007 booklet entitled *Ergonomic Guidelines for Manual Material Handling* from a reputable government source to guide intervention. (Sept. 29) |
| d. Develop impact and process objectives | Ability: By Nov. 2, 50 percent of participants in back injury prevention workshops for stockers demonstrate safe lifting techniques.<br><br>Accomplishment: By Nov. 17, 40 percent of stockers who attended workshop demonstrate safe lifting techniques during work. Environmental: By Nov. 2, 75 percent of Health and Safety Committee members are trained to instruct in back injury prevention. (Sept. 29)<br><br>Process objectives: See Gantt chart. (Sept. 30) |

| Steps & Activities[1] (number and time period) | Results Summary, with Completion Date |
|---|---|
| **ACT** | |
| 7. Take action (Sept. 29–) | |
| a. Tailor the intervention | Video meeting safe lifting criteria identified Oct. 6. Workshop agenda and presentation prepared and approved Oct. 20. First pilot with 6 stockers Oct. 13. Statistics too long and boring. Follow-up demonstrations were awkward and lengthy. Replaced presentation on statistics with handout and demonstration by participants with demonstration by Committee members for second pilot. Second pilot with 3 stockers Oct. 20. Most could pick out safe and unsafe but seemed to follow each other. |
| b. Make practical arrangements for the delivery of the intervention | Arrangements for location of workshop and showing video confirmed Oct. 6 (facilitated by Letecia). Posters on workshops in place on Oct. 13. Team members and Committee talk about workshops at lunch and breaks. Preparation and cleanup of workshop room shared by team and participants. |
| c. Develop evaluation measures | Sept. 29: Draft and test form to evaluate on-site lifting and carrying. Oct. 6: Revise form to include location; form found easy to use by 3 people. Oct. 13: Developed forms to record (a) timing, (b) interest (verbal and nonverbal) during pilot and interventions, and (c) ratings by participants of safe (thumbs-up)/ unsafe (thumbs-down) demonstrations. |
| d. Implement the tailored intervention and conduct evaluation | First workshop with 8 participants on Oct. 27 included Committee members as participants. Met timing; limited discussion. Second workshop with 10 participants Nov. 3 with Committee members leading discussions. Took 15 minutes longer; livelier discussion. Identification of demonstrated safe and unsafe lifting at end of workshop remained high. Workshop 1—7/7 correct; Workshop 2—8/10 correct. Observation, developing, and documenting lifting behaviors began Sept. 22. Posttest completed in week following each workshop. Committee members encouraged lively discussion and correctly demonstrated safe lifting to stockers. Two Committee members stated that they were ready to lead more workshops and others were willing to help them. All members of the Health and Safety Committee have indicated, individually and collectively, that the workshops are working well. |
| **EVALUATE** | Switched to project report. |

*Note*: 1. Steps 1–5 (Sept. 7–21) are not included; at evaluation, the team switched their documentation to the project report.

## Appendix 7.2:
## Approaches to Address Low Health Literacy

The basic measures health professionals can take to improve health literacy in their practice include identifying and supporting people with low literacy, and preparing and using materials written in a way that most people can understand. They also need to consider advocating for changes to improve health literacy in the health and education systems.

When working with groups that include older adults, immigrants, and the unemployed, the safest approach is to assume some will have low literacy and aim to provide information in **plain language**, language that they will understand the first time they read or hear it. When working with individuals, one simple question could identify those with low health literacy. Ongoing research studies and reviews with a variety of people with low literacy indicate that one question chosen from "use of a surrogate reader," "confidence with medical forms," or "difficulties understanding written information" were moderately effective for quickly identifying patients with limited literacy (Al Sayah, Majumdar, Egede, & Johnson, 2014; Powers, Trinh, & Bosworth, 2010; Sarkar, Schillinger, López & Sudore, 2011). The Agency for Healthcare Research and Quality (2014) provides four tested tools to measure an aspect of health literacy—individuals' reading comprehension in a medical context for English and Spanish speakers—for use in research, training, clinical, and program planning.

Supporting people generally and especially those with low literacy involves frequently asking them to tell you what they have learned from what you have said. This "teach-back" or "closing the loop" is a way to find out if you have provided the information in a way that is appropriate for them.

Working with people who have low literacy and low health literacy is a particularly valuable contribution that can be made by community health nurses and students working on a community nursing project. The online resource *Examples of Health Literacy in Practice* (Canadian Public Health Association, 2014) provides a range of examples from all areas of the country, and includes people of different ages and levels of health. The examples provide a guide for others to reduce the barriers to health by directly addressing low health literacy.

Plain language is especially important when preparing written content for people with low literacy. **Plain language** is communication your audience can understand and use the first time they read or hear it (Plain Language Action and Information Network, n.d.). The most common methods to achieve plain language are to use

- logical organization with the reader in mind
- "you" and other pronouns
- active voice
- short sentences
- common, everyday words
- easy-to-read design features

Even following these plain language methods will not work all the time. The approach that is likely to be the most successful would involve following the methods and consistently testing the content with your intended audience.

## References

Al Sayah, F., Majumdar, S., Egede, L. & Johnson, J. (2014). Measurement properties and comparative performance of health literacy screening questions in a predominantly low income African American population with diabetes. Retrieved from www.ncbi.nlm.nih.gov/pubmed/25082723

Agency for Healthcare Research and Quality. (2014). *Health Literacy Measurement Tools* (Revised). Retrieved from www.ahrq.gov/professionals/quality-patient-safety/quality-resources/tools/literacy/index.html

Canadian Public Health Association. (2014). *Examples of Health Literacy in Practice*. Retrieved from www.cpha.ca/uploads/progs/literacy/examples_e.pdf

Plain Language Action and Information Network. (n.d.). The Plain Language Action and Information Network (PLAIN). Retrieved from www.plainlanguage.gov/index.cfm

Powers, B., Trinh, J., & Bosworth, H. (2010). Can this patient read and understand written health information? Retrieved from www.ncbi.nlm.nih.gov/pubmed/20606152

Sarkar, U., Schillinger, D., López, A., & Sudore, R. (2011). Validation of self-reported health literacy questions among diverse English and Spanish-speaking populations. Retrieved from www.ncbi.nlm.nih.gov/pubmed/21057882

## Website Resources for Health Literacy and Developing Easy-to-Understand Health Materials

Agency for Healthcare Research and Quality, *Questions to Ask Your Doctor*: www.ahrq.gov/patients-consumers/patient-involvement/ask-your-doctor/index.html
This site encourages patients to ask questions at health visits because health depends on good communication. The site includes a Question Builder and short videos of patients and providers speaking about the importance of asking questions.

American Medical Association, *Health Literacy Video*: www.ama-assn.org/ama/pub/about-ama/ama-foundation/our-programs/public-health/health-literacy-program/health-literacy-video.page
This site provides informative and instructional videos related to health literacy.

BC Children's Hospital, *Health Topics*: www.bcchildrens.ca/KidsTeensFam/default.htm
This site provides links to family resources in various languages.

Best Start: www.beststart.org/resources/other_languages/index.html
This site provides support to service providers who implement health promotion programs for maternal, newborn, and early child development. Many resource pamphlets and posters have been translated into several languages, including Arabic, Chinese, Hindi, and Cree. *Note*: A fee is charged to order resources.

Canadian Public Health Association, *Health Literacy Portal*: www.cpha.ca/en/programs/portals/h-l.aspx

This website provides easy access to key information about health literacy in Canada for health professionals, researchers, and interested individuals. It features the Expert Panel on Health Literacy's final report as well as links to other key Canadian and international health literacy resources.

Centers for Disease Control and Prevention, *Health Literacy*: www.cdc.gov/healthliteracy

This CDC website provides information and tools to improve health literacy and public health. These resources are for all organizations that interact and communicate with people about health, including public health departments, health care providers and facilities, health plans, government agencies, nonprofit/community and advocacy organizations, child care and schools, the media, and health-related industries.

Harvard School of Public Health, *Health Literacy Studies*: www.hsph.harvard.edu/healthliteracy/

The Health Literacy Studies group provides links to an overview of health literacy with videos and presentations, research, policy reports, and detailed information and examples of preparing written material so it can be understood.

Institute of Medicine, *Health Literacy: A Prescription to End Confusion*: www.iom.edu/Reports/2004/Health-Literacy-A-Prescription-to-End-Confusion.aspx

This important document details the effects of limited health literacy and includes recommendations to reduce these effects.

MedlinePlus, *How to Write Easy-to-Read Health Materials*: www.nlm.nih.gov/medlineplus/etr.html

MedlinePlus, the National Library of Medicine's website for patients and their families and friends, includes easy-to-read health information and a resource page with tips on how to write easy-to-read materials.

Office of Disease Prevention and Health Promotion, *Health Literacy*: http://health.gov/communication/literacy/

This site provides an overview of health literacy, tools, reports/research, and related resources.

PlainLanguage.gov: Improving Communication from the Federal Government to the Public: www.plainlanguage.gov/

This website provides tips and tools to start and plan a plain language program. The site includes the Federal Plain Language Guidelines.

US Department of Health and Human Services, Centers for Disease Control and Prevention, *Simply Put*: www.cdc.gov/healthliteracy/pdf/Simply_Put.pdf

The Simply Put guide helps you to create easy-to-read materials using effective communication and design.

US Department of Health and Human Services, Office of Disease Prevention and Health Promotion, *Health Literacy Online*: http://health.gov/healthliteracyonline

This website provides a guide to writing and designing easy-to-use health websites.

# Chapter 8

# Ending Well—Step 8

N ow that the tailored intervention has been delivered, this chapter completes the project by analyzing the data, discussing the findings with the community group, and ending the project well. Analysis follows earlier phases that begin with gathering and summarizing the data, then making comparisons to other sources. These preliminary phases initiate a broader view of the data and encourage discussion of different interpretations with advisors and collaborators. The discussions within the team and with collaborators lead to the development of draft recommendations.

A highlight of the project is presenting and discussing the draft recommendations with advisors and the community group. The presentation demonstrates not only what was done and what was found, but also how the community was involved to identify issues and interventions that are relevant to them. The results of the discussions during and following the presentation are the basis for the recommendations included in the final project report.

To end well, consider what actions would help sustain the project. This includes providing the organization and community with a report and resources from your project work, and recognizing and thanking people for their support. The Supermarket Back Health scenario, continued from the previous chapter, illustrates how the team keeps organized as they work to bring their project to a good ending.

Another aspect to ending well is reflecting with the team on the lessons you have learned. This reflection assists each team member individually as well as helping everyone to feel positive about future teamwork.

## Learning Objectives

**Key Terms and Concepts**

analysis of evaluation data • ending well • limitations • presentation • recommendations • showing appreciation

After reading this chapter and answering the questions throughout the chapter, you should be able to:

1. Analyze the process and impact evaluation data.
2. Prepare and deliver a professional presentation on the project and findings to a group by following guidelines.
3. Draft and complete a project report that provides the process and resources for others to continue the project.
4. Promote sustainability by involving collaborators in the presentation and final plans.

5. Show appropriate appreciation for people who supported the project.
6. Reflect as a team and individually on what was learned about teamwork and working collaboratively with a community group.

## Ending Well

The final weeks of a project can feel hectic as team members focus on finishing their assigned tasks. Although completing tasks is important, an equally important part is taking care of relationships. Balancing tasks and relationships is the challenge in ending the project well. **Ending well** involves completing the project requirements and concluding relationships with community members, stakeholders, and team members in a professional and a meaningful manner. Ending well should leave the participants on the team and the collaborators from the community feeling that they did the best possible job, given the allotted time and available resources. For community health nurses, completing project requirements, including analyzing the data, drafting recommendations, presenting the results, and completing a project report, is all part of professional nursing practice.

## Evaluate Results and Complete Project (Step 8)

Step 8 is the final step in the project. The ongoing evaluation of teamwork (Step 9), described in Chapter 2, is brought to a conclusion in this chapter. Box 8.1 features Step 8 within the community project.

To complete the project on time, the team needs to complete the first three steps concurrently. When those three are complete, team members can conclude the relationship with the collaborators and, finally, with each other.

---

**SCENARIO: Supermarket Back Health**

The four nursing student members of the Supermarket Back Health team have three weeks to go before their final presentation. They have just completed the second workshop that included the training for members of the Health and Safety Committee. The student team and the Health and Safety Committee decide to work together on the final tasks. They identify the co-chairs for this last stage of the project: Letecia from the store, and Stephanie, a nursing student. Both realize they will have to be in constant communication to ensure that everything is completed.

**Discussion Topics and Questions**

1. How do you think the team is feeling with only three weeks to go in the project?
2. What is the benefit of working closely with the Health and Safety Committee at this point?

For suggested responses, please see the Answer Key at the back of the book.

## Analyze Evaluation Data (Step 8a)

**Analysis of evaluation data** involves the following phases: categorization, summarization, comparison, drawing inferences or conclusions, and making recommendations. **Recommendations** are suggestions for further action based on the analysis and interpretation of data. The analysis will provide information on whether the tailored intervention had an impact or not, or, in other words, whether it initiated the expected change in the community of interest. The other question, addressed by process evaluation, is whether the intervention was implemented as planned. The data used in the analysis come from the process and impact evaluation measures.

The data analysis is required for both the presentation of the project and the project report. Work on the report and presentation can begin earlier in the project but cannot be completed until you have finished the analysis.

The analysis of evaluation data follows a process similar to the analysis of the assessment data as explained in Chapter 5. However, the analysis of the evaluation data is perhaps more focused because you have already defined the criteria (for example, 30 percent of mothers will…) when you wrote the objectives.

Box 8.2 identifies the phases of analysis for the evaluation data. For additional explanations and examples of analysis, refer to Chapter 5.

---

BOX 8.1
**Step 8 in Completing the Community Health Nursing Project**

ASSESS
1. Orient to community project
2. Assess secondary data
3. Assess physical and social environment
4. Assess primary data
5. Analyze assessment data

PLAN
6. Plan action

ACT
7. Take action

EVALUATE
8. Evaluate results and complete project
   a. Analyze evaluation data
   b. Present the results for validation
   c. Draft and complete project report
   d. Conclude relationship with collaborators
   e. Conclude relationship with team
9. Evaluate teamwork

---

BOX 8.2
**Phases of Analysis for Evaluation Data**

*Categorize According to Process or Impact Objectives*
- Identify the data associated with determining the relevance to the community group and collaborative methods used to produce the intervention.
- Identify the data associated with each objective. Some data might be used with more than one objective.

*Summarize*
- Quantitative data: Tabulate the data and either perform calculations manually or enter data into a computer program and perform calculations electronically.
- Qualitative data: Determine themes by reviewing the comments from participants that may have been collected informally during the action or formally in an interview or focused discussion.

*Compare*
- Identify data gaps, inconsistencies, and omissions with team members, collaborators, and stakeholders.
- Compare to objectives.

*Draw Inferences or Conclusions*
After consulting with collaborators on the preliminary analysis, prepare conclusion statements about the following:
- Intervention: Relevance and collaborative production
- Objectives: Met or not met and the reasons they were not met
- Limitations of the project
- Sustainability of the intervention or project

*Make Recommendations*

The team holds a joint meeting with the Health and Safety Committee to plan what has to be done in the remaining three weeks. First on their list is the analysis of the workshop data, because they need this to prepare their presentation and complete their report.

They review the data collected so far. Of the 40 full- and part-time stockers, 26 (65 percent) attended either the pilot tests or the workshops. To evaluate the objectives for ability and accomplishment, they summarize information from the workshops in a table. They had a problem with the accomplishment objective at first, because the numbers did not add up correctly. After checking with the team, they identify and correct a duplication of some data. Table 8.1 presents the data that they collected during and following each workshop.

When the figures were in place, they compared the percentages to the criteria in the objectives. The following are the final impact objectives:

- *Ability objective*: By November 10, 60 percent of participants in back injury prevention workshops for stockers identify safe lifting techniques.
- *Accomplishment objective*: By November 17, 40 percent of trained stockers demonstrate safe lifting techniques during work.
- *Environmental objective*: By November 14, 75 percent of Health and Safety Committee members are trained to provide back injury prevention workshop to all shifts on a regular basis.

The results show that the ability of workshop participants to use the proper lifting techniques was greater than estimated; however, their application of these same techniques at work was much less than estimated. As discussed earlier, they feel the ability results at the end of the workshop were high because participants who didn't understand tended to follow others and the difference between the correct and incorrect demonstrations was too obvious. While discussing the disappointing results in transferring this knowledge to the workplace, the Committee members explain that 40 percent for the objective was probably too high, given the number of stockers with limited English skills, and the time to learn the skills and then apply them in their work. In addition, Stephanie states that when observing the lifting techniques on-site, they found two problem areas in the store. It was clear that stockers did not have sufficient room to lift and turn in two cramped spaces and consistently used the incorrect technique. Participants had also mentioned these problem areas in the feedback sessions. The team will include these limitations in the report.

## Present the Results for Validation (Step 8b)

Presenting effectively to community audiences is a necessary skill for community and public health nurses in all levels of practice (Quad Council of Public Health Nursing Organizations, 2011) and as a preparation for entry-to-practice (Canadian Association of Schools of Nursing, 2014). A community health nursing presentation could occur in a large auditorium to an audience of professionals and business people, or in the corner of a cafeteria while students or workers are having lunch. By learning and following the presentation guidelines, you will develop skills that will continue to evolve throughout your nursing career.

The **presentation** is the verbal and/or written delivery of prepared material to an audience. The final presentation for a student project can be in the community with your collaborators or in your educational institution as a finale for your course, or both. The presentations provide an opportunity for the team to display what it has learned and obtain feedback from a knowledgeable audience. You will find that the presentation

To determine the relevance of the workshop and video, they reviewed the comments made at the end of each workshop. The following is a sample of some of the comments:

"They made the lifts look easy."

"It makes sense to lift that way, but I would feel silly doing it if I was the only one."

"The video covered the kinds of lifting that I do."

"Maybe we could check out each other?"

"I don't know if I will lift right when we are busy."

The team members determine that the video and workshop showed techniques that were relevant to the stockers, and that safe lifting was catching on. However, they realize that more time and effort is needed to reinforce the continued use of proper techniques. They really appreciate that the Committee members will continue to promote and reinforce safe lifting and will seek to make changes to the problem areas. The meeting ended on a high note, with Letecia describing how she had come across three stockers practicing the lifting techniques on the loading dock during the night shift. She said they were embarrassed when she found them, so she did not think that they had staged it for her benefit.

**Discussion Topics and Questions**

3. What preparation would ensure that everyone collected observations of lifting and carrying techniques in the workplace in the same way?
4. Discuss the importance of meeting or not meeting the proposed percentage of an objective.

**Table 8.1: Key Results—Workshops 1 and 2**

| Evaluation Measure | Workshop 1 | Workshop 2 | Total Number (%) |
|---|---|---|---|
| Ability | 7/7[1] | 8/10[1] | 15/17[1] (88%) |
| Accomplishment | 2/7 | 3/10 | 5/17 (29%) |

*Note*: 1. Number of participants meeting the impact criteria/Number of workshop participants.

guidelines are similar to those used in preparing a health communication intervention, described in Chapter 7.

Project presentations in the community come before the completion of the report because you need the feedback to validate your findings and recommendations. If there is no opportunity to deliver a formal presentation, as an alternative, request an informal feedback session where you can present your data and get input for recommendations.

No matter where you give a presentation, you want it to move the minds and hearts of the audience closer to your point of view (KU Work Group for Community Health and Development [KU Work Group], 2013). The KU Work Group states that the following elements are key to a successful community presentation:

- *Right background*
  - Select and recruit desired audience
  - Know the presentation setting
  - Select the best format

- *Right preparation*
  - Clarify objectives
  - Develop the content
  - Select presentation method and visual aids
  - Practice

- *Right delivery*
  - Use notes
  - Convince audience
  - Invite interaction
  - Follow up

Although the sections on right background and preparation are listed and discussed separately, in practice there needs to be some overlap between them. The following section elaborates on the key aspects of developing a final presentation for the end of a community project.

### The Right Background

Before preparing the presentation, consider your expected audience, the setting, and then the format in which to deliver the presentation. The usual format is a computer slideshow or a poster presentation. We describe both in Table 8.2 and provide links to further information in the "Website Resources" for this chapter.

The audience may number from two or three to ten or more for slideshow presentations at an organization where the audience might include organizational staff, other community organizations recommended by the placement organization, collaborators, and community members. Although the overall audience for poster presentations at a college or university, nursing association meeting, or conference can be large, the number of people at each poster is usually limited to a maximum of 10 by the available space.

Ensure that the people you want to be at the presentation attend by sending them an invitation and/or personally inviting them. These invitations can be sent informally, such as by email, phone, or in person, or formally in a letter at least two weeks before the event. The invitation would include the date, time, place, parking availability, and other relevant information, such as the option of child care. If space is limited, ask people to confirm their attendance.

If your audience is going to be quite different from the people you have been working with, analyze the potential attendees with the help of your collaborators so that you can include their needs in your presentation plans. This means knowing their age range, education level, language ability, values, and cultural and ethnic background, as well as the depth of their knowledge about you and the project (KU Work Group, 2013).

Organizing the meeting place and equipment to provide a favorable environment for the presentation is essential. Preparing suitable background conditions includes organizing and inspecting the room, location, and equipment (KU Work Group, 2013). Visit the room to consider possible seating arrangements and the availability and functioning of equipment, including lighting. Request the type of equipment that is required for the size of the audience and that you will be comfortable using. Also inquire about the availability of technical support should problems occur during the presentation. Be certain that a person is available to open the room at the time of the presentation.

## The Right Preparation

The right preparation involves clarifying objectives, developing the content, selecting presentation method and visual aids, and practicing. One way to clarify the objectives is to ask yourself what you want the presentation to achieve. In particular, determine the purpose of doing the presentation at this time and what message you want to leave with the participants. Because the purpose of the project is to work with people to achieve community benefits, each presentation will have a motivational aspect to show appreciation to people who have contributed and to encourage participants to join or support the work of the project.

The best gift for the project team to receive at the end of the final presentation would be for the collaborators to declare that they will continue the project. Be certain that you are clear on what you want to have happen by the end of the presentation. To be the most effective, the presentation needs to do the following (Bender, 2000):

- Inform
- Entertain
- Touch the emotions
- Promote action (p. 42)

To prepare, decide on clear and concise messages, select delivery methods, and take time to practice your presentation (KU Work Group, 2013). Experienced presenters advise that you spend 80 percent of your preparation time on delivery and 20 percent on content (Bender, 2000). This 80/20 rule makes sense if you consider that you really do know "what" you want to tell the audience; the tricky part is "how" to tell it so that they will understand your message and be engaged by the presentation. A fundamental way to promote understanding is to use plain language in all your materials. Presenters stress that fewer, simpler words in the vocabulary used by audience members have the greatest impact (Bender, 2000). The "Website Resources" in the Appendix to Chapter 7 offer valuable links on preparing information using plain language.

To develop the content, first prepare an outline. The outline will guide the sequence of the slides in a slideshow and the placement of material on a poster (from upper left to bottom right). Box 8.3 lists the usual components of a presentation.

The opening of the presentation and the main feature in a poster must grab the audience's attention in the first few seconds. This can be done in various ways, for example, by (1) creating a strong mental image, such as ships sinking from an overload of people dying from smoking; (2) providing a bottom line message for the audience that answers "What's in it for me?" (e.g., "Why would you want to take part in this? Well, I'll tell you. If you join us you'll have fun and you'll learn job skills such as…"); or (3) citing something that you observed or heard about the audience or their community.

---

**BOX 8.3**

**Proposed Outline for the Final Presentation of a Community Project**

1. An introduction (start with something to grab the attention of the audience, such as a picture or a story from the action) to tell them what you are going to discuss
2. A background to the issue or situation
3. A description of what was done—the action
4. The results of the action
5. Your proposed options for what could be done now (recommendations)
6. A summary of what you have discussed
7. Any final points you want to leave with the audience

*Source*: Adapted from The Health Communication Unit, 2000; and KU Work Group for Community Health and Development, 2013.

In the body of the presentation, follow through with what you promised in the opening. Be objective. When presenting conclusions and recommendations, focus on a few options or actions, rather than promoting only one. When you promote only one action, the audience may feel the team is being directive and resent this. Recommendations can include suggestions for continuing the work; for example, teaming up with other community organizations with similar interests. When an educational institution organizes the project, one option is making arrangements for another student group to carry on with the project. Encourage members of the audience to offer suggestions.

The ending of the presentation and the conclusions in a poster (positioned in the bottom right corner) should be stronger than the opening (The Health Communication Unit, 2000). If you had a strong opening theme or a quote that worked, repeat it. Summarize your message. To leave the audience with an emotional message, tell them a story that is relevant (e.g., a new mother found friends when she asked for help, a girl shared how she learned to face up to a bully) and close with a call to action.

The end of the presentation is a good time to show public appreciation for the people who have assisted you. This recognition does not need to involve more than mentioning each person by name and saying a couple of words on how they helped.

Select a visual presentation method to augment your speech to help you to convey your message to both those who are familiar with the project and those who are not. By combining telling and showing, you increase the retention of material after three days by 55 percent over telling alone (Bender, 2000). Table 8.2 describes four types of

**Table 8.2: Types of Presentation Methods**

| Type | Disadvantages | Considerations |
|---|---|---|
| Computer slideshow presentation | – Requires computer program and knowledge to prepare presentation<br>– Need equipment and technical ability to display presentation<br>– May reduce interaction with audience | – Provides opportunity to easily use color, pictures, and graphics<br>– Can be printed and used as handout or poster<br>– Once prepared, is easy to modify |
| Poster presentation | – Limited space<br>– Requires considerable thought to identify and illustrate pertinent information | – Materials and costs range from the inexpensive handmade poster (for table or display board) to the expensive, professionally designed poster printed from a digital computer poster program<br>– Can be stand-alone or augmented by short verbal descriptions and responses to questions<br>– Can be left in location to reinforce message |
| Overhead transparencies | – Need projector, screen, prepared transparencies, and backup light | – Low cost but limits use of illustrative material<br>– "6 × 6" rule: 6 lines with 6 words each<br>– Use bullets with key phrases<br>– Use large (16+) bold serif-type font |
| Flip chart displays | – Requires flip chart and markers<br>– Needs to be prewritten by person with neat handwriting<br>– Need to check to ensure entire audience can see chart | – Easy to use and provides a record, but can be time-consuming<br>– "5 × 5" rule: 5 lines with 5 words each<br>– Use upper two-thirds of sheet |

presentation methods you could use. All four types add visual cues to your speech. Among the four types, the required equipment, knowledge, preparation time, and added benefits vary greatly.

You can combine the four types to enhance a presentation or for specific purposes. Flip charts, for example, can be used with a slideshow presentation to record comments. Links to specific guidance in preparing slideshow presentations and posters are found in the "Website Resources" at the end of this chapter.

The presentations can be augmented by visual aids such as handouts, posters, videos, or role-play. A handout of the slides or main points helps to reinforce your message and takes less time than the other visual aids.

Slideshows and/or a handout of slides guide the verbal presentation for audiences of various sizes and capabilities. With smaller groups (less than 10), or when participants have limited communication skills, a poster presentation or flip chart allows more opportunity to interact with the audience and adjust your delivery to their needs.

A slideshow presentation should be 15 to 20 minutes in length, including 5 minutes for questions. A good rule to follow is to present one slide per minute for the remaining time, not including the reference list. According to online tutorials (see "Website Resources"), it is important to keep the amount of information and animation per slide to a minimum. The most common problem with people new to presenting is that of providing too much information on slides. The discussion time will allow you to fill in more details.

Practice is essential for a good delivery. The following are suggestions to help you practice effectively: rehearse in front of a mirror, in front of your teammates, or with a video camera or tape recorder; read your script aloud, breathing and relaxing, with a clock, while maintaining eye contact, while paying attention to how your words are delivered, or by visualizing yourself doing the presentation (KU Work Group, 2013); also ask a community member to listen to you and identify any ideas or words that were unclear, not understandable, or confusing.

As you are preparing the presentation, try out your script with community members, especially if their first language is not English. Ask them if they understand the examples and invite suggestions for making the material easier to understand. You could try adding a picture of an activity related to the project to see if it might successfully replace a lot of written words.

Prepare the presentation material in sufficient time to have a rehearsal in the room and make adjustments before the actual presentation. For example, check that any visual displays or text are visible from the back of the room.

### The Right Delivery

The right delivery involves convincing your audience, inviting interaction, and following up (KU Work Group, 2013). Most of this section applies to slideshow presentations but is applicable to other presentations.

The main purpose of your presentation is to convince your audience that the points you are making are important. Your credibility begins with first impressions—of your clothing, statements, and manner. Clothing that is neat and attractive but not distracting adds to a favorable first impression. As discussed earlier, your opening remarks need to grab the audience's attention and create the impression that you have something significant to say and care about the audience (KU Work Group, 2013). First tell them what to expect and then follow up with your facts and ideas. Those beginning statements, facts, and notes should be accessible on your carefully prepared cue cards, with a main point on each card. Use large print and different colors to accentuate points. The cards will give you confidence and ensure that you know what to say from one minute to the next.

At the beginning and during a presentation, make the case that your topic is relevant to the audience. With a community project, emphasize that it was conducted in collaboration with the community and can be continued through collaboration. This reinforces the primary health care principle of community participation. The relevance of community collaboration to the project can be demonstrated by including the collaborators in the presentations. Their inclusion sends a strong message that the action was relevant to the community and that collaboration was productive. Not all collaborators will want to get up in front of an audience; however, some may be interested in building their skills in some other way, such as preparing materials, assisting with small group discussions, or organizing a meeting.

One purpose of a community presentation is to encourage community participation in making health decisions and involvement in your project, so take steps to engage the audience throughout the presentation. Making eye contact with members of the audience encourages interaction and conveys that you are interested in their reaction to your presentation. You will know from their response if they are following what you are saying or if you need to make adjustments. If your audience is not comfortable with eye contact, focus on an inanimate object or on the people who are more comfortable with direct contact.

To be involved and give input, the audience must understand your presentation. Provide pauses and time to think if you want answers to a question. Ask specific questions. For example, rather than ask "Are there any questions?" say "I would like to know what you feel about X. Take a minute to think about it, and maybe write down your ideas. Then I will ask you again."

Another way to get input is to ask members of the audience to discuss a question with the person beside them. That gives everyone time to think and gain confidence in voicing his or her ideas. Another option, when you want people to consider different options, is to arrange small group sessions. Small groups are particularly helpful for people with limited English skills.

Distribute team members and key informants from the community among the groups to explain the options in more detail. You can ask them to discuss specific points or list the points you have made in order of importance (The Health Communication Unit, 2000). Although you need to make a special effort to ensure understanding and to obtain feedback from multicultural groups, the effort is also worthwhile for all community audiences. Most community audiences will probably include people with a low to high range of knowledge and understanding of the issue. At the end of the session, have each small group report back the key points to the entire audience.

Consider the following tips when responding to questions from the audience (KU Work Group, 2013):

- Listen carefully.
- Repeat the question using the main ideas to ensure that you have heard it correctly and everyone knows what was asked.
- Show respect for the questioner.

- Encourage others to offer a viewpoint.
- Keep your answers short.
- Remain calm when dealing with difficult questions or situations. Admit when you do not know something and arrange to get back to the person. Identify common areas and the reason for your position if there are differences, and gently steer the discussion back to the main issues if an irrelevant issue is raised.

Above all, when giving a community presentation, bring out experiences that excited you and your fellow team members. Your excitement encourages others. Speak with personal conviction: show your emotions but keep them under control. When you want to solicit action, show that what you propose is important and possible (KU Work Group, 2013). When concluding your presentation, summarize and highlight your main ideas. End on a positive high note.

Immediately after a community presentation, be certain to capitalize on the enthusiasm that you have generated. Consider how you could encourage discussions with partners about their interests and how they could increase their involvement in this or other health initiatives. You want to (a) increase community participation in a community project, even if you are leaving; and (b) show support and appreciation for organization and community partners.

If the organization and collaborators want to continue the action, you could suggest that they have sign-up sheets that they can circulate or leave at the back of the room, and handouts and information for the next meeting. They can also leave posters and sign-up sheets in the reception areas of the agencies that are involved with the project. During the final presentation, the team can assist the collaborators by using the opportunity to recruit new people to the continuing project. Team members may find it much easier to advocate on behalf of others rather than for themselves. This gesture and the response to it can add to the impetus for the collaborators to continue on their own.

## Draft and Complete Project Report (Step 8c)

The project report, as introduced in Chapter 5, is a comprehensive account of a community nursing project and is integral to professional accountability in community health nursing practice (Community Health Nurses of Canada, 2011; Quad Council of Public Health Nursing Organizations, 2011). The project report explains the data-based rationale for the project, assessment findings, project plan, a record of how the intervention was delivered, and the project findings. The report summarizes the ongoing documentation of the project from work plans, weekly reports, and so on in a complete and concise way. The project report is a record that informs others about the work that has been done and its results, and gives recommendations about how to build on the work. The report can reach many people over time and contributes to the sustainability of the project.

Project reports are a valuable asset for community organizations because they provide detailed documentation on which the organization can build. Community health projects may extend over months or even years; responsibilities may change and organizations often have limited time and resources to allocate to pulling together the details and writing up projects conducted with a community group. These community initiatives,

Now that the data analysis is complete, the attention of the team turns to the final tasks of preparing the final presentation and report. So much to do, and so little time! They feel overwhelmed until they realize that a great deal is already completed.

They decide to emphasize three main points in the presentation: (1) safety training workshops are effective, (2) the Health and Safety Committee is trained to carry on with the workshops, and (3) conditions in the facility that affect safe lifting need to be addressed. Their evaluation shows that training is not sufficient by itself. For continued progress, changes in the physical environment and ongoing encouragement are required for staff to adapt safe back health measures into everyday work routines. They do not want the workshops to be dismissed or considered as the only solution to back health.

The expanded team assigns people to the tasks. The presentation subteam plans to adapt the presentation outline in Box 8.3.

Letecia leads the discussion on who will attend the presentation. The original list had 10 names, but the store manager has invited the district manager and wants other supermarket managers to attend. Letecia would like to invite representatives from the Health and Safety Committees in other stores, and another team member adds colleagues who provided the videos on

back health. They have to make decisions: the staff room had space for only 20 people, and they still need to include supermarket staff.

The team feels obligated to the people who provided the videos and to the supermarket staff; however, they want to include the others too. The Health and Safety Committee members propose that they set up a display in the staff room with the pictures and material from the presentation. That way all shift workers will have a chance to see it. The team feels that this is the best solution under the circumstances.

After two rehearsals they have adjusted their presentation to the times scheduled, and everyone in the expanded team knows his or her role. As the room is filling up for the presentation, they feel excited but not especially anxious. The audience enjoys the presentation and is ready to discuss how to promote a "back health culture" in the supermarket. Stephanie and Letecia propose four options, primarily involving the Health and Safety Committee:

1. Continue to offer workshops and reinforce safe lifting.
2. Address unsafe work areas (the Committee and management).
3. Offer rewards for people "caught" lifting correctly, or helping a co-worker maintain back health.
4. Distribute posters throughout the store demonstrating techniques pertinent to that area.

however, can assist others dealing with similar groups and issues. Project reports prepared by students can therefore make an important contribution to community practice.

The sections of the body of the report are shown in Box 8.4. The attachments can vary according to the project, but should include references and details of the intervention; data collection tools developed for the project, such as questionnaires, forms, and checklists; other resources; and tabulations of the evaluation data. (With some projects, a comprehensive assessment report could comprise the project report; see the Assessment Project Report form in Appendix A.3.3a.) Providing a written report of a project to the community organization is an expectation of professional practice. The report can be placed in a binder, folder, or USB key, and a copy of the report can become part of your professional portfolio.

You can begin drafting the project report as soon as you have summary information. It is preferable to begin filling in the information by the midpoint of your project.

After some discussion that recognizes the value of each of these options, the district manager asks how they can implement the workshops and other recommendations in each of the supermarkets in the district. The store managers quickly respond that they need to devote more staff time and money to health and safety. The district manager responds, "Okay, we can think about that. It might pay for itself through less sick time and better health for our employees!" A stunned silence occurs, then applause.

The response to the presentation overwhelms the team members. After the presentation, several managers ask how they can get nursing students to work on health projects in their stores. A public health nurse, who had provided resources, asks if she can have a copy of the report to use in her organization's Healthy Workplace Program.

**Discussion Topics and Questions**
5. Discuss how the workplace environment influenced the outcomes of the safe lifting workshops.
6. Explain how the presentation of results can be used to validate the findings.

**Table 8.3: Sample Outline for Final Presentation on Back Health**

| Elements and Time | Details | Responsibility |
|---|---|---|
| 1. Introduction: 5 min. | Pictures from the supermarket showing "before" and "after" shots of staff lifting | Health and Safety Committee (H&S) |
| 2. Background: 2 min. | The facts and figures on days off work due to back pain | Stephanie |
| 3. The action: 10 min. | The workshops—description | Denny |
|  | Demonstrations | H&S |
| 4. The results of the action: 2 min. | Ability and accomplishment objectives | Jose |
| 5. Options: 5 min. | Options on how to increase use of safe lifting techniques | Stephanie & Letecia |
| 6. Summary: 2 min. | What worked and what needs more work | Stephanie & Letecia |
| 7. Discussion: 4 min. | Feedback on options | Stephanie & Letecia, Store manager |

Consider the project report as a document that you complete as you go, rather than something you complete right at the end. This approach will help you become more efficient in your work and documentation.

The following material describes how to complete the six sections of the report: assessment, plan, action, findings, conclusions, and attachments. The academic course or organization specifies the length. Usually two to four pages, with attachments, are sufficient for a short-term project. This is similar to what you would expect in an executive summary for a lengthy report. The project report forms are provided in Appendix A.3.3a and A.3.3b.

**Assessment**
The first part of the report provides the information on the collection of primary and secondary data. You can complete this part of the report as soon as the issues for action

have been determined. The assessment section includes the following items:

- Background/introduction
- Key health issues of the population
- Community of interest
- Assessment methods

The background or introduction explains how the project originated. Usually two or three sentences are sufficient to achieve this. The key health issues of the population is a statement referenced from a reputable source or sources that indicates that the issue causes hardship, illness, or death and deserves to receive attention. Using the example of the multilanguage women living in a low-income apartment building (see Chapter 5), the key issues could include statistics to indicate that women living in poverty have a high rate of low-birth-weight infants. Although the team may have many statistics at this point, choose the two or three sources that are the most pertinent to make the point that it is worthwhile to work on this issue or problem. If possible, add a statistic that makes the issue key at the local or organizational level.

The community of interest describes the specific group of people, identified as needing improved services, who are the focus of the project. This group, identified through the assessment, may be different from originally intended. For example, the Multilanguage Project may have started with women who are pregnant or have babies less than one year in age, and then moved to include women with young children.

For the project report, condense the assessment methods and data. Table 8.4 provides an example of how to do this without losing the important elements. The example is again drawn from Chapter 5, Table 5.5, related to the multilanguage women living in a low-income apartment building. The assessment data provides the evidence for the priority action statement.

## Plan

The plan for the project report, as discussed in Chapter 6, can be completed near the end of implementation. The items in this section of the report are as follows:

- Priority action statement with supporting evidence
- Project goal
- Strategy and evidence-based intervention
- Impact objectives

The priority action statement and goal are simply transferred from the work plan to the project report. The intervention is described as planned, and references the health strategy and evidence on which it was based. List the impact objectives.

**Table 8.4: Example of Condensed Version of Assessment Methods and Findings**

| Original Assessment Report (Table 5.5) | Condensed Project Report |
|---|---|
| **Method: Timelines, Participants, Description** | **Assessment Methods: Sept. 10–Nov. 12** |
| Collection and review of secondary data: Sept. 10–Oct. 1 | Review secondary data and map community |
| Mapping neighborhood: Sept. 10–Oct. 1 Included food stores, laundry, bus stops, schools, post office, and so on | |
| Key informant interviews: Sept. 17–24 4 participants in total: 2 volunteers from building, 1 city support worker, 1 manager of multicultural organization | Four key informant interviews |
| Progressive inquiry: Sept. 24–Oct. 15 12 women from apartment building meeting in lobby | Progressive inquiry with 12 women meeting in lobby over 5 weeks |
| Questionnaire: Oct. 8–22 20 women from apartment building not meeting in lobby | Questionnaire with 20 women from building |

## Action

The action section explains how the intervention was tailored to the community group and delivered. For example, if the intervention was a health fair for older adults, describe the initiative in a few words and explain how you developed and pilot-tested the materials. Describe the event, the activities offered, key organizing details, the role of the team on the day, and so on. Refer to any evidence-based studies or reports that made a difference in how action was taken. This description of the intervention may be different in some respects from what you envisaged in planning.

Discuss how the project was evaluated. This is an updated summary of the process objectives from the timeline or Gantt chart completed in Chapter 6, and as modified during implementation in Chapter 7. Rather than listing separate activities according to date, group the activities into development and tailoring, implementation, and evaluation, with a time span indicated for each. Development and tailoring would include the adjustments you made following the pilot tests. The details of how you tailored the intervention for your community could be quite useful for others to follow. For each activity, include the actual number of participants who were involved. Complete the section with a description of your tailored intervention and refer to attachments.

## Evaluation

The evaluation section includes the following:

- Key findings
- Conclusions
- Limitations
- Sustainability
- Recommendations
- Relevance for community health nursing

This section draws on the process and impact evaluation. The usual format is to begin by giving the number and characteristics of the participants. Follow this with the results, tabulated by impact objective in a way that allows comparison to the measurement criteria identified for the objective. Process evaluation data, such as whether or not the intervention was implemented as planned, can be included in the conclusions, and possibly the limitations.

Conclusions are the interpretation of the results. When discussing reasons for the findings being as anticipated or higher or lower than planned, incorporate feedback from community members and stakeholders, and from the literature. This feedback provides validation for the conclusions.

**Limitations** of the project are factors that, to some extent, could reduce the ability of the intervention to achieve the desired results. In the course of delivering the tailored intervention, or when collecting evaluation data and analyzing results, you are likely to become aware of external factors that could compromise the intervention and affect the outcomes. Time and resources that interfere with participation can often be a barrier in short-term projects. This includes such things as equipment failure interfering with a presentation, or having insufficient time to reach people without Internet services. Or, you may find out too late that attendance has dropped off at your women's fitness group because of the weather or because participants do not like the instructor. Other factors may interfere with data collection or affect the accuracy of the data gathered in some way. Some factors might have been prevented; others not.

Analyzing why objectives were not met can be just as beneficial to community groups as identifying what worked. In research studies, limitations usually identify factors known to the researchers that would limit the generalizability of the results, such as small sample size. Projects on a smaller scale, such as those described in this text, tend to focus on improving practice for specific groups. While they may not have the rigor of research studies, they aim to document emerging practice (Association of Maternal Child Health Program, n.d.) and change practice in an incremental way. Such work is fundamental to community health nursing practice and paves the way for more definitive studies.

With regard to the sustainability of any health intervention, all you can report at the end of the project is what has been done to make continuation more likely; for example, the training provided to community organizers. Or you can provide evidence that has implications for continued action, such as how much people seemed to appreciate (or not) an intervention, and what the community organization has promised. Although you have considered sustainability from the beginning of the project, concrete results may not occur until some time after you leave the project.

The recommendations are based on the project findings and informed by responses to the presentation of results. Each recommendation proposes the continuation of what worked well, or suggests ways to make changes. For example, if the project showed that women who were learning English were comfortable learning in groups of four to six using pictures and plain language, you would recommend that approach. If, at the same time, you found they had difficulty concentrating when their children were in the same room, you would recommend making alternative arrangements for child care.

Base the sections on limitations and recommendations in the report on evidence and not speculation. The project reports and recommendations survive much longer than the feelings and experiences of the team members. For example, personality differences may have created friction in the project but are best addressed outside the report, after seeking advice from your advisors.

An important purpose of the recommendations is to identify policy changes that could further improve the health outcomes of the people involved in the project. Policy implications can be determined by asking "What could or should be done about this issue?" (Public Health Nursing Section, 2001, p. 315) beyond what we were able to accomplish. As with other recommendations, they need to be reasonable and strongly supported by the findings of the project.

Policy recommendations may address the need to remove barriers to health resulting from socioeconomic determinants such as poverty by adding resources or introducing legislation. For example, although low-income women can learn about the nutritional content of food and work together to buy food in bulk during a project, obtaining nutritional food will continue to be a challenge if food costs are higher than their income. Specific recommendations on what action to take based on the experience of working with the women would be useful to decision makers.

As well, policy change may be used to greatly enhance the value obtained from education and training. For example, health education strategies are used to change risk behaviors such as lifting incorrectly, riding a bicycle without a helmet, or texting while driving. Recommending changes to associated rules, regulations, or policies could help to drive change and reduce the cost and effort of providing education to increase effectiveness. For example, the policy could take the form of requiring back safety training every six months or fines for not using safety equipment.

At the conclusion of this section of the report, draw attention to the implications of the findings for community health nursing and the sponsoring organization. This is an opportunity for team members to reflect on what they learned during the project and to relate the learning to the relevant community/public health nursing standards or competencies. Community health projects involving teamwork contribute to practice learning in all the areas of assessment, planning, action, and evaluation, as well as collaboration, such as partnering and relationship building. As a team, identify two or three standards or competencies that were the most relevant to your work together.

To help ensure that the report is useful to the organization and meets other requirements (such as that of an educational institution), ask advisors and instructors to review draft material. For community health nursing students, obtain approval for the final report from the appropriate authority before submitting it to the organization.

## Attachments

Attach materials to the project report that help explain the report and further the work of the project. Since the purpose of the project is to promote change, include material, sorted into appendices, that you and your advisors feel would be useful to others. Reference materials for the report itself could consist of summary tables for the analysis of quantitative and qualitative data. As well, data collection tools used in progressive inquiry, pretest and posttest questionnaires, and focus group questions could help to explain the analysis of data in the report as well as save other groups who are continuing with the project considerable time and effort. A minimum requirement to include as an appendix would be a copy of your tailored intervention. We suggest you err on the side of being generous with the materials as long as you take the time to sort and organize them into appendices where they can be easily found.

The report does not include raw data, such as completed questionnaires, field notes, or materials that include the names of participants. As well, written and electronic working documents, such as weekly reports and work plans, are not included. Consult with your instructor and deal with this potentially revealing material according the policy of your facility.

You may have different options as to how you submit your project report. If you have several resources, they can be organized in a project binder or electronic file with different sections, such as assessment measures, graphs from assessment, evaluation forms, tabulations of results, and slides from the presentation. A comprehensive project report can facilitate steady improvement in the health of communities because practitioners are sharing information and are not continuously "recreating the wheel."

## Conclude Relationship with Collaborators (Step 8d)

Concluding the relationship with collaborators is an important aspect of teamwork (refer to the "ending" stage of team development in Chapter 2). This involves completing project work and thanking people who assisted the team in some way. In all project work there are written and unwritten requirements, especially in collaborative community health practice. Usually, project reports go through a formal approval process. All major players will receive a copy of the final project report and be invited to a formal presentation of findings. For community health nursing students, the team's supervisor or instructor needs to review and approve the report before distribution to ensure acceptable content.

**Showing appreciation** is recognizing and thanking people for the assistance they have provided. Although showing appreciation is a normal part of nursing practice, as well as good manners, in community health nursing it is especially important. Most of the people you contact during your project have no particular obligation to work with you or to help you. Whatever their motivation, what they do supports your work and benefits the community. Recognizing them reinforces their continued support for community health.

As the project draws to an end, take some time to determine who you want to recognize and how you will show your appreciation. Begin by listing all the people who have been involved and the contribution they have made. Next, consider the various options that you have for showing your appreciation. Box 8.5 provides some options to consider. Discuss the options with others who are familiar with the situation or the people on your list to determine which option would be the most appropriate.

Usually, teams have no difficulty identifying who should be recognized. They do have difficulty, however, ensuring that everyone is thanked appropriately in the final rush to complete a project. The "thank-yous" must be a designated task to ensure that the project ends well.

---

BOX 8.5

**Ways to Show Appreciation**

**Informal, Private**
- Phone call
- Email
- Verbal thank-you

**Formal, Private**
- Handwritten thank-you card
- Letter expressing appreciation with copy to manager (could be included in the person's work file)

**Public Recognition**
- Acknowledged verbally in presentation
- Active role in presentation
- Named in written record, such as agenda for presentation, or acknowledged in the report

---

After the excitement of the presentation, the four team members find it difficult to pull their thoughts together to complete the final report. The assessment section and most of the plan are complete, but the entire team needs to check out the draft description of the tailored intervention. They learn that commenting on one another's draft work makes the process move more quickly. As a team, they review the final draft with their advisors, make revisions based on feedback, and receive final approval. Feeling quite proud of their work, they hand a copy of the report to the Health and Safety Committee and store manager, and send one to the public health nurse who assisted them in obtaining the video. The Appendix to this chapter provides their final project report.

The team then considers what they have done, and need to do, to end their collaboration well. They had recognized all those who helped with the project at the slideshow presentation by reading out their names and asking them to stand, to a generous round of applause. The participants in the two pilot tests were recognized by including their names in the staff room display under the title of "Thanks to the workshop guinea pigs!" The store manager had provided valuable support, and they thanked him again for all he had done when they presented him with the project report.

As a final gesture, the team decides to write a letter commending Letecia for the consistent assistance she provided throughout the project and give a copy of it to the store manager. They hope that this will help her to get a full-time job working on health and safety, which is what she wants.

**Discussion Topics and Questions**

7. What is the value of the supermarket receiving a two-to-four-page project report?

8. How were people recognized for their contribution to the project?

## Conclude Relationship with Team Members (Step 8e)

As you are winding down your project, take time to reflect individually and as a team on what you have accomplished and learned. Individually, look back to what you felt as you started this project, and ask yourself "Did I learn what I wanted to learn? Did I learn what I expected to learn? Did I learn more than I expected to learn? What individual and group skills can I now add to my résumé? How did my team make a difference in the community?" As a team, review the high points and the low points, as well as your current stage of development as a team (see Chapter 2). Use the individual and team forms (see Appendix A.2.5–A.2.7) to evaluate yourselves. These evaluations, like work plans, are not a part of the report. They are considered confidential working documents.

Ending can be a time of celebration as well as a time of loss. Team members may start feeling sad when most of the tasks are completed and the work is done; others may have a delayed reaction to the loss. To assist people in recognizing what they have accomplished and preparing them to move on, take time to recognize the contribution that each team member has made. One team member may have found a talent for identifying key messages; another, for developing a role-play, and yet another, for preparing a slideshow presentation. When these previously hidden or taken-for-granted talents are recognized, people gain confidence to move on to new challenges.

You deserve a celebration at the end of the project. Plan a party, plan a trip, or plan on writing an article or giving a presentation on what your team has accomplished in collaboration with the community group. Community health groups and community health nursing need to hear about your accomplishments if we are to make a difference in the health of the population.

# Teamwork to the End

By now the team will have completed most of the project, which provides a strong incentive to bring things to a successful conclusion. The main challenges to the team at the end of the project are coordinating and allocating the many tasks, maintaining close communication, and evaluation. Ending well means ensuring that there are no loose ends, every task is completed, and every person has been properly treated and respected.

## Coordination and Allocation of Tasks

Coordination of activities as the project is ending is particularly important because much needs to be done in a short period of time. Multitasking becomes a necessity. The most effective use of time is to begin to prepare the final presentation and report at the same time as completing the evaluation and analysis. This means concurrent activity, with team members working alone or in small groups. As the tasks mount up—from determining invitation lists to analyzing evaluation data—it is easy to feel overwhelmed.

Team members may be sharing leadership functions, which shows maturity in the development of the team; however, one person, or at most two, needs to keep track of the deadlines. This will become even more important if the team has expanded to include collaborators. About three to four weeks before the end of the project, the team leader should make sure that the work plan is up to date, tasks are listed, and someone is assigned to monitoring completion. If deadlines are not being met, reassess priorities. There simply may be too many tasks for the time available. Determine what is a "necessity" and what is a "nicety." You need to drop tasks that are a nicety or refer them to collaborators. If a necessary task takes too long, scale it down so that it is manageable in the time remaining. For example, preparing a slideshow presentation can eat up a lot of time, especially if a team member becomes hooked on using all the animation features!

At the same time, it is important to focus on what is important and make sure it is done well. For example, the audience for the presentation may include people who have not been directly involved in the project but who can affect the future use of the intervention in the community. The team needs to consider that implication and seek advice from the instructor, agency representative, and relevant managers on what messages to impart at the presentation and how to frame them.

Coordination can be difficult at the end because team members may be feeling both sad about the end of the teamwork and rushed for time. One task for the team leader, with help from the instructor, is to monitor morale and work closely with individual team members to make fair and rational decisions to balance the welfare of the project and the people doing the work. Individual team members can also overextend themselves and may need to be "reined in" to avoid frustration for both them and the team as a whole.

## Communication

Lines of communication are usually well established by this time. However, as more people become involved, pay attention to the email distribution list to make sure it is kept up to date. Communication by email or phone becomes increasingly frequent now that the time available is short and last-minute changes are often necessary. For example, the team leader may learn that additional people need to be invited to the final presentation. Communicating last-minute changes, especially when team members are working on separate tasks, requires greater diligence in checking for and responding to messages.

Ending well means that the team members are satisfied by their accomplishments, the collaborators have gained from the experience, relevant resources have been produced, and most of those involved have positive feelings about the experience. Although there may be some feelings of regret because there was not enough time or resources to accomplish all that was planned, this is a time to appreciate what was done as positive and a movement in the right direction toward making a difference. In the most optimistic outcome, the organization and community members will continue the initiative and possibly collaborate on other projects. Both will eventually contribute to making a positive difference in the health of the population.

## Evaluation

The end of a project and an academic course usually requires an evaluation of team and individual functioning. The team agreement will help you to evaluate the team and document the results in the work plan or in forms provided by your course requirements. This is an appropriate time to review evaluations from earlier periods during the project, and identify where growth occurred and where challenges still exist.

Community health nursing can be immediately rewarding for some and a challenge for others, similar to other nursing clinical situations. This experience and reflection on the experience provides you with valuable insights on how to work with others to make a difference.

## Summary

After delivering the tailored intervention, the team has several tasks to complete before bringing the project to a satisfactory conclusion. They must analyze the data in terms of the objectives and make inferences in consultation with collaborators. Based on the draft results, they prepare and deliver a presentation on the project to the community group, taking the opportunity to validate what was learned and to consider recommendations. This feedback is added to the relevant sections of their project report. Once the report is reviewed, the report is provided to their organization to support continued work.

As well as completing the documentation of the project and communicating results, to end well the team members must bring the relationships that have developed over the course of the project to a satisfactory conclusion. Recognizing and reflecting on what was learned with others will assist with the sustainability of the project and the professional development of team members.

## Classroom and Seminar Exercises

1. What principles from primary health care and unique characteristics of community health nursing (see Chapter 1) are apparent in the preparation and delivery of the final presentation to the staff in the Supermarket Back Health scenario in this chapter?
2. Your team has just completed a heath education intervention to prepare children in an afterschool program to appropriately respond when confronted by unexpected smoke or fire. You have collected evaluation data on the objective "By November 15, 50 percent of children in the afterschool program can demonstrate the required three actions in the correct order when they see unexpected fire or smoke." The expected actions are: Get Out, Stay Out, and Call for Help (American Red Cross, 2014). Discuss the following questions in relation to the given situation:
   a. What would be an environment change that would support the objective?
   b. What are possible interpretations if the results are higher than expected?
   c. What are possible interpretations if the results are lower than expected?
   d. How would you decide what interpretations to include in your recommendations?
3. Your team has completed the collection of evaluation data on the use of three different methods of providing information on nutritional food to people who have difficulty speaking and reading English. Describe how your final presentation would vary if given to
   a. a community group in an area with many new immigrants
   b. lay workers who work with the community group
   c. health professionals who work with the community group
   d. the board of directors of a large health care organization providing services to the community group
4. Prepare an outline with timelines and responsibilities for the presentation to the Homeless Coalition based on the Improvement of Winter Services for the Homeless scenario (see Chapter 6).
5. Your team has the option of providing either a PowerPoint presentation or a poster of your project. Compare the pros and cons of each method.
6. Discuss how organizations and team members could use the project report in the future.

## References

American Red Cross. (2014). *Home fire safety*. Retrieved from www.redcross.org/prepare/disaster/home-fire

Association of Maternal Child Health Program. (n.d.). *Best practices program*. Retrieved from www.amchp.org/programsandtopics/BestPractices/Pages/BestPracticeTerms.aspx

Bender, P. (2000). *Secrets of power presentations*. Toronto, ON: The Achievement Group.

Canadian Association of Schools of Nursing. (2014, May). *Entry-to-practice public health nursing competencies for undergraduate nursing education*. Retrieved from www.casn.ca/en/123/item/6

Community Health Nurses of Canada. (2011, March). *Canadian community health nursing: Professional practice model & standards of practice*. Retrieved from www.chnc.ca/nursing-standards-of-practice.cfm

The Health Communication Unit, Centre for Health Promotion, University of Toronto. (2000). *Strengthening presentation skills*. Toronto, ON: Author.

KU Work Group for Community Health and Development. (2013). Making community presentations. *Community Tool Box* (Chapter 4, Section 5). Retrieved from http://ctb.ku.edu/en/table-of-contents/assessment/getting-issues-on-the-public-agenda/community-presentations/main

Public Health Nursing Section. (2001). *Public health interventions: Applications for public health nursing practice*. St. Paul, MN: Minnesota Department of Health.

Quad Council of Public Health Nursing Organizations. (2011). *Quad Council competencies for public health nurses*. Retrieved from www.resourcecenter.net/images/ACHNE/Files/QuadCouncilCompetenciesForPublicHealthNurses_Summer2011.pdf

Research and Education Unit (Cal/OSHA Consultation Service), Division of Occupational Safety and Health, California Department of Industrial Relations. (2007). *Ergonomic guidelines for manual material handling*. Retrieved from www.cdc.gov/niosh/docs/2007-131/pdfs/2007-131.pdf

US Bureau of Labor Statistics. (2003). *Workplace injuries and illnesses in grocery stores*. Retrieved from www.bls.gov/opub/mlr/cwc/workplace-injuries-and-illnesses-in-grocery-stores.pdf

## Website Resources

### Posters

Guidelines for posters can also be found using a search engine and typing in "Poster Presentation" site:edu.

Rose Sherman (2010), *How to Create an Effective Poster Presentation*: www.mc.vanderbilt.edu/documents/evidencebasedpractice/files/How%20to%20create%20an%20effect%20Poster%20Pres.pdf

*American Nurse Today* published the above article by Rose Sherman for nurses who are presenting a poster at a conference. The information also applies to students presenting a poster at the end of a project. The "Selected References" at the end of the article provide additional information.

### Slideshow Presentations

Tutorials and examples of slideshow presentations are available online from presentation software manufacturers such as Microsoft, the creators of PowerPoint®, and from providers (retailers) of PowerPoint®. As well, tutorials can be obtained from education sites by typing the following into a search engine window: "PowerPoint tutorial" site:edu. In addition, the following PowerPoint presentation listed below illustrates what to do and not do in a presentation.

Elizabeth (Liz) Diem (2011), *Presentation Tips*: http://chnresources.org/node/11

This PowerPoint presentation demonstrates graphically how to prepare a good presentation and illustrates what a bad presentation looks like.

## Appendix to Chapter 8

### Final Project Report

East Coast College, School of Nursing
Community Health Project in Collaboration with River
Street TruValue Supermarket

#### We Watch Our Backs!

December 1, 2014

Team members: Marie Lopez, Stephanie White, Denny
 Hoi, Jose Rupierez

Instructor: Janet MacWilliam

Agency representative: Ellen Maglacis

Agency manager: Joseph Offenbach

#### Assessment

*Background*: The Health and Safety Committee of the
supermarket had asked for a team of nursing students
to work on an injury prevention project with them. They
had figures indicating a high number of work-related
back injuries.

*Key health issues of the population*: A summary of grocery
store injuries and illness (US Bureau of Labor Statistics,
2003) identified grocery stores as one of the nine
industries in the US having more than 100,000 injury
cases in 2000. The most prevalent injuries were back
strains or sprains from lifting containers, boxes, crates,
and cartons. Store sick leave statistics are highest for
stockers and 70 percent relate to back injuries.

*Community of interest*: Stockers and Health and
Safety Committee working at River Street TruValue
Supermarket

*Assessment methods*: Review of statistics on injuries and
lost days of work; key informant interviews with four
Health and Safety Committee members; observation
and progressive inquiry with 12 stockers during two
night shifts

#### Plan

*Priority action statement with evidence*: Stockers have
potential for improved back health related to accessible
back injury prevention training. Evidence: injury
statistics for previous three years show back pain as

the most common cause for lost days of work, stockers
have the most lost days of work from back pain, no back
injury prevention training available to staff working
evenings and nights, Health and Safety Committee
willing to provide training

*Project goal*: Stockers have improved back health.

*Strategy and intervention, theory, evidence base*: Health
education strategy using intervention of a workshop
to demonstrate safe lifting techniques. Intervention
modeled on *Ergonomic Guidelines for Manual Material
Handling* (Research and Education Unit, 2007) included
video, demonstrations, discussions, and content tailored
to meet needs of supermarket staff and training for
Health and Safety Committee members.

#### Objectives

*Ability objective*: By November 10, 60 percent of
participants in back injury prevention workshops for
stockers identify safe lifting techniques.

*Accomplishment objective*: By November 17, 40 percent
of trained stockers demonstrate safe lifting techniques
during work.

*Environmental objective*: By November 14, 75 percent of
Health and Safety Committee members are trained to
provide back injury prevention workshop to all shifts on
a regular basis.

#### Action

*Preparation*, Sept. 21–Oct. 7: Conduct literature search
for evidence base, observe and document lifting and
carrying behaviors, acquire room and equipment for
workshops and final presentation.

Develop tailored workshop, Sept. 22–Oct. 27: Locate
training video; develop, test, and rehearse material for
workshop and evaluation forms. Two pilot tests (two
weeks apart) with total of 9 participants. Considerable
adaptations after first pilot; minor after second.

*Deliver tailored workshop and train Health and Safety Committee members*: Tailored workshop package (see attachments) consisted of pretest, introduction, discussion on experiences of back pain, 25-minute video on safe lifting, demonstration of safe lifting followed by rating of lifts in demonstration, discussion about ways to increase safe lifting, posttest; on-site rating of participants. First workshop, Nov. 3: 7 participants plus 3 Health and Safety Committee members; second workshop, Nov. 10: 8 participants, led by 3 Health and Safety Committee members

*Evaluation of on-site lifting*, Nov. 3–17: Evaluation of lifting by trained stockers

### Key Findings
*Process*: Delivered two pilots and two workshops as planned. 26/40 (65 percent) stockers attended pilot or workshop. Components of intervention delivered as planned after second pilot. Video of 25 minutes had appropriate techniques, was approved by participants in workshop

*Environmental objective*: Three of four members (75 percent) of the Health and Safety Committee demonstrated ability to provide safe lifting workshop as estimated.

### Conclusions
Rating of lifts during demonstration for ability objective was easier than expected. On-site demonstrations of safe lifting for appreciation objective were lower than expected, possibly because of barriers explained in limitations. Overall, the tailored workshops show promise for improving safe lifting and can be competently continued by the trained members of the Health and Safety Committee.

*Limitations*: Two areas of the store are too small for safe lifting techniques as identified through observation, ratings, and feedback from workers. Limited time and high activity in store could have reduced results.

*Sustainability*: Three staff members are trained to provide workshops and have led one workshop. Management is supportive in making changes to environment and to hiring staff to promote back health.

*Recommendations*: (1) Safety workshops be given to all staff on a regular basis, (2) have certain areas of the store assessed to determine necessary modifications for safe work movements, (3) offer rewards for people "caught" lifting correctly or helping a co-worker maintain back health, and (4) distribute posters throughout the store demonstrating techniques pertinent to that area.

### Attachments
(The following would be attached here: reference list, notes, and worksheets related to workshop, pretests and posttests and handouts, slides from presentation, tabulation of evaluation data.)

*Impact*:

**Key Findings Compared to Criteria**

| Evaluation Measures | Workshop 1 (*n* = 7) | Workshop 2 (*n* = 10) | # (%) of Participants | Estimated | Difference |
|---|---|---|---|---|---|
| Ability | 7 | 8 | 15 (88%) | 60% | ⇑ 28% |
| Appreciation | 2 | 3 | 5 (29%) | 40% | ⇓ 11% |

# Part 3

# Approaches for Working in Different Settings and Situations

Chapters 9 through 14 provide examples of community nursing practice during home visits, in school and rural communities, in public health, and during an emergency. These chapters illustrate different strategies relevant to community health nursing and indicate how nursing students could be involved in longer term programs. Chapter 9 describes the role of community health nurses in the home, provides an approach to conducting safe and effective home visits, and identifies the risk factors associated with older-age and single-parent families. The case studies within the scenarios illustrate the approach during home visits to older adults and a single mother. Chapter 10 describes an approach to community capacity building and statistics indicating the vulnerability of young adolescents and rural residents. The scenarios illustrate community capacity building in a school with young adolescents and in a rural community to improve access to food.

Chapter 11 examines the practice of community health nurses as they collaborate with communities to form coalitions and develop the commitment and resources of the community to take action on community health issues. In this chapter, the focus is on promoting physical activity in youth. Chapter 12 provides an introduction to the role of community health nurses in developing and providing support for healthy public policy. The scenarios illustrate public health collaboration with other health institutions and workplaces to develop Baby-Friendly policies. As with the previous chapter, the beginning practitioner is mentored by an experienced public health nurse.

Program evaluation is the focus of Chapter 13. The chapter describes the use of logic models and evaluates an innovative TB prevention program for foreign-born students. The program provides screening, treatment, and contact tracing and includes approaches to build a supportive environment for the students at risk. The scenario illustrates how students in an urban setting begin to develop evaluation skills at a flu clinic. Chapter 14 describes the four components of disaster and emergency management, and the role of community health nurses in each component. The scenarios follow teams in recruiting partner organizations serving vulnerable populations during prevention and mitigation, and response; and in recruiting and training additional nurses for a flu pandemic during preparation.

# Chapter 9

# Approaches to Community Health Nursing of Families at Home

This chapter builds on the skills and knowledge of working with groups in preparation for working with families in the home. Family is at the heart of caring for people in both illness and health. After introducing different purposes for providing nursing services in the home, and different approaches, theories, and concepts related to family home nursing, the chapter guides you through ways to engage families while conducting a safe home visit.

With the perspective of a community health nurse, you identify the family's existing strengths and supports, provide opportunities for new supports in the community, and collaborate with health professionals in the community. Tools, examples, and scenarios assist you in applying the information. The chapter content is illustrated in case studies involving a prenatal home visit, home visits in both an urban and rural area, and a long-term care home visit. They also illustrate the application of home health nursing standards and competencies. By the end of the chapter, you will have developed an effective approach to working with families in the home that you can expand and adjust as you gain experience.

## Learning Objectives

After reading this chapter and answering the questions throughout the chapter, you should be able to:

1. Apply what you have learned about working with groups to working with families in the home.
2. Identify the value of family home nursing approaches, theories, and concepts to community health nursing.
3. Identify and consider the sociodemographic factors related to family home health for vulnerable older adults and families with infants.
4. Develop an approach that builds relationships with families.

### Key Terms and Concepts

Calgary Family Assessment and Intervention Models: 15-minute (or less) family interview, circular questions, commendations • case finding • case manager or care coordinator • family • family as a component of society • family as a system • family as context • family as client • family diagrams: family circle, interaction diagram • family home nursing • home • home health care worker • home visit • referral • referred visit • service providers • vulnerable people

5. Develop an approach to conduct safe home visits, assist families in preparing plans, and link them to community resources.
6. Develop an approach to identify and collaborate with community organizations that support families.

## Building on the Community Health Nursing Process to Work with Families in the Home

The community health nursing process you learned as you worked with groups and communities in earlier chapters has prepared you well for working with families. Now you understand how to work as a team and follow a process, and are familiar with working in the unstructured environment of the community. The new aspects to learn in this chapter relate to the family, conducting home visits, and collaborating with other professionals and service providers in the community. **Service providers** are people who receive pay to provide services and include nurses, social workers, physicians, ministers, and house cleaners.

During assessment of the family, you identify the health concerns and strengths as you did with groups. The assessment is aided by family nursing approaches, theories, models, and concepts in addition to the broader approaches used with groups and communities. Each source of information supports the approach of the community health nurse in considering the needs and strengths of the family and linking the family to resources in the community.

Although this chapter emphasizes developing relations with families and with community organizations, rather than interventions with families, you will find most of the

---

**SCENARIO: Developing Case Studies for Home Visiting**

Cheryl is the manager of a home health care organization that provides nursing and other health professional and home support services to referred clients with acute and chronic illnesses living in rural and urban areas. Cheryl frequently discusses issues with Sharon, a public health nurse and supervisor of a branch office of public health in the same building, and with Ron, the outreach manager of a nearby community health center. The three managers agree that nurses seeking employment at their organizations are usually unsure about how to conduct home visits.

They decide to put together a guide for home visits as part of their orientation material, but do not feel that that alone will be sufficient. They want some way to focus on the diversity of approaches needed to nurse people in the home. Sharon recounts how they used the practice experiences of nurses in a workshop on new nursing standards. She suggests that they could involve

community health nursing students in developing case studies based on practice stories they collect during their clinical experience. Cheryl and Ron like the idea that the students will learn about different situations in home visiting and that the three organizations will have realistic material for their orientation. They each decide to organize a placement for a team of community health nursing students to work with experienced nurses who make home visits.

**Discussion Topics and Questions**
1. What experiences have you had with people receiving nursing care in the home?
2. What do you feel would make the experience of receiving home nursing care a positive or less positive experience?

For suggested responses, please see the Answer Key at the back of the book.

---

information on taking action familiar. The emphasis is on engaging people and initiating a change process that is relevant to them.

One area of difference in family home nursing is that you will be learning to visit people on your own or with a supervisor, rather than working together with a group. However, teamwork is still a factor in preparation, planning, and follow-up through weekly team meetings and Internet communication.

You will likely find it easier to learn about working with families than it was to learn about working with groups. Not only have you been prepared by working with a group, you can draw on your own experiences of family.

## Community Health Nursing of Families at Home

Home nursing with families is a combination of home health nursing, family nursing, and community health nursing. Home health nursing is also called "home care nursing" or "home visiting nursing" (see Chapter 1) and has been a practice in both the US and Canada since the late 1890s. The concept of family as the unit of care began to emerge in nursing school curriculums in the 1960s (Rowe Kaakinen & Harmon Hanson, 2014a).

Community health nursing includes family home nursing because community health nurses work across the continuum of care and where people live to promote health (Community Health Nurses of Canada, 2011). Community health nursing broadens the perspective of nursing in the home and with the family. The focus of this chapter is on the value and types of home visits with families, use of effective interviewing to engage family members, a process for conducting home visits that includes safety factors, linking families to community resources, and working collaboratively with other professionals and services working in the home. The "Website Resources" at the end of the chapter provide links to expand on family nursing and home nursing.

Definitions of both family and home have broadened and become more flexible to be consistent with present society. A **family** is defined as two or more individuals who identify themselves as members of the same family and depend on one another for emotional, physical, and economic support (Rowe Kaakinen & Harmon Hanson, 2014a). According to Wright and Leahey (2000, p. 70), "Families are who they say they are." The most important part of the family definition is that the members agree that they are family. Family can include a mother, father, children, and elderly or young relations living together; same-sex couples with or without children; or a homeless woman and her friend. **Home** is a place that provides shelter and some measure of safety. A home can be a house, an apartment, a residence, or a tent. For some people, home may be a homeless shelter, or a space under a bridge that provides more protection from the weather and other people than being out on the street.

All nursing care originated in the home. Although most nursing care of those who are ill is now provided in institutions, providing nursing care for at-risk or ill people at home remains an important strategy to reach vulnerable people. **Vulnerable people**, as discussed in earlier chapters, are those who have or are at-risk for poor health because of their race/ethnicity, socioeconomic status, geography, gender, age, disability status, sex, or gender (Centers for Disease Control and Prevention, 2014). The risk can arise from a developmental stage, such as pregnant women and newborn infants; unprotected sexual intercourse; exposure to infectious diseases, such as tuberculosis; social isolation; and factors associated with poverty, such as insufficient food, health care, and protection from heat and cold.

Home visits are often the only way to reach vulnerable people and therefore directly address the social determinants of access and equity. A **home visit** is the provision of community health nursing care to an individual or family at home (Stanhope, Lancaster, Jessup-Falcioni, & Viverais-Dresler, 2011). People may be restricted to their homes because of limited mobility from a disability, surgery, illness, or giving birth. Social isolation and poor mental health also limits people from seeking health care outside the home.

## Purposes of Community Health Nursing Home Visits

Community health nurses visit individuals and families at home for one of the following three purposes: (1) care of the sick and dying, (2) health promotion and illness prevention, and (3) case finding and referral. Each purpose is introduced below and elaborated later in case studies.

Home visits for the purpose of caring for the sick and for health promotion and illness prevention are initiated by a referral. A **referral** is a request or recommendation from one health professional or organization to another to provide a service to an individual or family. A **referred visit** to a home could result from a request by a health professional, organization, friend, neighbor, or family member within the home. For example, a doctor, school, or other social service organization can refer the family for a home visit. Case finding visits are usually initiated because of an organizational program or mandate.

### Care of the Sick and Dying

Care of the sick and dying is the major reason for a home nursing visit. People receive nursing care in the home because they are ill and have no family, or their family is unable to provide all the care they need. They may also choose to receive nursing care at home to maintain their independence and to avoid the usually higher costs of long-term care facilities.

Care of the sick at home is provided by home care services, which include home health and support services. Home health services include nursing as well as physical, occupational, and respiratory services by licensed health personnel. The predominant health professional in home care is nursing in both the US (National Center for Health Statistics, 2012) and Canada (Canadian Institute for Health Information, 2011). Personnel providing home support services assist with activities such as light housework and personal care (activities of daily living).

Home visits are largely conducted by nurses working for home health care organizations or, in some areas, organizations providing both primary care and home nursing services. In the US and Canada, home health care receives limited national funding and is delivered by nonprofit or proprietary (for-profit) health care organizations. Public health nurses conduct home visits for the care of the sick as part of a protocol for treating people with infectious diseases, such as tuberculosis or sexually transmitted diseases.

The need for home care in North America is expected to grow along with the expected increase in numbers of older people in both the US and Canada. In the US, those who are 65 years and older are expected to constitute 20 percent of the population by 2030

(National Center for Health Statistics, 2011). Canada expects a similar rise in the number of seniors (25 percent of the population by 2036) (Canadian Institute for Health Information, 2011).

The report of the National Center for Health Statistics (2011) on home health care states that the number of Americans receiving home health each day in 2007 was 1,459,900, a 7 percent increase since 2000. Most of the patients were 65 years or older (69 percent), women (64 percent), and lived with family or nonfamily members (68.5 percent). The Canadian Institute for Health Information (2011) estimates that 1 million Canadians receive home care at any given time; about 8 out of every 10 of these are seniors.

A fact sheet on age and socioeconomic status from the American Psychological Association (2014) identifies several factors related to poverty and older age: older people are among the most economically vulnerable groups, especially women, African-Americans, and Hispanics; have increased mortality rates for several physical and mental health diseases; have lower quality of life; and have smaller and less integrated social networks. Statistics Canada (2014) notes that studies have shown that the risk of health deterioration increases significantly when home care needs are not met, and some studies show that older adults who receive the most social support and professional home care services are less likely to be institutionalized. Consequently, the summary concludes that meeting the home care needs of individuals may encourage them to live in their homes for a longer period of time.

The information on home care utilization and the expected increase in the numbers of older people emphasize the importance of providing the appropriate home care for people who want to remain at home. Community health nurses have an important role to play in the well-being of the older population by advocating for appropriate funding for home health care and providing nursing care that includes the broader environment, such as promoting social support and links to community resources.

### Health Promotion and Illness Prevention

Home visits for health promotion and illness prevention are the primary focus for community health nurses employed by public health organizations. Frequently these visits deal with maternal, infant, and child health. Special programs might also include home visiting, such as a program to reduce falls in older adults.

National reports on births and the sociodemographics of mothers assist in understanding some of the issues related to caring for mothers and infants at home. Fertility rates for women under 30 has been decreasing, and for those over 30, increasing (Statistics Canada, 2013a). Similar trends are occurring in the US (Martin, Hamilton, Osterman, Curtin, & Mathews, 2013). The percentage of births to unmarried women (women who are not married or living common-law) has been fairly constant at approximately 33 percent for Canada (Statistics Canada, 2013b) and 40 percent for the US (Martin et al., 2013) over the last few years. In both countries, single mothers tend to be living in poverty, are less than 19 years of age, are of an ethnic minority, especially Aboriginal (Canada) or American Indian or Alaskan Native, and have less than a high-school education. These statistics for single mothers indicate that social and health programs are not yet reducing the number of "children having children" and raising them in poverty.

Child poverty is not decreasing in the US and Canada (Anderson Moore, Redd, Burkhauser, Kassim Mbwana, & Collins, 2009; Campaign 2000, 2014). Poverty affects the mother and child throughout their lives: for the mother, through poor maternal nutrition, reduced mental state, and lessened ability to manage child care; and for the child, through low birth weight, chronic ill health, and poor learning (Crawford, 2008; Larson, 2007).

These statistics related to the effects of poverty on mothers and children have implications for home visits. Families living in poverty have multiple requirements for community support, including education, health promotion, and links to community resources.

### Case Finding and Referral

**Case finding** are contacts initiated by a health care organization with people in their home or the community to offer health care and referrals to reduce a risk factor. For example, a public health department or community health center may decide to conduct outreach visits to isolated older people, homeless people, or families living near a hazardous dump site. Case finding is frequently used during an emergency to identify and refer people at risk.

When the contact is to screen for families at risk, such as mothers having difficulty caring for children, short and specific assessment tools for the mother and infant often guide the visit. In other situations, extensive assessment tools may be required by agencies or funding bodies. Before these tools are used, the nurse is expected to spend some time conversing with the family members to gain some understanding of their experiences and explain the tool before launching into the assessment.

Case finding is particularly important during an emergency, such as a power outage due to a heat wave, ice storm, earthquake, or flooding. Without electricity, people may try to cook or heat using unsafe equipment for the house, such as a barbecue, and those who are dependent on mobility devices, such as wheelchairs, will be unable to use the elevators in apartment buildings. People in these situations need to be contacted at home, assessed for risk, and, if necessary, referred to a shelter facility. Preparations to assist vulnerable people during an emergency are described in Chapter 14.

Visits based on case finding and referrals usually occur because a person or family meets defined criteria. Ways of approaching people about a possible health risk when the contact is unexpected are discussed in "Addressing Challenges during Home Visits," later in the chapter.

## Advantages and Disadvantages of Home Visits

Several authors have pointed out that home visits have both advantages and disadvantages for families, community health nurses, and the health care system (Clark, 2008; Rowe Kaakinen & Harmon Hanson, 2014b; Stanhope et al., 2011). Home visits provide both the context of the home visit and the involvement of family to increase the impact of nursing care in the home. Community health nurses doing home visits have the opportunity to focus on the family; develop a relationship; observe the physical, social, and emotional environment surrounding the client/family; and work with the family to identify their strengths and address specific needs and potential health problems. In other words, the home environment encourages collaboration in the development of realistic nursing care and plans with the family.

Economically, home care services for older adults can alleviate demands for hospitalization, reduce readmissions and the likelihood of institutionalization, and can be more cost-efficient than residential care (Statistics Canada, 2012). Home visits also help prevent fragmented care for specified groups, such as infants who are vulnerable because of poverty, social risk, or prematurity (Kearney, York, & Deatrick, 2000).

Home nursing visits are not able to meet the needs of all the people who would like to receive nursing care at home (Clark, 2008; Rowe Kaakinen & Harmon Hanson, 2014b; Stanhope et al., 2011). For example, some home care patients might need "24/7" nursing care to be able to remain at home. Frequently the number of hours of care and type of services are limited by government restraints. This limit on services places a burden on people who are ill, on their families, and on professional caregivers. Families may prefer more formal surroundings or be overburdened by providing care in the home.

The National Alliance for Caregiving in collaboration with AARP (2009) identified that more than three in ten US households (31.2 percent) report that at least one person has served as an unpaid family caregiver within the last 12 months, most caregivers are women (66 percent), and a third care for two or more people. The report identifies that, on average, caregivers spend 20.4 hours per week providing care, and caregivers who live with the recipient spend 39.3 hours per week providing care.

In Canada, a survey of Canadians over 45 in 2014 indicates that 26 percent participate in providing care to an aging relative or friend (Canadian Medical Association, 2014). The Canadian Institute for Health Information (2011) reports that almost all seniors receiving home care (97 percent) have informal caregivers: 33 percent are spouses, and 50 percent are children. Caregivers experience stress in their role, as the number of hours they provide each week increases: 8 percent report stress at 10 hours or less per week, 17 percent report stress at 11 to 20 hours, and 32 percent report stress at 21+ hours (Canadian Institute for Health Information, 2011).

For community health nurses, home visits are more time-consuming, create difficulty in maintaining professional distance, raise safety concerns related to the home and neighborhood, and are subject to more interruptions and distractions (Allender, Rector, & Warner, 2010; Stanhope et al., 2011). Community health nurses can find home visits stressful because equipment or consultations with others are not immediately accessible, clients are diverse and have a multiplicity of problems, and situations are constantly changing.

The advantages and disadvantages to clients, community health nurses, and the health care system emphasize the need to capitalize on the advantages and minimize the disadvantages of home visits. Certain actions can address some of the disadvantages of home visits for community health nurses and promote health and injury prevention in the home. The first is supporting nurses while they learn to develop collaborative relationships with families and service providers in the community. Developing health-promoting practices with families requires time and considerable reflection. Health-promoting practices include changing the focus from working with one person to working with the whole family, and moving from an emphasis on disease or behavior modification to a focus on helping the family deal with the socioenvironmental aspects of health (Hartrick, 1998).

This change to focusing on the family, rather than just the client, benefits the client, family, and nurse. The approach fosters a caring environment for the client and family where each person's perspective is considered when making plans that include connecting to appropriate community resources. At the same time, the community health nurse is in a supporting role to foster family problem solving.

Moving to a family focus also assists practitioners new to the home environment to maintain a professional distance. Over-involvement can arise from long-term involvement with a family in the home and from feeling responsible for all the care that is provided. Signs of over-involvement include accepting or giving gifts, providing too much personal information, or feeling that you are the only professional who can provide the appropriate care to that family (College of Registered Nurses of Nova Scotia, 2012). The nursing association in your jurisdiction likely provides guidance on maintaining professional boundaries.

Another action to improve home visiting for community health nurses is to provide procedures and support for effective and safe nursing care in the home. Home visits are distinguished from other sites used in the provision of community health nursing care by the intimacy and privacy of the situation. The privacy of the home visit also means that the nurse is more exposed to unsafe situations in both the neighborhood and the home itself. Safety procedures during home visits are included in the section "Home Visiting Process," below. These measures are particularly important for nurses doing home visits because they usually conduct visits alone. Support from peers and guidelines for community health nurses will encourage the maximum health benefit for families receiving nursing home visits.

## Approaches to Family Nursing in the Home

**Family home nursing** consists of using the community health nursing process with family and family members to build on their strengths to address their concerns. Community health nurses working in the home have the advantage of adding family nursing approaches, theories, concepts, and frameworks to their knowledge of the community.

Family nursing identifies four different approaches for working with families. The four approaches are: (1) family as the context or structure, (2) family as client, (3) family as system, and (4) family as a component of society (Rowe Kaakinen & Harmon Hanson, 2014a). These approaches have evolved from different perspectives of family and provide a lens for considering a family in different situations.

**Family as context** is the traditional approach used with families and places the individual first and the family as second. Alternate labels for this approach are "family-centered" or "family-focused." With this approach, the community health nurse might ask the individual, for example, if the change to a diabetic diet will affect the rest of the family, or if efforts to quit smoking would be supported by the rest of the family.

**Family as client** places all family members in the foreground and assesses how each person is affected by the health event of one family member. This approach is usually used in primary care clinics in the community where families are seen over time by general practice physicians or nurse practitioners. Using this approach, a community health nurse might ask a family member who has just become dependent on a wheelchair and other family members how the change has affected the family, who is available to assist with transfers, and who has the most difficulty with the change.

**Family as a system** focuses on family interactions. This approach assumes that when something happens in one part of the system, such as a family member becoming ill, other parts are also affected. This approach developed from the specialty of psychiatric and mental health nursing. Questions based on this approach might involve changes between siblings if, for instance, one is allergic to nuts, or a change in relations between parents if a teen girl becomes pregnant.

**Family as a component of society** includes the family unit as one of the institutions of society, along with health, education, religious, and financial institutions. The approach focuses on the interface between the family and community agencies. Questions based on this approach might be about family relations with the school if a child has been charged with Internet bullying or the use of community support programs for families of alcoholics.

Each of the four approaches could be used at different times and situations. The most usual practice for community health nurses is to combine the approaches of family as client, family as a system, and family as a component of society. Importantly, family members who are ill or stressed benefit from approaches that recognize and mobilize family support. The questions used in each of the approaches help to identify both the family issues and family strengths.

Community health nurses are able to blend these approaches and consider ways to make home visiting more effective and efficient. For example, they can group together families with similar characteristics, such as being in the same stage of family development, or families dealing with a confused family member, for planning and intervention purposes. The purpose of grouping is to identify common concerns and strengths that apply to most families in the group and thereby identify promising practices, and then further tailor the practice for each family. The grouping can be within a community health nurse's caseload or within a team. The approach is similar to working with a group except that the families do not interact with each other.

## Theories, Models, Frameworks, and Concepts in Family Nursing

According to Rowe Kaakinen and Harmon Hanson (2014a), the interaction of theory, practice, and research creates a synergy, which leads to improved quality of care. For example, community health nurses are particularly interested in the family's social support system, which is included in the external and context portions of Wright and Leahey's (2013) family structure and the family-as-a-component-of-society approach. The four types of supportive behaviors—emotional, instrumental, informational, and appraisal (Heaney & Israel, 2008)—are usually provided by different people. Family members often provide each other with emotional support, such as empathy, love, trust, and care. Family and home care support staff can provide instrumental or practical support, such as preparing meals, cleaning house, and transportation. Health care professionals, family, and friends can provide informational support, such as education and referral resources in the community. Family, close friends, and home health care staff can provide appraisal or feedback support. Community health nurses need to learn about the family so they can assist them in connecting with people to meet each type of social support need.

The Calgary Family Assessment and Integration Models is one of the top three national and international family models. The **Calgary Family Assessment and Intervention Models** (Wright & Leahey, 2013) are based on a systems model that includes a structural, developmental, and functional assessment and has unique intervention features, such as the 15-minute (or less) family interview, and stresses the importance of commendations. Some aspects of the Calgary Family Models and approaches are used throughout this chapter.

## Community Health Nursing Process with Families at Home

As with assessments of individuals, groups, and communities, the community health nursing process with families at home is used to identify health concerns and strengths, and plan and take action to improve the health of the family. The use of the community health nursing process with families at home depends on the family situation, the purpose of the home visit, and the expected number of home visits. For example, community health nurses may see mothers with infants when they are first discharged from the hospital for one or two visits, families with a disabled child for one or two months, and families dealing with a chronic illness for several years.

Many of the families who are visited by nurses are struggling to survive as well as care for a family member who is ill. These families may have just arrived in the country, may not speak the language, may be poor, or may in other ways be dealing with unknown difficulties. When working with these vulnerable families, community health nurses are expected to learn about their cultural practices, especially as they relate to children. They are also expected to consistently engage in reflection, as described in Chapter 2. Although an interpreter from the cultural community could assist with obtaining the family history, building an ongoing relationship requires that the family and nurse converse directly. Suggestions for using plain language are given in the Appendix 7.2.

The following sections prepare you for conducting home visits. The first explains how to develop therapeutic relations with the family using Wright and Leahey's (2013) 15-minute (or less) family interview. The second outlines a step-by-step procedure for conducting a safe home visit. The third provides practical information on finding community resources for the family.

### Developing Therapeutic Relationships with Families in the Home

Home visiting provides the opportunity to build a health-promoting relationship with families, even when the relationship is short term. This relationship is fostered by privacy, a sense of intimacy, a relaxed environment, and continuity of care in the home environment. A synthesis of qualitative studies indicates that building and preserving relationships with clients in the home is at the core of home nursing (McNaughton, 2000).

Guidelines for establishing professional, collaborative relationships with families are adapted from Wright and Leahey's (2013) brief family interview. Janice Bell (2012), editor of the *Journal of Family Nursing*, states that the use of this interview technique has spread throughout the world and seems to instill a sense of competence and confidence in even the novice practitioner. The **15-minute (or less) family interview** has six key instructions: (1) begin the therapeutic conversation with a purpose that can be accomplished in 15 minutes or less; (2) use manners to engage or re-engage the family; (3) assess key areas of internal (e.g., family composition, relationships), external (e.g., extended family, larger systems), and context (e.g., ethnicity, social class, religion, environment) structure and function (e.g., activities of daily living, communication, problem solving, beliefs); (4) ask three key questions; (5) commend the family on one or two strengths; and (6) evaluate usefulness and conclude (Wright & Leahey, 2013). This interview process focuses more on the family as client and family as a system.

Wright and Leahey's (2013) 15-minute (or less) interview is a unique and powerful tool to initiate change in families because it integrates task-oriented care with an inter-active purposeful conversation, and recognizes and affirms the family's illness and health experiences. The most therapeutic aspect of the interview is showing compassion and recognizing family strengths in the form of commendations (Bell, 2012; Bell & Wright, 2011; Moules & Johnston, 2010). The goal is not to determine problems but to under-stand the family's view of the world. Wright and Leahey (2013) identify how the interview differs from social conversation. In the home, the differences in the interview include

- acknowledgement of the patient's and the family's skill in managing health problems.
- encouragement to practice how they will handle interactions differently in the future.
- routinely consulting with family and patients about their ideas for treatment and discharge.

**Begin with a Purpose**

When preparing for the interview, choose a topic that can be adequately discussed in 15 minutes or less. Conversations in the brief family interview are purposeful and time-limited and acknowledge and affirm people (Wright & Leahey, 2013). Explain the purpose of the interview and check to see if the purpose is acceptable to the family. Adjust the topic if necessary.

Before beginning the interview, try and position family members so that everyone can see each other. You will likely find that sitting around a table works better than sitting in a living room, because a table often encourages conversation. In other circumstances, you may be grouped around a family member who is receiving care. You want people to be comfortable, as well as focused on the discussion or the care you are providing. If some family members are unable to be present, have someone explain why they are unable to be present and their role in the family so you have a more complete picture of all family members. During the discussion, ask how the person might feel about dif-ferent topics throughout the discussion.

Allow some time for the family to become oriented to you and what you want to discuss or do. In other words, go slowly. Watch body language and wait until people are settled before you start.

**Use Manners to Engage or Re-engage the Family**

Using manners helps to establish a collaborative relationship and builds trust and understanding. When you contact people to arrange the visit, give your name, role, and the name of anyone who may accompany you. As well, when first meeting people face-to-face, introduce yourself and provide your title (e.g., "I am Jean Roland, a student nurse working with home care. This is my advisor, Vicky, a home health nurse"), establish eye contact, provide the reason for contacting them, and invite their participation in the care (Wright & Leahey, 2013). As you meet other family members or friends, continue to introduce yourself and others the same way. If possible, invite their participation. For example, "Hi, Jake. My name is Jean Roland, a student nurse working with public health. I've been working with your mother and younger sister to try to figure out an easier way to feed your sister. Do you want to watch? Maybe you'll have some ideas."

Another aspect of a collaborative relationship is fulfilling promises and being honest (Wright & Leahey, 2013). If you say that you will do some task, ensure that you remember to do it within the time period stated. If you are not able to perform the task, or forget, be honest. When asked for a favor, be honest and inform people as to what you can and cannot provide. This needs to be done in a manner that is noncritical and clearly provides limits. For example, if you are asked for a ride, say, "The organization has quite strict rules. I am not able to take anyone anywhere in my car," rather than "I cannot take you to the store because I do not have time right now." The latter response suggests that at other times you would be willing to take the person in the car.

You also need to establish boundaries in a collaborative relationship. For example, refreshments or gifts may be considered appropriate by the family, and the nurse could be considered unsociable if the offers are not accepted. A middle ground could be to accept the offer of refreshments at the end of the visit if time allows rather than the beginning (Wright & Leahey, 2013). This shows a willingness to accept hospitality while indicating some boundaries on the interaction. Gifts, especially expensive gifts, are not acceptable in a professional relationship. The spirit of giving needs to be recognized, and possibly a smaller token such as food can be substituted. When family members talk about what you have done for them, emphasize how they have helped you gain a greater knowledge about working with families.

### Assess Key Areas of Internal, External, and Context Structure and Function

Mapping of family members and relationships within the family and with the community greatly assists with the assessment and your understanding of the family's connections (Wright & Leahey, 2013). If this is not the first visit, similar information may have been collected in an admission form. However, the use of family mapping diagrams provides a visual depiction of the family and greatly facilitates a collaborative effort. If the situation is appropriate and there is no map of the family, you are encouraged to initiate one on your first encounter with a family. If there is a map available, review it and possibly update it with the family.

Two types of family mapping diagrams are typically used in family nursing: the genogram and the ecomap. The genogram depicts the family tree. It includes three generations: the parents, siblings, and offspring. The ecomap is a visual representation of the family in relation to the community, and indicates the nature and quality of relationships (Wright & Leahey, 2013). The symbols and instructions for genograms and ecomaps are provided in most community health and family health texts. Genograms and ecomaps can help the community health nurse sort out difficult or complicated relationships.

An alternative, simplified system is proposed that uses two **family diagrams** that are completed in three phases, either during one visit or perhaps over two or three visits, depending on the family situation. The first diagram is called the family circle and the other the family interaction diagram. Together they help to provide a picture of the family's connections for both the family and the nurse. The **family circle** indicates the family members and family and friends who frequently relate to them. An **interaction diagram** indicates the people who are physically and emotionally available to the family according to frequency of contact and category of relationship. Involving the family in developing the diagrams is a strategy that quickly engages family members and sends a clear message that you are interested in them as a family (Wright & Leahey, 2013). Completing these diagrams with families who do not speak the same language as the nurse will be difficult, but is worth pursuing. Possibly another family member, a friend, or an interpreter can assist in obtaining the information for the mapping. Often, if the family understands the symbols used in the map, the symbols can be pointed to during discussions to be sure that the relationships are understood.

Phase 1 involves mapping the relationships with family and friends using the family circle, a simple hand-drawn diagram. The family circle quickly identifies the people in the family and the people important to the family (Thrower & Walton, 1982) and can be included in every first encounter you make with a family. The family circle will probably take the family only a few minutes to complete.

Introduce the idea by drawing a large circle to represent the family as it is now and by saying "As a health professional, I am interested in you, your family, and the people who are important to you." Invite all available family members to take part in completing the circle. Ask the family members to draw smaller circles for women or squares for men to represent themselves and the people important to them—family and others. The size of each circle or square indicates the person's significance or influence. Ask them to include the person's age and name in the middle of the square or circle. People can be inside or outside the large circle, touching or far apart. Encourage them to include people whom they would call upon if they needed help. There are no right or wrong circles.

The result is a family circle that is a schematic diagram of a family system completed by family members (Thrower & Walton, 1982). Date the family circle and additions or revisions. The diagram can then be used as a point of discussion about family connections and the support provided by different people. An example of a completed family circle is shown in Figure 9.2.

If the family will be seen for more than one visit, ask them to draw a circle around the people who live with them. The symbols for the people in the household are then placed in the inner circle of the family interaction diagram in Figure 9.1. The various circles in the family interaction diagram are explained in Figure 9.1.

Phase 2 involves mapping interactions to include the people in the family circle who interact with the ill family member or caregiver each week. The people are included in the family interaction diagram in the middle circle and in one of the four categories. Not all these people may have been included in the family circle. Because of the broad definition of family, the distinctions between family and friends may be blurred. Service providers are those who receive pay to provide services.

After completing the inner and middle circles, the nurse and family will be able to clearly see the number of people who interact with the family often and the importance of these people to the family. Some categories, such as community organizations, may not be involved at all and could be a potential source of support for the family. The family interaction diagram allows the family and nurse to objectively see what connections the family has and, if needed, what sources of support could be expanded.

Phase 3 involves mapping the people who interact with the family less often than weekly. Checking with the family will reveal whether the interaction diagram is complete. When the family interaction diagram is first completed, the start and completion dates should be indicated. As changes occur, such as a death, birth, or someone leaving home,

**Figure 9.1: Family Interaction Diagram**

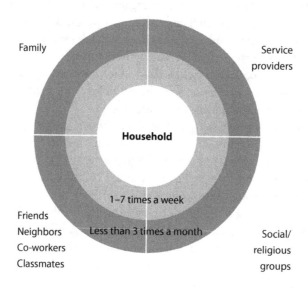

**Instructions for Completing Figure 9.1**

The family interaction diagram consists of three circular areas indicating different frequencies of interaction among people and the categories of people involved in the interactions.

The diagram is an adaptation of an ecomap developed for use with elderly persons by Moyer, Jamault, Roberge, and Murphy (1998). People in the inner circle live in the same household and interact daily. People in the outer two circles interact less frequently and are divided into categories. *Inner circle*: The people who are in the household are shown in the inner circle. A square is used for a male; a circle is used for a female. Age and name are included. If a person from the household has died, this is shown with an X through the appropriate gender symbol, and a date of death is included. Pets may be included in this circle. *Middle circle*: This circle includes people with at least weekly contact with the person requiring care or the primary caregiver. The same symbols apply. Four categories are used to indicate the source of support for personal care and community living needs such as shopping and banking: family, friends and neighbors, informal clubs and groups, and service providers from the community. These four

categories are shown as four quadrants. The quadrants are not meant to be absolute, but do give an indication of the sources of support to measure the ability to live alone. They could be used to show areas of strength and weaknesses, where support is weak and needs to be bolstered, and potential sources of support. Connections to the person requiring care or to the caregiver are provided by different types of lines. An unbroken line means a face-to-face interaction. A line made with dashes means the contact is not usually face-to-face. When contact is usually made by telephone, email, or letter, a T, E, or L, respectively, is used with the dashed line. An arrow in one direction or another means that the visitor always comes to the home or the person always makes the visit. Arrows in both directions indicate that there is visiting both ways. A line with crossed lines is an indicator of negative emotions attached to the relationship. *Outer circle*: The four categories in this area include people who interact with the family household less than once a week. The system of recording the social connections is the same as that used in the middle circle.

the changes can be added in another color to keep the diagram up to date. New connections, such as joining a self-help group, also need to be added. As new health practitioners encounter the family, the diagrams can be used to orient them to the family situation.

The act of completing the family interaction diagram together is almost more important than the final diagram. By working with the family to complete the diagram, the community health nurse builds rapport with the family, and the family gains a different perspective on how they function.

### Ask Three Key Questions

The nurse engages the family in therapeutic conversation to help each family member understand and express the meaning of common and unique experiences. The conversation, although purposeful, is more free flowing than an interview to allow new ideas to emerge. This means that when questions are posed, answers are not cut off prematurely by opinions or conclusions. For example, in a family living with a confused elderly grandparent, the nurse would seek each family member's experience and perspective on living with someone who is confused and continue with more detailed questions to clarify what was said. This approach is consistent with considering the family as client.

When you ask questions in a certain way, you encourage family members to talk about their experience with illness or the family's illness story. **Circular questions** are open-ended questions where one question leads to another to reveal explanations for problems (Wright & Leahey, 2013). This means that the nurse asks a question, such as "What has it been like for the family living with _____ (name of person) having this condition?" and allows each person time to think and respond. The nurse's response should indicate some understanding of the family's experience and encourage further discussion. The drawing out of these illness stories requires an attitude of "listening to learn" and is an art as well as ethical practice (Bell & Wright, 2011).

As a general guide, some possible questions (adapted from Wright & Leahey, 2013) follow:

- What is it like to live with someone who has _____ (name condition)?
- What makes it easier or more difficult?
- What has the family done that has made it easier for you?
- What has worked for your family in the past? What has not worked?

In the home, a major issue is the burden on caregivers. Often caregivers can be putting forth a tremendous effort to the detriment of their own health. When caregivers have the opportunity to converse about the effect the illness has on their lives, they are better able to sustain and conserve family relationships (Tapp, 2001). Various questions related to caregiver burden need to be included with every visit.

The nurse opens up possibilities in these conversations by providing information from different sources, linking the family with other community resources, or using other means such as literature to stimulate discussion. The purpose is to clarify what has been taken for granted and to discover new patterns to promote family health and healing by considering the family as a component of society.

Four nursing students were asked to prepare a case study explaining the use of the 15-minute family interview. For their clinical experience, they were assigned to the postnatal home visiting team in public health and given the opportunity to observe the approaches of different public health nurses as they visited families of new infants living in urban and rural areas. By the third week, they were starting to conduct parts of the visit, and by the sixth week, they had each done all parts of a full visit under the supervision of the public health nurse.

On their way to the home visits, the students had the opportunity to ask the public health nurses about their use of the family interview. They kept field notes of what they observed and learned from the public health nurses, communicated by email after each clinical day, and prepared drafts of the case study, which they reviewed with the nurses. After six weeks, they completed the case study to be used for orientation and training.

## Case Study Using the 15-Minute (or Less) Family Interview with a Single Mother

Nancy, a new public health nurse, arrives at Julie's home to conduct a second postnatal home visit. Nancy is feeling a bit nervous because she is to do this visit alone, rather than with the nurse who did the first visit. Nancy remembers what the nurse told her: "Pay attention to the diagrams. They are like the family's life story and help them see things more objectively, and, of course, help us to get a picture of the family better than any photograph!"

Julie invites Nancy in. Nancy introduces herself, explains that she is there to conduct the second visit with Julie and her family, and tells her why the nurse she saw before is unable to be there. Julie proudly shows off

her month-old son, who is sleeping in a crib in the next room, and her daughter Lea, who is on the floor playing. Nancy explains that she would like to talk to Julie for a few minutes before she weighs the baby. Julie nods and they sit down at the table in the kitchen.

Nancy pulls out the family circle diagram that Julie completed at the first visit. She asks Julie to tell her about the people indicated in the diagram. Julie points to the circles of herself and two children and says they are the only ones now living in the home. Nancy asks her to draw a circle around the three of them. Julie's family circle is displayed in Figure 9.2.

**Figure 9.2: Julie's Family Circle, February 10, 2014, March 2, 2014**

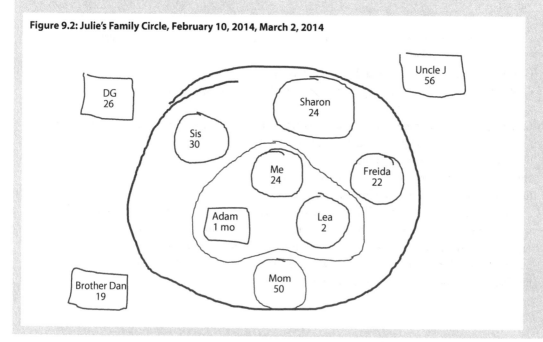

Julie then starts talking about her friend Sharon and how much she does for her, along with her mom and sister. She mentions two other friends but not as much. Nancy senses that they are both now relaxed and asks Julie if they could complete another diagram (Figure 9.1) that shows how often people are involved with the family. Julie seems to enjoy filling in the diagram and asks Nancy questions about how to indicate different ways of connecting with people. Figure 9.3 displays Julie's completed interaction diagram.

Nancy moves on in the interview and asks Julie how she is feeling about being on her own with two children. Julie says that she feels much stronger now without DG, whom she asked to move out six months ago. She appreciates the help she gets from her mom, sister, and friends and helps them in return when she can. Nancy gathers from the conversation that Julie interacts with someone outside the house on most days. During the conversation, Nancy notices that Julie is keeping an eye on Lea and easily substitutes a fork that has fallen off the table with a toy.

When Nancy points to the diagram and asks about involvement with community groups, Julie comments that her social worker had asked the same thing. Julie says she just does not have the time right now. Nancy mentions that a group of young mothers meets at the nearby community health center, which also has a clothing exchange program. Julie laughs and says that will be a good reason to go because she has to get some clothes for her boy. All the clothes that she and her friends have are frilly and pink!

Nancy brings the interview to an end by saying that Julie is really showing responsibility for her children by her actions, keeping up her relations with family and friends, and maintaining a positive attitude about herself. Julie seemed a bit taken aback after Nancy's statements, but then says, "Yeah, I guess you are right. Everyone says I am like that punching doll that keeps popping back up!"

**Discussion Topics and Questions**

3. What assistance did the circle diagram provide in the interview?
4. Discuss how Julie might have felt at the end of the home visit if Nancy had arrived and concentrated on weighing and testing the baby and asked about what he was eating.

**Figure 9.3: Julie's Interaction Diagram, March 2, 2014**

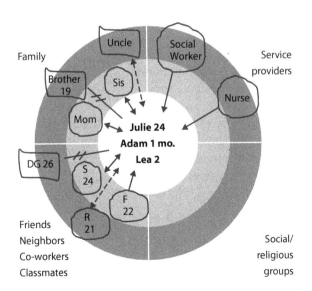

### Commend the Family on One or Two Strengths

During the conversations the nurse commends family members on their functioning. **Commendations** are observations or reports of strengths, resources, or competencies that have occurred over time and are reflected back to the family during the discussion (Wright & Leahey, 2013). Wright and Leahey emphasize that commending the family and individuals on their strengths is an important role of the nurse and state that at least one or two should be offered in each 15-minute family interview. Commending is providing affirmation support. Porr (2015) found that when public health nurses engaged single mothers in a positive manner and offered verbal commendations, the mothers' defensiveness was reduced and the process of relationship building was improved.

Examples of commendations are: "I see that everyone in your family has a part to play in the care of grandmother. You all work together" and "Children at four can be a handful, but I notice that when the baby starts crying, Eric starts gently rocking the crib. It's great that you have found something that makes him feel that he can help." In contrast to commendations, compliments are usually based on something that is displayed once and is more likely an attribute rather than a sustained behavior. Wright and Leahey (2013) state that families experiencing ongoing illness, disability, or trauma suffer from feeling that they have nothing positive left, and need to receive as many sincere commendations as possible.

### Evaluate Usefulness of the Interview and Conclude

At the end of the discussion, you might find it useful to conduct a round-robin. Ask each person to relate how they felt about the discussion and move on to the next person without discussion until everyone has spoken. After a short discussion about the responses, sum up what you felt was accomplished, ask for any additions, and then move to planning.

The next steps involve planning and taking action on what was decided during the interview. Possibly a family member will agree to take notes. Encourage the family to identify who is going to do what and when they are going to do it. Offer suggestions only at this point, if you are asked, so it is their plan rather than yours. Conclude your part of the interview by confirming arrangements that involve you.

## Home Visiting Process

Each home visit includes four phases: preparation, arrival at the home, conducting the visit using the 15-minute family interview described above, and completing visit follow-up after leaving the home. Home visits begin with initial preparation for the visit and end with the completion of activities related to the visit, those of documentation and evaluation. For families receiving more than one visit, the end of one visit initiates planning for the next, and the cycle does not end until discharge.

The list below provides the phases and activities of a home visit, adapted from Allender and colleagues (2010) and Wright and Leahey (2013), and includes activities to increase the safety of the visit.

A.  PREPARE FOR HOME VISIT
1.  Study referral, record, or other information on family, review relevant literature, and consult with staff or team members if unfamiliar with type of visit or location.

2. Contact family to
   a. set up appropriate time for home visit to increase availability of family members and reduce interruptions;
   b. obtain address and directions to home; and
   c. ask if there are any particular issues or concerns in the neighborhood that you should know about. For example, if the neighborhood is considered dangerous, visit in the morning and/or with an escort.
3. Ensure your organization has accurate information about you, including your visit schedule with phone numbers, vehicle description and license plate number, mobile phone number.
4. Plan a route to the home and prepare maps, or use the GPS (Global Positioning System) in the vehicle.
5. *Equipment*: Ensure you have maps for the area and bus routes, sufficient gas in the car, a whistle for alerting others, and that your phone is fully charged and has emergency number on speed dial.
6. *Prepare self*: Dress modestly or wear uniform with name tag. Do not carry a purse or wear expensive jewelry. Know organizational policy about potentially dangerous situations, discuss or role-play possible situations with colleagues, and learn personal defense techniques.
7. Collect relevant health care equipment and information.

B. ARRIVAL AT HOME
8. Park vehicle as close to the home as possible. Check the address. Avoid dark areas and loitering groups. Walk directly to the home, keeping one arm free.
9. Make your arrival known with a sharp knock or use doorbell (even when door is open), and give your name, role, and organization name.
10. Do not enter until you know that your contact family member is present and you feel comfortable.

C. CONDUCT THE HOME VISIT
11. Begin process for 15-minute (or less) interview (see previous section). If a refreshment is offered, request that it be shared at the end of the visit.
12. Leave if you feel threatened or if the environment does not allow you to establish a relationship.
13. Provide or complete nursing care, such as dressing changes, review of medications, health promotion, provision of the format for a family agreement (see Box 9.2), or other purpose of visit.
14. Conclude visit by making future plans as needed for timing of the next visit, referrals to other resources, or discharge.
15. Thank family for working with you.

D. COMPLETE VISIT FOLLOW-UP AFTER LEAVING HOME
16. Report to organization at the end of the clinical day.
17. Document home visit in a timely manner.
18. Review information from visit to follow through with plans, including next visit, referrals, or discharge.

19. Report and discuss with supervisor any threatening or difficult behavior during visit.
20. Note family needs or interests that are consistent with those of other families and pass these on at team meetings.
21. Complete a self-evaluation of home visit. (This list can be used as a checklist.)

## Addressing Challenges during Home Visits

One of the first difficulties you may encounter when arranging the first home visit is that the people in the home may not be aware that they have been referred for a home visit. One reason may be that the referring person did not inform the family, or the family did not understand or forgot. Often women who have had their first baby are referred for a home visit as part of a maternal–infant program, and people with continuing health problems will usually be referred to home care after being discharged from hospital. In these situations, where there is a recognized health concern, usually an explanation by the community health nurse at the initial phone call will reassure the person that the visit is appropriate. If people are still concerned, they could be given the phone number of their physician to check on the need for the visit.

In contrast, making visits for the purpose of case finding can be challenging. These visits might be conducted based on a referral from a family member or neighbor who is concerned about a person or family's well-being. Another reason is to identify people for a particular reason, such as to find isolated elderly people or people living in houses that contain lead-based paint. The case finding visits often require what is called in business and sales a "cold call," in that the person has not been notified or prepared in any way for the contact. If a cold call by the community health nurse or the person's physician to arrange a visit is not effective, going directly to the home is necessary. In this situation, the community health nurse would attempt to include family members, the manager of the building, or neighbors to introduce the community health nurse to the person or family. If this approach is ineffective, and the concern or need for contact continues, another approach is to involve other services, such as social services or, in an emergency, the police.

During the home visit, you might need to deal with some disturbances. Disturbances can involve differences between family members, family members under the influence of alcohol or drugs, and the presence of strangers (Allender et al., 2010). In the first two situations, the community health nurse does not become personally involved and usually leaves the situation with the suggestion of arranging another visit. If physical harm is a concern, call 911 once you are out of the situation. Always maintain a clear route to the nearest exit. When people unknown to the community health nurse, such as neighbors and friends of the family, cause distractions during the visit, inquire about their relationship to the family and whether they should be present. The community health nurse may find that they provide valuable support to the family or that the family was too distracted to think about asking them to leave.

Developing a therapeutic relationship with the family during a safe home visit is the goal of home visits. Once the relationship with the family is initiated, it needs to be nurtured by building on the family strengths and linking the family to community resources that will support the development of family strengths.

Four post-RN (RN to BScN) student nurses prepared the following two case studies depicting case finding experiences. The examples are a blend of experiences described by community health nurses and the student nurses' own experiences while learning about family home visits.

*Case Study 1*

The nurse felt anxious as she drove down the rutted driveway to the farm house. She had been told that the older woman and her son who lived there were rarely seen by the neighbors in the village or at the church. She had tried to phone to make an appointment, but didn't get an answer or even an answering machine. She knocks at the door, but gets no answer. She is about to leave when she sees someone moving in the barn and decides to start there. The man greets her with a gruff "What do you want? We aren't buy'n." The nurse greets him and asks if he is Mister Conrad. He nods and she introduces herself, informs him of where she works, and her reason for making the visit. She asks if she could talk to him and his mother. The man reluctantly agrees, but says that they will have to meet upstairs because his mother cannot manage the stairs anymore. The mother is sitting in her room, and they bring in more chairs so they can complete the assessment. Part of the discussion includes questions about limitations of movement, getting out of the house quickly in an emergency, and use of community services.

When the nurse asks the woman if she gets out of the house, the woman's eyes well up with tears. She says she is so lonely now that she can't get out. She used to enjoy going to church, the library, and attending women's meetings. Her son tries to stop her talking by saying that they don't accept any charity. The nurse does not argue with the son but continues on with the assessment. At the end, she describes a couple of community programs in the area. The community health nurse explains that one program is designed for people

who are limited to the house to have an opportunity to discuss their interests and concerns with a home visitor, and another is a mobile book lending library. The man admits that it upsets him to see his mother looking sad most of the time. When the nurse asks if someone from the community health center could visit again, the son agrees.

*Case Study 2*

In an urban low-cost housing unit, a nurse conducts an interview with an older couple to complete the family home risk assessment. The woman is smiling and answers most of the questions; the man has only given one-word responses. On the nurse's way out, the woman explains that her husband recently found out that their car is not working and cannot be repaired. They cannot afford another car. The community health nurse asks, "What has it been like living with your husband recently?" The wife explains that before this happened with the car, he had been getting quieter but now he hardly talks to her at all. She was surprised that he had said anything at their meeting. She adds that she really misses the conversations they used to have. The nurse asks a few more questions, and suggests that maybe they could meet with a health professional at the Center or someone could visit them at home. The woman's face brightens. She says, "Oh, could someone come here again? I would really like that. I can't get him to go out."

**Discussion Topics and Questions**

5. In Case Study 1, what actions by the community health nurse helped to gain some positive feelings from the son?

6. In Case Study 1, what home health nursing competencies (Community Health Nurses of Canada, 2010) or home health nursing standards (American Nurses Association, 2014) would be the most relevant?

7. In Case Study 2, what family nursing approach(es) and methods were used by the community health nurse?

## Collaboration in Home Visits

For clients receiving home care services, the other services involved are usually indicated in the client's record. The coordination of services for patients living in a specific area or with designated conditions are often managed by a health care professional called a home care **case manager** or **care coordinator**. A case manager in home care is a registered health professional who has responsibilities that include designating the type, frequency, and duration of services that are provided in the home. A case manager is usually a Registered Nurse but may also be a physiotherapist, occupational therapist, speech-language pathologist, social worker, dietitian, or psychologist (Ontario Ministry of Health and Long-Term Care, 2007). Depending on the jurisdiction, case managers may be employed by a government organization that assigns contracts for home nursing visits, or a part of the home care organization providing the services. The case manager for a family receiving home care would be the person to contact about home services involving other service providers.

Nursing students and beginning practitioners develop knowledge and skills in interprofessional collaboration by identifying and learning about the service providers in the practice area. Interprofessional collaboration means interacting and working together effectively to improve the health of clients. A basic understanding of the scope of practice of the different professionals can be obtained from journals, texts, websites of professional associations, discussions, and home visits with other professionals.

Professionals who could be involved with families receiving care in the home are social workers, physical therapists, occupational therapists, psychologists, general or family practice physicians, and medical specialists. Because of the dispersed nature of practice in the home, case conferences organized by the case manager may not be feasible. Alternatively, interactions may be facilitated by Internet conferencing or secure digital devices and programs. Recent work with electronic records could possibly support collaboration by providing current health care information.

The most prevalent paid worker in the home is the home health care worker. A **home health care worker** is an unregulated care provider with basic training in providing personal care and household tasks in the home. Job titles for a home health care worker include home health care aid (HHA), personal support worker (PSW), or service support worker (SSW). The educational preparation of home health care workers varies in different areas, but mainly involves learning basic personal care skills, communication skills, and home management skills, including meal preparation, doing laundry, and housecleaning. Home health care workers are usually in a home for at least an hour to provide a specified task, such as assistance with a bath, or for longer periods to complete several tasks, engage in social interaction, or provide respite for the caregiver. Home health care workers are supervised by a person, usually a nurse, from their employment agency.

Home health care workers are a valuable part of the home health care team because they spend more time in the home and often have a closer relationship with the family. They can provide valuable information on how the family functions, and can promote the care plan if they understand it. Collaboration with the worker will ensure that the family is being supported in a consistent manner and is not receiving mixed messages. Other workers and technologists with specific training, such as respiratory technologists and child development workers, can also be involved in specific home care situations and can contribute to the home health care team.

In addition to knowledge about the different service providers, a collaborative practice requires skill in interpersonal relations and communication. These are the same skills needed to effectively function on a team, whether the team is composed of people from the same or different professions. The development of team skills is explained and applied in Chapter 2. In home care, written documentation is particularly important because the team has few if any opportunities to meet.

Opportunities to collaborate with other service providers can emerge from dealing

## BOX 9.1
## Examples of Interprofessional Collaboration to Reduce Falls in the Home by Older Adults

In a systematic review of interventions to reduce falls by the elderly in the community, Marks (2014) identified several interventions that have some empirical support. The interventions could be delivered in the home or referred to an appropriate health care organization in the community.

Interventions for the home:
- A comprehensive multifactorial risk assessment
- An individualized treatment plan
- A comprehensive multifactorial management plan
- Exercise, muscle strength training, endurance building exercises, balance training
- Education
- Home safety inspection and home modifications

Referrals to health professionals in the community:
- Anti-slip shoe devices and multifaceted podiatry to patients with specific foot ailments
- First eye cataract surgery and pacemakers in patients with cardio-inhibitory carotid sinus hypersensitivity
- Vitamin D supplementation
- Withdrawal of psychotropic medications

In home health care, screening for multifactorial risk of falling would involve a health professional who has received training in using the appropriate assessment tools and analyzing the results. The health professional may be from the home care organization or from a specialized fall prevention program. Home health professionals and workers would contribute to the assessment, especially if the person has difficulty communicating.

Once an older person at risk of falling is identified, the case manager would prepare a treatment plan that would be tailored to the needs of the family by nursing, physiotherapy, and occupational therapy. The physiotherapist would design an exercise program consistent with best practice guidelines and instruct the person and family members how to carry out the program. The occupational therapist would conduct the home inspection and supervise the modifications. The community health nurse would prepare and deliver evidence-based educational materials on fall prevention to the person and family. Once the exercises and home modifications are in place, the nurse and home health worker would continue to work with the client and family to provide education and support in maintaining the fall prevention program. The case manager or the community home health nurse would provide the results of the assessment to the person's general practitioner, and discuss relevant referrals and medication changes.

If the fall prevention program is delivered through an official public health organization, the same health professionals could be involved, but the manner of screening and ongoing monitoring and support would be different. Elderly people could be recruited to the program through referrals from hospital emergency departments, physician offices, or families or by self-referral. The organization would probably work in collaboration with organizations in the community, such as churches and older adults' apartment buildings and organizations. Once people at risk are identified, the four components of the program—exercises, hazard reduction, review of psychotropic medications, and coordination of activities—would be instituted in the home. The community health nurse working for the public health organization would probably continue to provide the educational portion of the fall prevention program to the client and family for a certain number of home visits.

---

with difficulties faced by a single family or a problem faced by many families. When working with a family of a premature infant, a community health nurse would be collaborating with the parents, a child development worker, and a social worker. For a family member who is disabled and therefore restricted in performing activities of daily living such as walking, talking, eating, bathing, or working, a different collaboration team would be involved. An example of interdisciplinary practice to reduce falls by elderly persons is provided in Box 9.1.

BOX 9.2
**Agreement for Ellie's Family**

Date: November 11, 2015
Requirement: Provide Ellie with exercises, as indicated by the physiotherapist, four times a day.
People involved: Mom, Dad, Jean, Roger, Jessica

*Schedule*:
**Assignment for Ellie's Exercises**

| Time | Monday | Tuesday | Wednesday | Thursday | Friday | Saturday | Sunday |
|------|--------|---------|-----------|----------|--------|----------|--------|
| Breakfast | Jean | Roger | Dad | Jean | Roger | Dad | Jean |
| Morning | Mom & Jess | Mom & Jess | Mom & Jess | Mom & Jess | Mom & Jess | Roger | Dad |
| Afternoon | Mom & Jess | Mom & Jess | Mom & Jess | Mom & Jess | Mom & Jess | Dad | Jean |
| Evening | Roger | Dad | Jean | Roger | Dad | Jean | Roger |

*Action*: At the indicated time, work with Ellie to perform the required exercises for 20 minutes. Check beside name when complete. Tell Mom if Ellie liked the exercises or if there were any problems.

*Evaluation*: Once a week by physiotherapist and family

*Reward*: Family will have their "weird" pizza (pizza with peanut butter and olives) on Sunday night if everyone completes exercises

Signatures _____    _____

## Using Contracts or Agreements in the Home

Agreements or contracts are a valuable tool in community health nursing in the home. Agreements or contracts among families, community health nurses, and/or service providers are a collaborative way to set goals and work toward these goals. The contracts include four characteristics: partnership and mutuality, commitment, format, and evaluation (Allender et al., 2010). The agreement identifies who will be partners, what action they commit to doing, what format they will use to specify the details, and how the agreement will be evaluated. Everyone who is involved needs to review a draft of the agreement. An agreement lays out what is to be done by whom and must be easy to manage or it will not be followed. Once the use of an agreement has been introduced, the family may use it in other situations.

Above is an example of how a collaborative agreement can be used. A small child, Ellie, in a family of four children and two parents, needed specific exercises at least four times a day. The physiotherapist was prepared to train the family members and monitor the child's progress. In preparation, the community health nurse worked with the family to draw up an agreement. Roger, the 12-year-old son, drew up the schedule. The agreement is displayed in Box 9.2.

The physiotherapist taught the exercises to the mother, who demonstrated them to the other family members. After a week, the physical therapist came in to assess the progress and was pleased with the results. She asked them to continue in the same way for another week, and then the length of the sessions or the frequency might be changed.

The mother was pleased because she did not need to remind anyone to work with Ellie. Everyone seemed to enjoy the time alone with the child. The family celebrated by having a favorite meal together.

## Finding Community Resources for Families

Once community health nurses come to know the community, they know what organizations provide services and resources and how to access these resources. This knowledge is a precious resource for community health nurses and is not easy to write down or pass on to others because it frequently changes. The community health nurses' relationships or partnerships with the people in community organizations are necessary to support individuals and families who want to live independently at home. Since these organizations and the staff often change, precise information is not always as important as using a process to investigate what is currently available.

The process used in assessing the physical and social environment in the community health nursing process includes (a) observing and mapping the physical and social environment, and (b) interviewing key informants with the purpose of finding useful resources for families. Observing and mapping of an area can be done in the same way as for a group, using windshield surveys, Internet mapping programs, and paper maps of an area that include the location of various health and social services. The most useful approach to finding specific resources is to ask for suggestions from key informants and check back about what you have found on municipal and social service websites. The challenging part is finding which municipal or regional website has the most comprehensive listings, with descriptions. That website will also likely provide links to related websites. Once you have located an organization providing the relevant resource, you then might need to consider the distance and accessibility to public transportation if the family needs to attend a program or obtain materials.

Another approach is to conduct an Internet search for national/state/provincial associations for a specific disease, such as heart and stroke, asthma, or mental health. These organizations usually provide very useful information and links to local organizations. Often a search of those local websites or a call to the office will be invaluable in providing information and supportive resources for the family.

As a student or new employee, start seeking resources first through organizational staff. Note the names of people who are identified as the "go-to people," or the person who can answer all your questions or knows where to find an informant if they can't. Be polite and considerate as you approach these people. You may not realize that you sound abrupt when you feel anxious about asking people for assistance. Ask first if they would be willing to help you find information about the community for your clients and, if so, ask what timing and method of communication works best for them. For example, ask them if they like short conversations at lunch or break, or emails or texting at different times of the day. People might say, "I always check my emails first thing in the morning and only look at the immediate ones at the end of day" or "I take phone calls and respond to emails at noon and at the end of the day. I cannot be distracted while I am on a home visit." Continue to be polite by thanking them for any information and letting them know, later on, how things worked out.

## SCENARIO: Case Study on Finding Community Resources

Three nursing students were assigned to work with home health nurses in the long-term home health care program and to develop a case study on finding community resources. The students usually went on home visits with the same nurse, but occasionally with others. They also had an opportunity to go on home visits with a physiotherapist, an occupational therapist, and a social worker.

The students decided to use progressive inquiry to gather information on how to find community resources for families. After asking the home health nurses how long it had been since they graduated and how long they had worked in the community, they started progressive inquiry with three questions: "What community resources are needed by most people? How easy or difficult has it been for you to find these resources? What advice do you have for new nurses about finding resources?" Each student asked the questions in a way and at a time that fit with the practice style of the home health nurse. Some asked the questions while they were driving, some at lunch, some at the end of the day. They each had a smartphone or mobile Internet device to check out websites right away.

At the end of the day, they wrote up their information and sent it as an email attachment to the other team members. They included how the questions worked and what they had found, and suggested questions for the next round if they were working with the same person. They used Internet teleconferencing to make their decisions about the next set of questions. After six weeks, they had each talked to three to six home health nurses, for a total of ten. They also asked the other health professionals about their sources of information. They used the data they gathered to prepare the following case study on finding community resources to be used for orientation and training purposes.

## Summary

Community health nurses conduct home visits for people with acute or chronic illness and those at risk for illness to build family capacity and promote health and healing. Community health nurses add family nursing approaches, theoretical models, and concepts to their community perspective to assess, plan, act, and evaluate their nursing practice with families in the home. These family theories and approaches reinforce that a professional relationship with a family is collaborative and characterized by mutual respect, an understanding of the family structure and dynamics, and a reflective process.

Nurses working in the home start with the narrow end of the telescoping lens to consider how a particular family can be supported and linked with community resources. They work closely with other service providers in the community to coordinate the support provided to families. Then, as community health nurses, they consider the common needs faced by families they serve and advocate with families or on their behalf to health care agencies and governments. Community health nurses work with families as they develop their capacity to thrive in the community.

## Case Study on Finding Community Resources

Ten home health nurses were interviewed over six weeks, and four practitioners from physiotherapy, occupational therapy, and social work were consulted, about finding community resources. The home health care practitioners shared their ideas with three nursing students who accompanied them on home visits to older adults with chronic health conditions living in a rural and urban area.

The first question to the home health nurses asked about the community resources needed by most people. The initial responses were very specific to medical care, such as pharmacies that do home deliveries, blood sugar/glucose meters, and mobility aids. The students were able to quickly find answers to these responses by using the Internet and the local directories, and by asking the other health professionals and clerical staff.

When the home health nurses were asked about the ease or difficulty in finding resources, and for advice to new nurses, the responses were varied. The nurses felt that physiotherapists and occupational therapists helped with mobility in the home, and social workers, along with other aspects of their role, could assist with finding funding for equipment and renovations. Where the home health nurses had difficulty was in finding resources for getting people to doctor appointments, community social and fitness programs, the library, and community events. Without the opportunity to readily get out, the nurses felt that patients limited their horizons and became more and more housebound, with fewer social contacts.

The students conducted an Internet search using the term "senior transportation." For the city and rural area of Ottawa, Ontario, they found a guide that includes buses that lower for walkers and wheelchairs, transportation for people with disabilities, and a rural shopping service (Council on Aging of Ottawa, 2014). In Jefferson City, Missouri, they found the website of a nonprofit organization that provides transportation for senior citizens, people with disabilities, and the rural general population in 87 districts in the state (OATS, Inc., 2013). In other words, transportation services might be available for people with mobility challenges through municipal and charitable organizations, such as the local cancer association. However, when public transportation is not available, transportation needs to be arranged through family and friends.

The advice the home health nurses had for new nurses was to accept and admit that you do not have all the answers about community resources, but to tell the person that you will find out and get back to them. The other advice was that most people, and especially those who have been limited to their home, are not going to immediately act on the information you provide. Most are going to feel at least a bit afraid of venturing out. They suggested that a family interview might be useful to initiate family involvement in organizing activities outside the home so that the person can be eased into activities.

### Discussion Topics and Questions

8. What challenges would you expect home health nurses to have in finding community resources?
9. What could make it easier for home health nurses to find community resources?

## Classroom and Seminar Exercises

1. Respond to the exercises below using the 15-minute (or less) family interview (Wright and Leahey, 2013) with a family you know:
   a. Plan an interview using the following outline:

      1. Family names (use fictional names):
      2. Most likely health concern facing family:
      3. Most likely meeting location:
      4. Your introduction of yourself and the discussion:
      5. Diagram of family circle
      6. Interaction diagram
      7. Three questions for the family:
      8. One or two commendations for the family:
      9. Your conclusion for the interview:

   b. Discuss the reasons for your choice of answers to items 3 to 9.

2. Using your own practice or experience, develop the following:
   a. Examples of how caregivers react when asked about their own health
   b. Examples of collaboration in home visits
   c. Examples of when early collaboration could have reduced later problems

3. Identify a local unsafe area, and change or augment the safety measures given in the home visiting process list based on that area.

4. Write an agreement to include all family members in a family of four (with two adults who smoke) to reduce environmental tobacco smoke in the home.

5. Discuss where transportation is included in the social determinants of health and primary health care.

## References

Allender, J., Rector, C., & Warner, K. (2010). *Community health nursing* (7th ed.). Philadelphia, PA: Lippincott Williams & Wilkins.

American Psychological Association. (2014). *Fact Sheet: Age and socioeconomic status.* Retrieved from www.apa.org/pi/ses/resources/publications/factsheet-age.aspx

American Nurses Association. (2014). *Home health nursing: Scope and standards of home health nursing practice* (2nd ed.). Silver Springs, MD: Author.

Anderson Moore, K., Redd, Z., Burkhauser, M., Kassim Mbwana, M., & Collins, A. (2009). Children in poverty: Trends, consequences, and policy options. *Child Trends, 11.* Retrieved from www.childtrends.org/?publications=children-in-poverty-trends-consequences-and-policy-options-april-2009

Bell, J. (2012). Making ideas "stick": The 15-minute family interview [Editorial]. *Journal of Family Nursing, 18,* 171–174.

Bell, J., & Wright, L. (2011). Creating practice knowledge for families experiencing illness and suffering: The illness belief model. In E. Svavarsdottier & H. Josdottier (Eds.), *Family nursing in action* (pp. 15–52). Reykjavik, Iceland: University of Iceland Press.

Campaign 2000. (2014). *Canada's real economic action plan begins with poverty eradication: Report card on child and family poverty in 2013*. Retrieved from www.campaign2000.ca/reportCards/national/2013C2000NATIONALREPORTCARDNOV26.pdf

Canadian Home Care Association. (2014). *Family caregivers*. Retrieved from www.cdnhomecare.ca/content.php?doc=223

Canadian Institute for Health Information. (2011). *Health care in Canada, 2011: A focus on seniors and aging*. Retrieved from https://secure.cihi.ca/free_products/HCIC_2011_seniors_report_en.pdf

Canadian Medical Association. (2014). *14th annual report card on health care*. Retrieved from www.cma.ca/En/Lists/Medias/2014_Report_Card-e.pdf

Centers for Disease Control and Prevention. (2014). *Minority health*. Retrieved from www.cdc.gov/minorityhealth/populations/atrisk.html

Clark, M. (2008). *Community health nursing* (5th ed.). Upper Saddle River, NJ: Prentice Hall.

College of Registered Nurses of Nova Scotia. (2012). *Professional boundaries and the nurse-client relationship: Keeping it safe and therapeutic*. Retrieved from www.crnns.ca/documents/ProfessionalBoundaries2012.pdf

Community Health Nurses of Canada. (2010, March). *Home health nursing competencies Version 1.0*. Retrieved from www.chnc.ca/competencies.cfm

Community Health Nurses of Canada. (2011, March). *Canadian community health nursing: Professional practice model & standards of practice*. Retrieved from www.chnc.ca/nursing-standards-of-practice.cfm

Council on Aging of Ottawa and OCTranspo. (2014). *Choices: Seniors' transportation*. Retrieved from www.coaottawa.ca/documents/2014_Transportation_CHOICES.pdf

Crawford, M. (2008). *The elimination of child poverty and the pivotal significance of the mother*. Retrieved from www.ncbi.nlm.nih.gov/pubmed/19009739

Hartrick, G. (1998). Developing health promoting practices: A transformative process. *Nursing Outlook, 46*(5), 219–225.

Heaney, C., & Israel, B. (2008). Social networks and social support. In K. Glanz, B. Rimer, & K. Viswanath (Eds.), *Health behavior and health education: Theory, research, and practice* (4th ed., pp. 189–210). San Francisco, CA: Jossey-Bass.

Kearney, M., York, R., & Deatrick, J. (2000). Effects of home visits to vulnerable young families. *Journal of Nursing Scholarship, 32*(4), 369–376.

Larson, C. (2007). *Poverty during pregnancy: Its effects on child health outcomes*. Retrieved from www.ncbi.nlm.nih.gov/pmc/articles/PMC2528810/

Marks, R. (2014). Falls among the elderly: Multi-factorial community-based falls-prevention programs. *Journal of Aging Science, 2*, e109. doi:10.4172/2329.8847.1000e109

Martin, J., Hamilton, B., Osterman, M., Curtin, S., & Mathews, T. (2013). Births: Final data for 2012. *National Vital Statistics Reports*. Retrieved from www.cdc.gov/nchs/data/nvsr/nvsr62/nvsr62_09.pdf

McNaughton, D. (2000). A synthesis of qualitative home visiting research. *Public Health Nursing, 17*(6), 405–414.

Moules, N., & Johnston, H. (2010). Commendations, conversations and life-change relationships: Teaching and practicing family nursing. *Journal of Family Nursing, 16*, 146–160.

Moyer, A., Jamault, M., Roberge, G., & Murphy, M. (1998). *Designing and testing individual and community-based interventions for the elderly in need using action research* (Publication no. M98-05). Ottawa, ON: University of Ottawa, Community Health Research Unit.

National Alliance for Caregiving in collaboration with AARP. (2009). *Caregiving in the U.S.* Retrieved from www.caregiving.org/data/Caregiving_in_the_US_2009_full_report.pdf

National Center for Health Statistics. (2011). *Home health care and discharged hospice care patients: United States, 2000 and 2007.* Retrieved from www.cdc.gov/nchs/data/nhsr/nhsr038.pdf

National Center for Health Statistics. (2012). *Characteristics and use of home health care by men and women aged 65 and over.* Retrieved from www.cdc.gov/nchs/data/nhsr/nhsr052.pdf

OATS, Inc. (2013). *Public transportation system.* Retrieved from www.oatstransit.org/

Ontario Ministry of Health and Long-Term Care. (2007). *Community Care Access Centres: Client services policy manual.* Retrieved from www.health.gov.on.ca/english/providers/pub/manuals/ccac/ccac_6.pdf

Porr, C. (2015). Important interactional strategies for everyday public health nursing practice. *Public Health Nursing, 32,* 43–49.

Rowe Kaakinen, J., & Harmon Hanson, S. (2014a). Family health care nursing. In J. Rowe Kaakinen, D. Padgett Coehlo, R. Steele, A. Tabacco, & S. Harmon Hanson, *Family health care nursing: Theory, practice, and research* (5th ed., pp. 3–30). Philadelphia, PA: F.A. Davis.

Rowe Kaakinen, J., & Harmon Hanson, S. (2014b). Theoretical foundations for the nursing of families. In J. Rowe Kaakinen, D. Padgett Coehlo, R. Steele, A. Tabacco, & S. Harmon Hanson (Eds.), *Family health care nursing: Theory, practice, and research* (5th ed., pp. 67–104). Philadelphia, PA: F.A. Davis.

Stanhope, M., Lancaster, J., Jessup-Falcioni, H., & Viverais-Dresler, G. (2011). *Community health nursing in Canada* (2nd Can. ed.). Toronto, ON: Elsevier Canada.

Statistics Canada. (2012). *Seniors' use of and unmet needs for home care, 2009.* Retrieved from www.statcan.gc.ca/pub/82-003-x/2012004/article/11760-eng.htm

Statistics Canada. (2013a). *Fertility: Overview, 2009 to 2011.* Retrieved from www.statcan.gc.ca/pub/91-209.x/2013001/article/11784-eng.htm

Statistics Canada. (2013b). *Live births, by age and marital status of mother, Canada* (Table 102-4507). Retrieved from www5.statcan.gc.ca/cansim/pick-choisir?lang=eng&p2=33&id=1024507

Statistics Canada. (2014). *Canadians with unmet home care needs.* Retrieved from www.statcan.gc.ca/pub/75-006-x/2014001/article/14042-eng.htm

Tapp, D. (2001). Conserving the vitality of suffering: Addressing family constraints to illness conversations. *Nursing Inquiry, 8*(4), 254–263.

Thrower, S., & Walton, R. (1982). The family circle concept for integrating family systems concepts in family medicine. *Journal of Family Practice, 15*(3), 451–457.

Wright, L., & Leahey, M. (2000). *Nurses and families: A guide to family assessment and intervention.* Philadelphia, PA: F.A. Davis.

Wright, L., & Leahey, M. (2013). *Nurses and families: A guide to family assessment* (6th ed.). Philadelphia, PA: F.A. Davis.

## Website Resources

### Family Nursing

Canadian Association of Perinatal and Women's Health Nurses (CAPWHN): www.capwhn.ca/en/capwhn/About_CAPWHN_p3185.html

CAPWHN is a new organization representing women's health, obstetric, and newborn nurses from across Canada. The website provides very useful links to associations providing services relevant to the family, including obstetrical, neonatal, women's health care, breas-feeding, and Canadian Perinatal Programs, and related provincial, territorial, national, and international programs.

Family Nursing Resources: www.familynursingresources.com/

This website is produced by L. Wright and M. Leahey to provide written and digital resources related to their Calgary Family Assessment and Intervention Models.

International Family Nursing Association (IFNA): internationalfamilynursing.org/

The IFNA website and the association seek to act as a unifying force for family nursing globally. The website provides ways to become involved in online exchanges and webinars, attend conferences, and download resources.

Journal of Family Nursing (JFN): http://jfn.sagepub.com/

JFN is a peer-reviewed quarterly journal of nursing research, practice, education, and policy issues, as well as empirical and theoretical analyses on the subject of family health. Its interdisciplinary, international, and collaborative perspectives examine cultural diversity and families across the life cycle.

D. Westera (2010), *Family Assessment in Community Health Nursing Practice*: www.ucs.mun.ca/~dwestera/community.html

This 10-minute YouTube clip introduces a 26-minute video on family nursing and family nursing models from the perspective of frontline community health nurses.

## Home Health Nursing

Saint Elizabeth: www.saintelizabeth.com/

Saint Elizabeth's website includes their history as a visiting nursing organization in Ontario since 1908 and expansion across Canada, newsletters with tips and resources for family caregivers, a variety of programs, and ingenious use of Internet services to support and stay connected to their staff.

Victorian Order of Nurses (VON): www.von.ca

VON's website includes the history of their formation and development in Canada since 1897 and an extensive list of links to organizations associated with home care, nursing, health care, and seniors. The history and links are provided in "About VON."

Visiting Nurse Associations of America (VNAA): www.vnaa.org

VNAA represents home and hospice nursing organizations in over 40 states. The site offers educational resources, including guidelines and webinars.

D. Westera (2010), *Home Visiting in Community Health Nursing*: www.ucs.mun.ca/~dwestera/community.html

This 9-minute YouTube clip introduces a 26-minute video on the home visit from the perspective of a home health and public health nurse.

# Chapter 10

# Approaches to Community Capacity Building

················································································································

Community capacity building expands on the collaborative process used in short-term projects in its application to longer term health promotion projects with population groups and communities. Although collaboration is emphasized in earlier sections, in capacity building, collaboration is expected to lead to or begin with leadership by the community. The purpose of community capacity building is to work with communities to provide an environment where the community can develop skills and knowledge, recognize their strengths, and work together to deal with their challenges. Although capacity building may lead to a change in health behavior, the emphasis is not on individual behavior change, but on encouraging community action.

Two vulnerable groups, young adolescents and rural residents, are featured in this chapter as appropriate recipients of community capacity building. An examination of the social context of young adolescents, represented by youth ages 11 to 15 years who are attending schools in the US and Canada, indicates how vulnerable youth are to disruptions in family, peer, and school support. The scenario on building school capacity illustrates how a school could provide opportunities for youth to work together and to speak out on ways to improve the school climate. The scenario on community capacity building in a rural area illustrates how nursing students and new practitioners use a community capacity–building process to increase the availability of healthy food.

## Learning Objectives

After reading this chapter and answering the questions throughout the chapter, you should be able to:

1. Apply what you have learned about working with groups to working with communities.

2. Explain the use of community capacity building as a health promotion strategy in community health nursing practice.

### Key Terms and Concepts

collaborative partnerships • community capacity • community capacity building • community health • dialogue • early adolescence • food security • rural • sense of community: membership, influence, integration and fulfillment, shared emotional connection • transparency

3. Identify the concepts, theory, and practices associated with community capacity building.
4. Identify the characteristics of two vulnerable populations: rural and remote communities and young adolescents attending school.
5. Develop an approach to establish relationships with communities.
6. Develop an approach to work according to the community's direction and time frame.

## Building on Work with Groups to Work with Communities

Your understanding of how to work with groups and the community health nursing process from the previous section provides a foundation for working on capacity building in communities. However, building the capacity of a community is likely to take much longer than with a group. The focus, moreover, is on the community learning to work together rather than on health education leading to behavior change. As well, the leadership role is held by the community.

The longer time frame of community capacity building means that each phase of the community health nursing process might extend for months rather than weeks. With the longer time frame, the community health nursing process will cycle within each phase. Figure 10.1 illustrates these cycles within the process.

**Figure 10.1: Phases and Cycles within the Community Health Nursing Process**

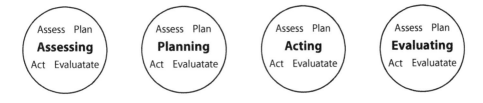

Assess  Plan  **Assessing**  Act  Evaluatate

Assess  Plan  **Planning**  Act  Evaluatate

Assess  Plan  **Acting**  Act  Evaluatate

Assess  Plan  **Evaluating**  Act  Evaluatate

Given the long time frame, nursing students and new practitioners would be involved in only one phase, or even one aspect of a phase, of the process. What is important is to be aware of the overall process and the cycle within the phase you are working on. By thinking of what occurred before you joined the program, where it is now, and where you would like it to go in the future, your involvement will be beneficial both to you and the future of the program.

The focus on facilitating capacity for community members to work together requires some change in attitude. In community capacity building, the emphasis is on the process used to bring together community members from across geographical areas or different interest groups to solve common problems. This emphasis requires that the community takes the lead. Otherwise, they are less likely to be involved. For example, the community may be interested in reducing speeding on local roads, rather than a health provider agenda such as smoking reduction or increasing exercise or immunization. For health providers, this means that the emphasis is on engaging people and being transparent, rather that feeling pushed to accomplish something within a short time frame. **Transparency** means being open about what you are doing, how you are doing it, and why it is important so that others are aware of this and feel free to respond.

Teamwork remains important, although team discussions and decisions involve ways to engage and motivate people on behalf of the community, rather than motivating people to improve their own health. The team is also important for keeping up one another's morale. Community change occurs gradually, or in fits and starts. Small successes, such as an increase in attendance at an event or recruiting an influential person to the advisory group, need to be celebrated.

## Community Capacity Building

Most communities have people, groups, and organizations that have come together over the years to make changes, such as building a library, establishing a park, or starting an annual community event. The community members who have carried out these initiatives are likely involved because they like working with others to benefit the whole community; they are not primarily concerned with their own well-being or that of their family and friends. Initiatives to encourage this civic-mindedness provide some structure through demonstrating a process and providing support. Newer community-driven models of community development, such as community capacity building, extend beyond the older models of community development or organization that are more externally driven and may implicitly accept the status quo (Minkler, Wallerstein, & Wilson, 2008).

**Community capacity building** is a strength-based approach of working with people that identify as members of a shared community to engage in the process of community change (Minkler et al., 2008). Community capacity building starts where the people are (Nyswander, 1956) and increases when community members work together effectively to: (1) "develop and sustain relationships," (2) "solve problems and make group decisions," and (3) "collaborate effectively to identify goals and get work done" (Mattessich & Monsey, 1997, p. 61).

Many different terms are used in community health and development. The following are those most pertinent to this chapter: "community," "sense of community," "community health," and "community capacity." A community is a group of people who share a common place, experience, or interest (KU Work Group for Community Health and Development [KU Work Group], 2014). A community defined by location can be a neighborhood, village, reserve, town, city, or country. A community of people can also be defined by race or ethnic background, such as Norwegian communities in northern Minnesota, or Asian communities in Vancouver and Toronto; by religious affiliation, such as Mormon communities and Muslim communities; by employment, such as the military and health care workers; and by experiences, such as dealing with a physical or mental disability, or suffering from grief and loss. Communities based on similar interests include business, advocacy, sports, and recreation.

The easiest communities to consider are those based on location, such as a neighborhood, town, or rural area. However, not all neighborhoods or towns would be considered a community; they may share a location, but the residents may not feel that they are related to one another. A sense of community comes from not only living in the same location, but also developing similar ways of thinking or behaviors over time.

A **sense of community** embodies the social attachment of individuals and reflects the social engagement and participation within communities (Statistics Canada, 2010). Social isolation tends to be detrimental to health, while social engagement and attachment are associated with positive health outcomes and support an upstream approach to preventing illness and promoting health (Statistics Canada, 2010). Possibly the easiest way to find if there is a sense of community in a location is to ask if people see themselves as distinct from the larger society and part of the local community.

**Community health** refers to the well-being of each person in a community (KU Work Group, 2014). Community health means considering the health of everyone within the larger community, including people living in poor areas, people living in apartments, single mothers, people with a disability. **Collaborative partnerships** are connections forged by people or groups from across the community to improve the health of a community. Collaborative partnerships need to include the people who can make a difference. For example, a collaborative partnership to reduce underage drinking would need to include bar owners, liquor and beer outlets, educators, and the police, along with youth. **Community capacity** refers to the ability of community members to make a difference over time and across different issues (KU Work Group, 2014). Capacity isn't demonstrated by one successful outcome, for example, developing a walking path or erecting a public water fountain. Rather, capacity builds from having a sense of community, consistently taking action together, and learning from experience so that working together for community health is normal behavior. Community capacity would then be manifested in the development of a network of walking paths, convenient public toilets and water fountains, and a skateboard park, all of which are used consistently by community members.

Community capacity building is the process used to identify, strengthen, and link a community's tangible resources, such as community members' skills and resources and local service groups, and intangible resources, such as a sense of community. Community capacity building is an important strategy used by community health nurses; however, it is a very lengthy and time-consuming process. As the Public Health Nursing Section (2001) points out, it is best used in combination with other interventions.

## Concepts, Theories, and Frameworks in Community Capacity Building

The concepts used in community capacity building help to explain the fundamental values of the approach. A main purpose of community capacity building is to strengthen the sense of community and community capacity. The most popular and relatively unchallenged theory on sense of community was developed by McMillan and Chavis (1986) and identifies the following four components (Fremlin, 2014):

- **Membership** is feeling a part of the community, identifying with the community and sharing common practices and symbols.
- **Influence** is present when individual members can make a difference by having a say in the group and when the group is having an effect on its members.
- **Integration and fulfillment** of needs occurs when members are able and willing to help one another and receive help in return.
- **Shared emotional connection** is the commitment and belief that the community has (and will continue to share) a history, common places, shared events (both good and bad), time together, and similar experiences.

A sense of community is nurtured when people feel that they are part of change in the community. Community capacity building is based on the premise that "change is more likely to be successful and permanent when the people it affects are involved in initiating and promoting it" (Thompson & Kinne, 1999, p. 30). Minkler and colleagues (2008) state that a good issue for change must be winnable, simple, specific, unifying, involve the community in a meaningful way, affect many people, build up the community, and be part of a larger plan. Relevance would underlie both peoples' willingness to participate and their feelings of ownership. If the issues that are raised are not relevant to them, they will neither participate nor take ownership. Ensuring that issues remain relevant will increase active participation and feelings of ownership.

Participation means that the community is engaged in creating a healthy community and better quality of life (National Association of County and City Health Officials, 2014). Participation levels will differ for members of the community. For some, participation might mean working in partnership; for others, it might mean having control over all decisions. A good way to determine different levels of participation is by using Arnstein's (2006) ladder of participation, shown in the middle column of Table 10.1.

Approaches to increasing a sense of community, participation, and ownership include Freire's (1972) three-stage listening-dialogue-action approach. Listening means being receptive and supportive. **Dialogue** is the art of "thinking together" (National Association of County and City Health Officials, 2014). It involves transcending individual perspectives to discover a larger resolution: a "we" result. It does this through a combination of

1. awareness of one's own assumptions, in a way that allows them to be held lightly, as well as deliberately.
2. skills of listening that clarify and validate other perspectives, rather than beat them down, producing better mutual understanding.
3. the art of holding differences together in a way that allows shared understanding to emerge.

**Table 10.1: Levels of Citizen Participation**

| Category | Ladder | Amount of Citizen Control |
|---|---|---|
| Degrees of citizen power | Citizen control | People control all decision making. |
| | Delegated powers | People have some areas for which they control the decisions. |
| | Partnership | Decision making is collaborative. |
| Degrees of tokenism | Placation | A minor change is made in plans in response to feedback from people. |
| | Consultation | People are asked which of a few options they would like. |
| | Informing | People are told what is going to happen. |
| Nonparticipation | Therapy | Professional directs changes. |
| | Manipulation | People are exploited. |

*Source*: Adapted from Arnstein, 2006 [1969]; and Goeppinger & Hammond, 2000.

When there is shared understanding, there is greater likelihood of true shared agreement (National Association of County and City Health Officials, 2014).

Different frameworks are available as guides for building community capacity. Many, such as the KU Work Group for Community Health and Development's (2014) *Building Capacity for Community and System Change*, provide a process for working with large communities. The KU model has five basic parts: (1) community context and planning, (2) community action and interventions, (3) community and system change, (4) risk and protective factors and widespread behavior change, and (5) improving more distant long-term goals.

A guide for smaller, more localized initiatives, entitled *Building a Healthy Community to Take Action in Health Promotion* (MACS-NB & Boivin, 2011), was developed from work in small communities. The guide is used as a framework for this chapter and has five stages:

1. Drafting or sketching a portrait that resembles us
2. Finding the rallying idea
3. Planning and putting into action
4. Maintaining the momentum
5. Evaluation

Although many of the stages are similar to the community health process, the steps in each stage slant the process toward building capacity. For example, five of the six steps in the first stage of drafting a portrait emphasize community strengths: identifying what people like, identifying the strengths, identifying the resources, identifying the needs and challenges, identifying the leaders, and identifying the octopuses (well-connected people). In the second stage, that of finding the rallying idea, the last two steps are developing a clear message and sharing the idea. Box 10.1 illustrates how important it is to know the community when you prepare and share the message.

BOX 10.1
**The Message Is in the Song**

*Helping Health Workers Learn* (Werner & Bower, 1982) describes training women in an African village to work with others to help reduce baby deaths caused by diarrhea. The workers had been unable to convey the importance of regularly giving water to the babies with diarrhea to keep them hydrated. Then they noticed how the women loved to sing and dance, and decided to include the message about water in a song. The women loved the song, and the number of babies dying from dehydration was greatly reduced.

The guide for building a healthy community provides possible actions and questions for each step to help gauge the sense of community and determine which issues will rally the community (MACS-NB & Boivin, 2011). The stages are illustrated later in the scenarios involving a school community and a rural community.

## Community Capacity–Building Practice

In community capacity–building practice, community health practitioners, often called organizers, work with and between people, groups, and organizations to identify and use the resources they have for the betterment of the community. They build capacity by providing particular types of services, programs, and goods that help community members feel like a community and address their health issues (Ontario Prevention Clearing House, 2002).

The complete practice of some community health practitioners, such as social workers or community developers or organizers, is composed of community capacity building. For community health nurses working for a public health organization or a community health center or organization, community capacity building will often be only a part of their practice. The other parts could consist of health teaching, immunizing, or running medical clinics. These multiple roles of the community health nurse can be confusing for community members who are unfamiliar with the social determinants of health. People may ask, "Where is the health in what you are doing?" For example, nurses could be working with community groups on controlling street traffic, obtaining legal assistance, or building a playground. On the surface, these activities do not appear to be directly related to health, although they do relate to the determinants of health. Community health nurses need to take time to explain how community capacity building can be as important to the health of the community as other public health or medical services directed at preventing specific diseases.

Although most community health nurses are building community capacity part time, they can include the concepts in all their relationships within the community. This requires using dialogue that encourages a sense of community and community action. Dialogue is the skillful interaction between people that develops shared understanding as a basis for trust, ownership, true agreement, and creative problem solving (National Association of County and City Health Officials, 2014). During dialogue, a leader moves from a totally receptive listening role to a position that starts challenging the people to look critically at their beliefs in what has been called a problem-posing approach (Wallerstein & Bernstein, 1988). Being challenging does not mean that community health nurses and others impose ideas on a group, such as wanting to address poverty, rather than a more manageable project, such as a clothing exchange. It does mean asking questions and introducing other ideas, issues, perspectives, or underlying problems.

Be prepared for people to take time to think about your information and questions. For example, I was engaged in participatory research with mothers of adolescent girls (Diem, 2000). As part of the discussion, I asked if they felt their daughters had to deal with discrimination. A couple of women responded quickly with "No, not like I had." However, the next time we met, a few mentioned how they had come to realize that a son was favored over a daughter and how girls still do not have as much freedom as boys.

Discussion and dialogue also offer hope and a vision that will inspire the community. The challenge includes encouraging and supporting community residents to take action on the issues that they have identified.

## Communities with Vulnerable Populations

Vulnerable populations may be designated as at-risk, underserved, or another term indicating that they are in some way more apt than the general population to become ill. In the US, the following vulnerable populations are designated as priority populations (Agency for Health Care Research and Quality, 2014): racial and ethnic minority groups, low-income groups, women, children (under age 18), older adults (age 65 and over), residents of rural areas, and individuals with special health care needs, including those with disabilities and those needing chronic or end-of-life care. In Canada, one organization designates vulnerable populations as those that include children, Aboriginal people, older adults, persons with disabilities, racialized and immigrant groups, and injured workers (Canada without Poverty, 2014). Certainly those affected by a combination of vulnerabilities, such as an Asian woman with diabetes living with a low income, or an Alaskan Native adolescent, would have increased risk for poor health and would require compensatory action by the health care system.

Vulnerable populations are often accessed through communities. The access point in the community could be a homeless shelter, a community health center, or a school because the people you want to reach live near that location and use those services. In the next section, we discuss the characteristics of two types of communities: school communities and rural and northern communities. Although the approach to building capacity follows the same process, the two types of communities provide a range of features to consider when tailoring the approach to different situations. The discussions and scenarios related to the two types of communities reinforce the need to develop an open and supportive role in working with communities.

## School Communities

Schools are the prime civic center for children from about age 5 to 18 throughout most of the world. In past centuries, children developed and contributed to the family through farm work or assisting in the family business. Now children acquire most knowledge and skills by attending school. Schools are an institution of society that provides the opportunity for children from a variety of backgrounds to attain the resources and guidance to prepare them to earn a living and contribute to society. Schools also help to define a community.

Elementary or primary schools for younger children are usually located close to where students live. High, or secondary, schools for older children often receive students from several elementary schools. Other schools, called middle schools, serve children in grades 7 to 9 or 10. Although the smaller elementary schools are easier to consider as part of the community, all schools have the potential of becoming a center for the community.

Schools might provide nursery schools programs, afterschool programs, and additional sports and recreation programs outside school hours.

The World Health Organization (WHO, 2014a) identifies adolescence as the period between childhood and adulthood that is second only to that of infancy in terms of the rate of growth and development. Early adolescence is particularly challenging. **Early adolescence** begins with puberty, between the ages of 10 and 14 years, and includes cognitive, emotional, sexual, and psychological transformation (United Nations Children's Fund [UNICEF], 2011). UNICEF states that early adolescence should be a time when children have a safe and clear space to come to terms with these many changes, unencumbered by having to perform adult roles and with the full support of nurturing adults at home, at school, and in the community. Early adolescence is also a time of considerable risk during which social contexts exert powerful influences. A nurturing environment provides opportunities for early adolescents to learn a wide range of important skills that can help them to cope with the pressures they face (WHO, 2014a).

Since its inception in 1983, the Health Behaviour in School-aged Children (HBSC), a WHO collaborative cross-national study (Currie et al., 2012), provides key insights into the health-related behaviors of hundreds of thousands of young people ages 11, 13, and 15 years in many parts of the world. The fifth international HBSC report focuses on social determinants of health and provides a full description of the health and well-being of young people growing up in 39 countries and regions across Europe and North America through data collected from the 2009/2010 survey. The report includes data from each country and region, a summary of research related to groups of indicators, analysis of the results, and policy recommendations.

The HBSC report (Currie et al., 2012) includes four types of indicators:

1. Social context, specifically relating to family, peers, and school, which often serve as protective factors
2. Health outcomes, with indicators that describe current levels of health and well-being
3. Health behaviors, relating to indicators that are potentially health sustaining
4. Risk behaviors, relating to indicators that are potentially health damaging.

Since capacity building has the potential to increase the protective factors provided by peers and school, this section focuses on those factors in the social context indicator.

According to the HBSC report (Currie et al., 2012), establishing peer friendships is a critical developmental task for young people, since friends provide a unique social context for the development of essential social skills, afford different kinds of social support, and help young people face new situations and stressful life experiences. One of the items on the survey asked students if they had three or more close friends of the same gender. The positive responses from 11-year-old boys and girls in the US and Canada ranged from 82 to 89 percent; the responses from 15-year-olds ranged from 75 to 83 percent. These responses were average or slightly above average compared to other countries. The report states that a positive experience at school can support the development of close friendships and recommends school programs that involve multiple social contexts.

A positive school experience is considered a resource for health and well-being, while a negative experience may constitute a risk factor, affecting students' mental and physical health (Currie et al., 2012). The survey asked how much the students liked school. It also asked about their perceived school performance and support from classmates. The report states that liking school has been identified as a protective factor against health-compromising behaviors including bullying, sexual risk-taking, and tobacco, alcohol, and drug use. In response to the item on liking school, 27 to 47 percent of 11-year-old boys and girls in Canada and the US responded that they liked school a lot. This dropped to 19 to 24 percent for 15-year-olds. These responses from the two countries showed the definite decline by age, as in other countries, but were below average when compared to the others. The proportion of students who perceived their school performance as good or very good as compared to their classmates for both countries was 73 to 82 percent for 11-year-olds, and 59 to 70 percent for 15-year-olds. These responses showed some decline by age as in other countries, but were above average compared to others. The proportion of students in both countries who agreed or strongly agreed that their class-mates are kind and helpful was 62 to 66 percent for 11-year-olds and 49 to 56 percent for 15-year-olds. The decrease by age was similar to other countries, but the responses for this item in North America were much below the average.

In the analysis of the items related to schools, affluence or high family income was associated with positive responses. After a review of the literature, however, the editors (Currie et al., 2012) conclude that strengthening relationships between young people and their classmates and teachers can develop self-efficacy, and young people with high self-efficacy are more willing to invest in learning to overcome difficulties. The school environment can therefore be used to bolster young people's resources and, in turn, develop positive health and education outcomes irrespective of family affluence.

The report concludes the school section by stating that school perceptions worsen with increasing age across countries and regions, with liking school, perceived academic achievement, and, to a lesser extent, classmate support decreasing, and perceived school pressure increasing (Currie et al., 2012). The report indicates that there is a systematic pattern of schools increasingly not meeting students' basic psychological needs from ages 11 to 15 and the pattern reflects the mismatch between the environment in middle and secondary schools and young people's needs. The report states that at an age when students would benefit from greater connectedness with their teachers and a more supportive school climate, the opposite occurs. School organization tends to become more depersonalized from primary and middle to secondary school, with different teachers for different subjects and, in many countries, different student groups for each subject, stratified by academic level and school.

Community/public health nurses working in schools can help identify and address health and social issues at the level of individual students, staff, and families, as well as factors that affect the whole school. In a report to maximize the role of public health nurses in school setting, the Community Health Nurses Initiatives Group (2013) identifies that public health nurses in schools bring a unique perspective to health and well-being to address barriers to healthy growth and development, social inclusion, academic achievement, literacy, and obtaining food, as well as language and culture. The unique perspective integrates both asset-based approaches, such as social competence skill building, and risk reduction/prevention strategies in their practice. This perspective also underlies the social determinants of health.

The perspective of community health nurses working in schools and the conclusions and recommendations of the HBSC report reinforce the need for building capacity within schools. A positive school climate, sometimes called school culture or school

As a public health nurse and as a faculty clinical instructor, Bev has worked in schools for several years and supervised student nursing teams at the Eastvale Public School for the previous four years. The school has almost 600 students, ranging from kindergarten to grade 8. As Bev talks to the principal about plans for the fall, the principal recounts the successful nursing student projects that had been completed so far: a healthy eating project with grade 3 classes, a two-year anti-bullying project with grade 5 classes, and healthy sexuality with grade 7 classes. Almost in passing, the principal mentions discussions with the teachers about increasing unrest among the students in grades 6 to 8. When Bev asks what this means, the principal says it is hard to pin down except that the teachers feel that there are more outbreaks of anger and that fewer students join the school clubs and activities. Bev proposes that a nursing student team with male and female students work with the senior classes to explore the students' strengths and issues. The principal really likes the idea and knows that she can easily recruit teachers and students to work with the team.

The student team looks forward to working with the senior classes. They remember the difficult experiences and mood swings they had when they were that age. In preparation for their first meeting at the school, they review the information on capacity building, the social context part of the HBSC report (Currie et al., 2012), and the school's website to prepare questions to ask the principal, teachers, and students.

At the first meeting with the principal and teachers, the team asks about a statement on the school's website: "The student population is culturally and linguistically diverse, with many students speaking a third language." One teacher, who immigrated from Somalia 10 years ago, indicates that the majority of the students originate from the Middle East, Africa, and South Asia. Then the team leader asks how the students who transfer to the school manage, since the website indicates that students from three primary schools transfer to Eastvale for grades 7 and 8. The question generates a lively discussion among the teachers, with most indicating that the transfer students have difficulty getting used to the school because the school is much bigger, they are often separated from their friends, and students who have been in the school longer have their own circle of friends. They also mention that perhaps the school does not do enough to welcome students from different cultures. At the end of the meeting, the team feels that they are off to a good start by demonstrating the team's interest in the school and identifying that the teachers want to improve the students' school experience.

**First Step in Drafting a Portrait of the School**

For the first step in drafting a portrait of the school (MACS-NS/Boivin, 2011), the team seeks answers to the following questions: "What are the students' preferred activities? Where do they gather? Who are they with? What makes them happy? What do they like to celebrate? What do they like to eat?" To find these answers, the team forms three subteams. Two males are on one subteam and focus on talking to boys during gym classes, at lunch, and in the play yard. The other two subteams arrange opportunities for observation and interaction in the classes, play yard, lunchroom, and afterschool groups. Each subteam seeks out students to collaborate with them in each location. After each interaction session, the subteam records the responses from students and collaborators in field notes.

After two weeks they feel that they are starting to get an idea of what students like, how and where to approach them, and also have the beginnings of a group of student collaborators. They also realize that they are missing input from the transfer students, especially those in grade 7. By asking around, they find those students gathered in quiet corners of the hallways and lunchroom. After the team explains why their views are important, the transfer students gradually start talking. Their responses are quite different from previous responses and most relate to experiences they had at their primary schools, such as multicultural events with food and dancing, and opportunities for their parents and family members to be involved in school activities, such as playing chess and needlework groups. The team is able to recruit a few transfer students to work with the other collaborators.

## Steps Two and Three in Drafting a Portrait of the School

As the team moves to the next steps, they realize that they need to involve the teachers and hopefully some of the parents. Using the six steps of drafting a school portrait, they work with their school advisors and Bev to prepare a list of key informant questions to determine what the teachers and principal like, and the strengths, resources, needs and challenges, and leaders and octopuses of the school. Each team member arranges to interview at least one teacher from grades 6, 7, or 8 with a student collaborator over the next few weeks. They also find out that they can meet with parents when they come for parent-teacher interviews.

After determining what the students, parents, teachers, and principal like, the team and collaborators find that the process for gathering information on strengths and resources goes much quicker. One student collaborator suggests using the bulletin board in the main hallway for people to post their ideas on strengths and resources. The team and collaborators take turns staffing the bulletin board and record comments if people are reluctant to write their ideas. The remaining team members ask about strengths and resources during their informal interactions with students.

## Step Four in Drafting a Portrait of the School

To identify the needs and challenges, the team asks for 30 minutes alone with the students in each of the nine grade 6, 7, and 8 classes. They want to spend as much time as possible getting feedback from the students, but also to tell them about the positive things they have found so far. In addition, they distribute the written questions in the classroom as well as verbally asking people to respond. Students can choose to hand in their responses or not. They work in their small groups with their collaborators to identify the main needs and challenges.

The next week, the team and collaborators take time to summarize their results from the students, teachers, and parents. They do not do an in-depth analysis, but want to get some sense of where the different groups stand in terms of positive aspects and needs.

## Steps Five and Six in Drafting a Portrait of the School

The final two steps are to identify the leaders and the "octopuses," well-connected people. The team and collaborators draw up a preliminary list of leaders and octopuses from among the students, teachers, and parents. They fan out through the school to ask if the list of leaders is accurate. During their consultation with students, teachers, and parents, they add some people's names and remove others.

As the final involvement with the school, the team asks the advisors, Bev, the collaborators, and the principal how and where to present the portrait of the school. The collaborators suggest that the information could be posted inside an outline of a portrait frame in the main hallway. The advisors and principal concur, as long as the people identified as leaders and octopuses agree to have their names included.

The team and collaborators stand back and look at the portrait of Eastvale Public School. Having completed this first stage, they hope that the building of capacity of the school community will be carried on. Even if that does not happen as they envision, they know that the work they did in asking, listening, and recording what people had to say about the school will provide long-term benefits.

## Discussion Topics and Questions

3. How were students included in the capacity building?
4. How did the team include information from the HBSC report (Currie et al., 2012) in the approach?
5. How did the team manage to use consistent questions and approaches when they were working in different locations?

environment (similar to a sense of community), is associated not only with higher academic achievement but also with better self-reporting of students' health, well-being, and health behaviors. Recommendations to promote a positive school climate include identifying and promoting young people's special interests and skills to acknowledge that schools value the diversity they bring, especially for marginalized students; providing students with a voice within the school community; and using a variety of learning and teaching strategies, possibly suggested by students, to better promote student engagement. These recommendations are consistent with capacity building.

Community capacity building in a school can start in one classroom, with a group meeting at the school, or with a parent-teacher association, and be for a short time or expand over time. For example, a small primary school in Vermont instituted the Safe Routes to School (SRTS) Program (see Box 1.4 in Chapter 1) over three years to bring the school and community together to improve the health and well-being of children by enabling and encouraging them to walk and bicycle to school. Other school and community initiatives could involve developing a community garden, keeping a local park clean and safe, or partnering with a school in another country. The important aspect for school capacity building is that the action brings students together to interact and make decisions. Students then have the opportunity to feel they belong and can contribute to the school and community.

## Rural, Northern, and Remote Communities

Rural and northern communities develop their own culture based on their history, geography, and major occupation. This culture affects the health status of rural residents and the role of the community health nurse working in those areas. Rural and northern communities have usually been formed by self-reliant and independent people determined to eke out a living from the land (Keating, 1991; Leipert & Reutter, 1998). Their pioneering spirit allowed them to harvest natural resources such as crops, domestic animals, fish, minerals, or trees to support the economic growth of the country. This spirit also encourages a strong sense of community.

In Canada, rural and small town (less than 10,000 inhabitants) refers to the population living outside the commuting zones of larger urban centers (Canadian Institute of Health Information, 2006). For purposes of health care services in the US, Rural-Urban Commuting Area (RUCA) codes classify subcounty areas on a scale representing urbanization, population density, and daily commuting (Rural Assistance Center, 2014). **Rural** is defined as an area that is sparsely populated and outside daily commuting distance to a large urban center.

In both countries, areas of greater isolation exist. In Canada, these areas include the three northern territories and the northern parts of the larger provinces. In the US, these frontier areas are located in the west, a part of the country where individual counties tend to cover a large geographic area, and in Alaska. Remote and frontier areas are far from health care, schools, grocery stores, and other necessities (Rural Assistance Center, 2014). These isolated communities are often characterized by severe climatic conditions and either great distances between areas of habitation, lack of road access, or road access only at certain times of the year (Leipert & Reutter, 1998).

One important factor of living in rural, northern, and remote communities is the difficulty of obtaining healthy food. People who have sufficient healthy food are said to have food security. **Food security** has three aspects: (1) availability of food in sufficient quantities and on a consistent basis, (2) sufficient resources to obtain appropriate foods for a nutritious diet, and (3) appropriate knowledge of basic nutrition and care, as well as adequate water and sanitation (WHO, 2014b). Transportation costs, storage costs, insufficient resources for public water and sewage, and limited sources of information about the preparation of healthy food all contribute to limited food security in rural and remote communities.

Another issue related to rural and remote communities is that young adults often migrate to urban areas, leaving behind an aging population (North Dakota State University, 2014). On the other hand, people may choose to locate to rural areas because of a preference for a safe, friendly, family-focused routine associated with a small-town way of life. These shared values illustrate a strong sense of community and can be promoted as quality-of-life incentives to bring people back, as well as keep them (North Dakota State University, 2014).

Rural areas are frequently associated with right-wing politics, traditional family values (Keating, 1991; Leipert & Reutter, 1998), and less experience in dealing with differences and change compared to people living in more urban areas. The culture can mean that male preferences dominate in both the community and the delivery of health care (Leipert, 2005, 1999; Leipert & Reutter, 1998). Other groups in the community, notably women who are elderly, lesbian, disabled, or First Nations, suffer from lack of appropriate health and social programs (Leipert, 2005). Often a major part of the nursing role in rural areas is to work with women to develop programs that are appropriate for them and their families.

## Health Status of Rural, Northern, and Remote Populations

According to the US Census Bureau (2010), 19.3 percent of the US population live in rural areas. Similarly, Canada was close with 18.9 percent of the population living in rural areas in 2011 (Statistics Canada, 2013). Compared with their urban counterparts, rural residents in the US are more likely to have chronic conditions and be older, poor, in fair or poor health, less likely to receive recommended preventive services, and more likely to report having deferred care due to cost (Agency for Health Care Research and Quality, 2014). They must deal with several barriers to health care, including a reduced number of physicians, dependence on small, underfunded hospitals, few services for people who have limited English proficiency, and difficulty with transportation (Agency for Health Care Research and Quality, 2014).

Similar findings are apparent in Canada. The Canadian Institute of Health Information (2006) reports that, generally, rural residents of Canada are more likely to live in poorer socioeconomic conditions, have lower levels of education, exhibit less healthy behaviors, and have higher overall mortality rates than urban residents. On the positive side, rural residents feel a strong sense of community belonging, in greater proportions than their urban counterparts. The report offers some success stories that could be used for community health interventions: occupational health and safety programs focused on rural-based industries such as farming, fishing, logging, and mining, and rural-friendly

Bev is working from a sub-office in West Selkirk County, a large rural county that takes over an hour and a half to drive to from the city center. Bev raises the concern with the rural program that many of the older and poorer county residents have limited access to healthy, affordable food, since the closest supermarket is an hour's drive away. Bev receives approval to initiate a capacity-building strategy based on improving access to healthy food in the county and is encouraged to seek outside funding, since additional staffing and resources will likely be needed.

### Stage 1: Draft Portrait that Resembles the Community

Bev begins drafting a portrait of the community by telling people that she is asking questions to help them see the county's strengths and resources, challenges, and leaders so they can decide if there is sufficient interest and commitment in the community to get a food project off the ground. Right from the beginning, she has support from a variety of people: the coordinator for the county's food bank, public health inspector, and dietitian, and the county councillor who brings in representatives from the rural advisory board, seniors' council, and the local media. Bev brings these collaborators together as an advisory committee to determine the needs and challenges, leaders, and well-connected people. The committee quickly identifies the need for increased access to healthy, affordable food. One immediate challenge is storage for donated food, because the food bank lacks a freezer. Most of the leaders and well-connected people are already at the table, but when Bev asks "Who else should be involved in this committee?" several others, including ministers, leaders from women's groups, and farmers, are mentioned.

### Stage 2: Find the Rallying Idea

A local newspaper article on the portrait of the county provides quick results; the food bank is the grateful recipient of a commercial-type freezer. The momentum might have stopped there, but Bev and the committee have other health benefits that they want to see. They envision a series of cooking events at different locations in the county where residents can prepare food together, learn about healthy food, eat the food, and take food home for future meals. They hope these food events will also build community capacity and connections among people.

The committee discusses possible names for what they want to do and a rallying idea. Bev suggests taking the ideas to the people and finding out what they would like. She is able to recruit volunteers from the high school and first-year students from the nursing program to poll county residents at fall fairs, farmers' markets, and churches over four weekends. The students find that the rallying idea of "Country Kitchen" works for everyone and that almost all the residents welcome the idea of a country kitchen, and want to know when it will start, and what they can do to help.

When the committee meets, they soon have a name for their initiative, West Selkirk Country Kitchen, and a clear message: Cooking together and eating together, learning new recipes, getting nutritional tips, and having fun in the kitchen. The name of their committee is the West Selkirk Country Kitchen Committee, which is quickly shortened to The Kitchen Committee. The local paper and radio station quickly pass on the latest developments.

### Stage 3: Planning and Taking Action

The Kitchen Committee draft a work plan. Most are familiar with planning and have often worked together. The plan includes applying for funding, hiring a coordinator, recruiting and training volunteers, requesting use of community kitchens from community groups, requesting food donations from local famers and residents, recruiting participants, and implementing and evaluating the plan. Once the plan is completed, Bev can see opportunities to involve a student nursing team in implementing it and requests a team from the nursing program.

The four-member nursing student team takes a couple of weeks to orient themselves to the county and to learn about the West Selkirk Country Kitchen. One of them has a car, and they spend a day finding the villages, schools, recreation centers, and churches that Bev has indicated may be involved in the Country Kitchen. They feel a bit overwhelmed with the size of the area, and decide to print off a map for each of them so they can find places that people mention.

They have a bit of difficulty understanding the capacity-building aspect of the Country Kitchen, even after Bev reviews the previous stages. They wonder, but don't ask Bev, why public health doesn't simply put on a series of demonstrations on how to cook healthy foods. Bev indicates that they can start learning about the community by helping her to recruit volunteers and community kitchens at meetings of community groups throughout the county. At the first meeting at the Hawthorne Community Center, Bev takes the lead in describing the ideas involved in the Country Kitchen and what their involvement might be. She then asks for their thoughts and sits back in her chair. Some agree to become involved, and some disagree. Bev doesn't speak again until everyone in the group has had a chance to talk. As she looks around the group, Bev summarizes the discussion by saying that some can see the value of being involved with the Country Kitchen, while others are concerned about detracting from their own efforts at the community center. At a break in the discussion, Bev thanks the group for taking the time to listen to her proposal, provides the chair with her contact information, and says that she hopes to hear from them regarding their decision in the next couple of weeks. After the meeting, Bev explains to the team that she knew that this group was going to be the most challenging and encourages the students to discuss how she conducted the session.

The team works with the newly hired coordinator to plan and deliver the training for volunteers. They also prepare evaluation questions for use during the event with Bev. The team is able to attend the first event of the Country Kitchen and take turns helping out in the kitchen, serving, observing, and asking the evaluation questions. At the end of the day, they admit that they are amazed by everyone's enthusiasm and excitement. They observed women learning about different foods and ways to prepare the foods, and they saw the care shown to older people as they were picked up and driven to the event, provided a meal to eat with their neighbors, and given food to take home. They admit that they now appreciate the value of capacity building, because they now also feel a part of the community and are sad to leave.

### Stage 4: Maintaining the Momentum

Once the student team finishes and the paid coordinator takes over the management of the planned events, Bev has more time to consider different options to offer to the Committee to maintain the momentum of the Country Kitchen. The Committee looks again at the vision and the preliminary evaluation conducted

by the student team and decides to add more locations and different themes according to the season, such as organic cooking and gardening, homemade fast foods, and gifts in a jar for Christmas.

An ongoing concern is organizing transportation for mothers and older adults. One Committee member suggests that the different recreation centers and churches take this on for each area. The suggestion is met with a pause until the person offers to form a subcommittee to take over the organizing. That offer is met by applause.

The chair of the Committee then looks around at the members and starts identifying the unique contributions of each person. Others add to the accolades. Although people often look embarrassed, they are also pleased. They plan to hold a celebration party twice a year.

### Stage 5: Evaluating

Although the Committee is collecting and reviewing evaluation comments from each event and monitoring participation figures, they feel that a formal evaluation will help them in determining their direction and meeting their goals. Luckily their requirements meet with the needs of a master's student in nursing who wants to evaluate a community capacity–building initiative for her thesis. The master's student works closely with the Committee to find answers for the following questions (MACS-NB & Boivin, 2011): "Have you accomplished what you set out to do? What worked well and what could be changed? What results did you obtain? What lessons can you draw from the experience? How did your work affect your community?"

### Discussion Topics and Questions

6. How did Bev's discussion with the Hawthorne group incorporate the three aspects of dialogue (awareness of one's own assumptions, skills of listening, and allowing for different perspectives until a shared understanding emerges)?

7. What aspects of community capacity building do you feel the team came to appreciate?

8. What made the experience of working on different aspects of the Country Kitchen worthwhile for the team?

approaches in disease prevention and health promotion in the areas of smoking reduction, increase in consumption of fruits and vegetables, and obesity.

## Working in Rural Communities

Community health nurses working to build on the capacity of community groups in rural areas face a particular opportunity as well as a challenge. The opportunity derives from the strong sense of community usually seen in rural areas. The challenge is for new community health nurses to become oriented to the rural area and to gain the trust and acceptance of community members.

It is helpful to know that the land of a state or province is divided into various areas with defined boundaries. The most common, in approximate order of increasing geographic size, is municipality or township, county, and state or province. The usual description of a county is that it is a geographical unit of administration intermediate between the larger state or province and the smaller township or municipality. The jurisdiction of each unit will be similar within the same state or province, but is likely to vary between states and provinces and countries.

Determining the boundaries of a rural area is part of the early assessment. This would include the names of the county administrators, the location of their office, and their responsibilities. As these boundaries become known, further assessment would involve determining whether the people living in the county identify with being a resident and are concerned about county matters. For example, there may be many people who decide to be reclusive and have minimal contact with the community. They would meet one aspect of being a community by sharing the same location, but lack the relational ties that bring people together to work on common issues.

Examples of community capacity–building initiatives with women used by public health nurses in northern British Columbia are an informal women's coffee group and a women's wellness day (Leipert, 1999). In a small northern Ontario mining town, the author and a colleague worked with women in the community to determine a community project. The women decided that they wanted something for women like the community hunting and fishing show for men. The events they decided on included discussion groups on menopause, parenting adolescents, and child care; displays of household and kitchen merchandise; and a fashion show of casual clothes. The women continued the events on their own. Community health nurses need skills and knowledge to identify issues that will bring rural community groups together and support them while they make changes to improve their community.

## Summary

Successful community capacity building involves engaging community members in planning and carrying out community initiatives. For community health workers, including community health nurses, the two most important approaches are to use dialogue to engage people and a process that requires their active involvement. Community members become engaged when the dialogue is open to a variety of viewpoints, helps to clarify and validate different perspectives, and seeks a shared understanding. The process of building community capacity begins with defining the strengths, challenges, and leadership in the community and progresses through planning, taking action, and evaluation.

The pertinent sociodemographic and developmental characteristics of two vulnerable groups of people, early adolescents and rural residents, illustrate approaches and the process of community capacity building with different populations and situations. The process not only involves community members at every stage, but it also provides a direction and purpose so community members feel that their effort is worthwhile and will benefit the community.

## Classroom and Seminar Exercises

1. Discuss how the community health nurse's role (Bev's involvement) changed over time in the rural scenario and how this change fit or did not fit with concepts related to levels of participation and community capacity building.
2. Identify how community capacity building in the following situations would differ:
   a. In an urban setting compared to a rural area
   b. Working with younger people as compared to older people
   c. Working with low-income people as compared to those with higher income
3. Take one of the following issues and identify how community capacity building would differ from a health education approach:
   a. Teenage pregnancy
   b. Women's or men's health
   c. Parenting practices
4. Describe a community group you are familiar with and explain which circumstances faced by the group could best be dealt with by using community capacity building.
5. Take one of the issues or circumstances described in question 4 and identify what actions you would take to involve the community in drafting a community portrait.

## References

Agency for Health Care Research and Quality. (2014). *National healthcare disparities report, 2013* (Chapter 11, Priority Populations). Retrieved from www.ahrq.gov/research/findings/nhqrdr/nhdr13/chap11.html

Arnstein, S. (2006 [1969]). A ladder of citizen participation. *Journal of the American Institute of Planners, 35*, 216–224. Retrieved from http://lithgow-schmidt.dk/sherry-arnstein/ladder-of-citizen-participation.html

Canada without Poverty. (2014). *Vulnerable populations*. Retrieved from www.cwp-csp.ca/resources/vulnerable-populations/

Canadian Institute of Health Information. (2006). *How healthy are rural Canadians?* Retrieved from https://secure.cihi.ca/free_products/rural_canadians_2006_report_e.pdf

Community Health Nurses Initiatives Group. (2013). *Healthy schools, healthy children: Maximizing the contribution of public health nursing in school settings.* Retrieved from www.chnig.org/documents/News%20Attachments/School%20Health%20Policy%20Paper.pdf

Currie, C., Zanotti, C., Morgan, A., Currie, D., de Looze, M., Roberts, C., & Barnekow, V. (2012). *Social determinants of health and well-being among young people. Health behaviour in school-aged children (HBSC) study: International report from the 2009/2010 survey* (Health Policy for Children and Adolescents, No. 6). Copenhagen: World Health Organization Regional Office for Europe. Retrieved from www.euro.who.int/__data/assets/pdf_file/0003/163857/Social-determinants-of-health-and-well-being-among-young-people.pdf?ua=1

Diem, E. (2000). Balancing relationship and discipline: The pressing concern of mothers of early adolescent girls. *Canadian Journal of Nursing Research, 21,* 87–103.

Freire, P. (1972). *Pedagogy of the oppressed.* New York: Herder and Herder.

Fremlin, J. (2014). *Identifying concepts that build a sense of community.* Retrieved from www.senseofcommunityresearch.org/research/updates/identifying-concepts-that-build-a-sense-of-community

Goeppinger, J., & Hammond, R. (2000). The renaissance of primary care: An opportunity for nursing. In J. Hickey, R. Ouimette, & S. Venegoni (Eds.), *Advanced practice nursing: Changing roles and clinical applications* (2nd ed., pp. 175–189). Philadelphia, PA: Lippincott Williams & Wilkins.

Keating, N. (1991). *Aging in rural Canada.* Vancouver, BC: Butterworths Canada.

KU Work Group for Community Health and Development. (2014). Our model of practice: Building capacity for community and system change. *Community Tool Box* (Chapter 1, Section 3). Retrieved from http://ctb.ku.edu/en/table-of-contents/overview/model-for-community-change-and-improvement/building-capacity/main

Leipert, B. (1999). Women's health and the practice of public health nurses in northern British Columbia. *Public Health Nursing, 16*(4), 280–289.

Leipert, B. (2005). *Rural women's health issues in Canada: An overview and implications for policy and research.* Retrieved from http://pi.library.yorku.ca/ojs/index.php/cws/article/viewFile/6074/5262

Leipert, B., & Reutter, L. (1998). Women's health and community health nursing practice in geographically isolated settings: A Canadian perspective. *Health Care for Women International, 19*(6), 575–588.

Mattessich, P., & Monsey, B. (1997). *Community building: What makes it work.* Saint Paul, MN: Amherst H. Wilder Foundation.

McMillan, D., & Chavis, D. (1986). *Sense of community: A definition and theory.* Retrieved from http://mc7290.bgsu.wikispaces.net/file/view/McMillan_1986.pdf

Minkler, M., Wallerstein, N., & Wilson, N. (2008). Improving health through community organization and community building. In K. Glanx, B. Rimer, & K. Viswanath (Eds.), *Health behavior and health education: Theory, research, and practice* (4th ed., pp. 287–312). San Francisco, CA: Jossey-Bass.

Mouvement Acadien des Communautés en Santé Du Nouveau-Brunswick (MACS-NB) & Boivin, N. (2011). *Building a healthy community to take action in health promotion.* Retrieved from www.ohcc-ccso.ca/en/webfm_send/560

National Association of County and City Health Officials. (2014). *Public health infrastructure and system: Dialogue.* Retrieved from www.naccho.org/topics/infrastructure/dialogue/overview.cfm

North Dakota State University. (2014). *Center for community vitality.* Retrieved from www.ag.ndsu.edu/ccv/documents/building-a-sense-of-community-in-your-town

Nyswander, D. (1956). Education for health: Some principles and their applications. *Health Education Monographs, 14*, 65–70.

Ontario Prevention Clearing House. (2002). *Capacity building for health promotion: More than bricks or mortar.* Retrieved from www.opc.on.ca

Public Health Nursing Section. (2001). *Public health interventions—Applications for public health nursing practice.* St. Paul, MN: Minnesota Department of Health.

Rural Assistance Center. (2014). *What is rural?* Retrieved from www.raconline.org/topics/what-is-rural/faqs#goldsmith

Statistics Canada. (2010). *Community belonging.* Retrieved from http://www.statcan.gc.ca/pub/82-229-x/2009001/envir/cob-eng.htm

Statistics Canada. (2013). *Canada's rural population since 1851.* Retrieved from www12.statcan.gc.ca/census-recensement/2011/as-sa/98-310-x/98-310-x2011003_2-eng.cfm

Thompson, B., & Kinne, S. (1999). Social change theory: Application to community health. In N. Bracht (Ed.), *Health promotion at the community level* (2nd ed., pp. 29–46). Thousand Oaks, CA: Sage.

United Nations Children's Fund (UNICEF). (2011). *The state of the world's children 2011.* Retrieved from www.unicef.org/adolescence/files/SOWC_2011_Main_Report_EN_02092011.pdf

US Census Bureau. (2010). *2010 census urban and rural classification and urban area criteria.* Retrieved from www.census.gov/geo/reference/ua/urban-rural-2010.html

Wallerstein, N., & Bernstein, E. (1988). Empowerment education: Freire's ideas adapted to health education. *Health Education Quarterly, 15*, 379–394.

Werner, D., & Bower, B. (1982). *Helping health workers learn.* Berkeley, CA: Hesperian Foundation.

World Health Organization (WHO). (2014a). *Adolescent development.* Retrieved from www.who.int/maternal_child_adolescent/topics/adolescence/dev/en/

World Health Organization (WHO). (2014b). *Food security.* Retrieved from www.who.int/trade/glossary/story028/en/

# Website Resources

### Community Capacity Building

Asset-Based Community Development (ABCD) Institute: www.abcdinstitute.org/

The ABCD Institute at Northwestern University is built upon three decades of community development research by John Kretzmann and John L. McKnight. The Institute develops tools to mobilize communities and to help identify and develop community assets. The site also links to research papers and best practice information on community development.

Health Nexus: http://en.healthnexus.ca/topics-tools/community-engagement

Health Nexus has evolved from the former Ontario Prevention Clearing House, which provided community development and health promotion resources for over 25 years. The community engagement website includes resources for collaboration, healthy communities, leadership, network mapping/network development, partnerships, and technology and socialmedia.

Mobilizing for Action through Planning and Partnerships (MAPP): www.naccho.org/topics/infrastructure/mapp/

MAPP is a strategic approach to community health improvement. The MAPP tool was developed by the National Association of County and City Health Officials (NACCHO) in cooperation with the Public Health Practice Program Office, Centers for Disease Control and Prevention. This site provides tip sheets on various aspects of MAPP, such as a very practical tip sheet "Engaging the Community," which is found under Tools on the home page.

Ontario Healthy Communities Coalition, and Canadian Healthy Communities: www.ohcc-ccso.ca/en/what-we-do, and www.chc-csc.ca/

Both websites provide many examples and resources for community development and capacity building, including the guide *Building a Healthy Community to Take Action in Health Promotion*, developed by the Mouvement Acadien des Communautés en Santé Du Nouveau-Brunswick (MACS-NB) and N. Boivin (2011).

### School Capacity Building

Environmental Youth Alliance (EYA): www.eya.ca

EYA is recognized as a leading agency in youth engagement through environmental education and community grassroots action projects. The Programs and Projects section of their website provides descriptions of community gardens, school projects, obtaining food, and other projects.

World Health Organization, *School and Youth Health*: www.who.int/school_youth_health/gshi/hps/en/

This website defines the characteristics of a health-promoting school and provides resources for health-promoting schools generally and specifically in areas such as nutrition, physical exercise, and sun screening.

### Rural Information and Rural Nursing

Canadian Association for Rural and Remote Nursing (CARRN): www.carrn.com/articles.htm

The CARRN website provides interesting articles on the experiences of nurses providing care under difficult geographical situations and conditions.

Rural Information Center (USDA): http://ric.nal.usda.gov/ http://ric.nal.usda.gov/rural-health-0

This page on the Rural Information Center website provides links to websites related to rural health. The website has an interactive atlas to identify small towns and rural areas in each state.

Rural Nurse Organization: http://rnojournal.binghamton.edu/index.php/RNO

This US organization provides an online journal of rural nursing and health care with free access to abstracts.

# Chapter 11

# Working with Coalitions

· · · · · ·  · · · · · · · · · · · · · · · · · · · · · · · · · · · · · · · · · · · · · · · · · · · · · · · · · · · · · · · · · · · · · · · · · · · · · · · · · · · · · · · · · · · · · · ·

Practicing community health nursing within a primary health care framework requires a broad vision and long-term perspective. The focus of this chapter—working with coalitions—provides insight into the nature and time scale of this collaborative community activity and identifies the role community health nurses can, and do, play within coalitions. Part of the network of professional relationships in the community, coalitions are integral to community health nursing practice (Community Health Nurses of Canada, 2011; Quad Council of Public Health Nursing Organizations, 2011). Empirical research shows that today's practitioners are engaged in forming coalitions, supporting their work, and evaluating their function and health impact (MacLellan-Wright et al., 2007; Schoenfeld & MacDonald, 2002). Given the broad scope of coalitions, a practitioner usually works as part of a program team with management guidance and support; however, within the coalition, the community health practitioner represents community/public health and is the human face of the organization.

Bearing in mind that the life of a coalition is measured in years, not weeks, nurses may not gain experience in this aspect of community work as part of their nursing education. So, how do nurses acquire the knowledge and skills for this practice? Typically, students spend days in a clinical setting, albeit over a three- to four-month period, and the practicum may not coincide with observable coalition activities. To complicate matters even further, by definition, coalition work extends outside the boundaries of an organization. Coalitions are likely to involve various professions and disciplines, and different sectors of the community. These partnerships can involve delicate negotiations—this is not a role for the novice.

This chapter introduces the conceptual foundation for coalitions within population health promotion and provides an orientation to their structure and function from formation through action and evaluation. The scenarios illustrate the bridging role of the public health nurse between public health and a coalition to promote physical activity with school-age children and youth. Throughout, there are many examples to show how community nurses can acquire the competence to contribute to coalitions and address specific local needs while promoting broader community participation and resources to support community health.

There is nothing like being part of a coalition to understand this complex process of cross-community collaboration, and students and beginning practitioners can bring considerable knowledge and skills to the experience. As discussed in Part 2 of the text, Chapters 3–8, student teams use the community health nursing process in guided clinical practice to apply knowledge of ecological theories of health and gain experience in collaborating with communities. Forming a coalition has similarities with team build-ing, albeit on a larger scale. Bringing together groups and agencies is more complex than bringing together individuals and moves more slowly, but the principles are the same. The same is true of the monitoring and evaluation of the foundational work and the imple-mentation of community-based interventions. All to say that the principles and practi-ces in this text can be adapted to the time scale and realities of working with coalitions.

---

**SCENARIO: Physical Activity in School-Age Children and Youth**

Mary completed her undergraduate degree through distance learning two months ago and has just moved to the city to take up a health department position. She is excited and nervous about the new job—promoting physical activity in school-age children and youth. A keen skier, Mary has competed in national competitions and, when at university, was the assistant director of activities at a summer camp for boys and girls. She thinks her sports background and experience in working with young people helped her to get the job.

Mary is assigned to the school-age health program. She will work closely with a mentor, Jean, an experienced public health nurse, who has represented the health department on various community groups and coalitions.

Physical activity has been a component of health department programs for many years, and a new mandate clearly identifies physical activity promotion across the age span as a key strategy for the prevention of chronic disease and injury. A review of all relevant programs—walking programs for older adults, fall prevention, prenatal classes, heart health—is underway to identify common elements and develop a comprehensive physical activity strategy. The anticipated announcement of new funding for the primary prevention of chronic disease provides an impetus to move quickly.

Lately, coalitions have been a requirement for federal funding. Several community partners, including the local school board, have expressed interest in forming a community coalition around increasing physical activity in school-age children and youth. The health department has a lot of experience with coalitions and is seen as a community leader because of its regional focus.

"I find it difficult to get my head around the size of the programs here," says Mary. "Back home, one nurse was responsible for everything to do with children, from prenatal programs to school health. This is so complicated." Jean helps Mary put together a work plan (see Table 11.1) for the next few months and advises, "Take it a step at a time." She explains that working together will give Mary a chance to find her way around the health department and meet future team members while preparing the ground for the school-age physical activity initiatives. "Also, you will be helping me with the coalition. That is the way I learned about coalitions, by being part of one," says Jean.

Mary thanks Jean for her help in putting together the work plan—this is another skill she needs to practice. "I have a lot to learn," she says. "We all do," says Jean. "Working in the community means lifelong learning. On the physical activity front, you have arrived at a very important time; we have focused on injury prevention with children for a long time. Suddenly everyone is ready to promote fitness. At least we have something to build on. When you talk to the programs, get a list of their community contacts. This will help to identify potential partners. By the time you finish, you will know the health department very well and be an expert on fitness promotion with children."

# Learning Objectives

After reading this chapter and answering the questions throughout the chapter, you should be able to:

1. Discuss the concepts, principles, and evidence base for using coalitions to promote community health.
2. Describe community capacity–building approaches to facilitate the formation and development of a coalition.
3. Share epidemiological data with a coalition to support a needs assessment.
4. Document and communicate the actions of a coalition.
5. Evaluate the effectiveness of a coalition.

**Key Terms and Concepts**

coalition • coalition sustainability • community-based intervention • community capacity • community capacity building • social capital

**Discussion Topics and Questions**

1. Read "Creating Safe Routes in a Rural Community" (Centers for Disease Control and Prevention, 2014a, p. 12, available from www.cdc.gov/nccdphp/dch/pdfs/health-equity-guide/activeliving.pdf). Identify the health issue(s) addressed by the coalition, and discuss whether or not capacity building is an intended outcome.

2. Thinking about your community, what characteristics would you look for in the leader of a coalition to improve services for developmentally disabled adults? Identify three potential sources for such a leader.

For suggested responses, please see the Answer Key at the back of the book.

**Table 11.1: Work Plan**

| Work Plan | | | |
|---|---|---|---|
| **Activities** | **Results** | **With Whom** | **By When** |
| Interview program team leaders about physical activity component. | – Written summary of physical activity across programs<br>– Know key players<br>– Feel confident, understand the program | Team leaders<br>• injury prevention<br>• school-age health<br>• older adults' programs<br>• prenatal program<br>• heart health | May 6 |
| Learn about coalitions.<br>• Review best practices.<br>• Attend coalition meetings.<br>• Talk to experienced practitioners. | – Review of literature—two or three useful reference articles<br>– Understand how coalitions work | Jean to arrange | May 12<br><br><br>May 17 |
| Review evidence-based literature on benefits of physical activity in school-age children and intervention strategies. | – Annotated bibliography, key articles, reviews<br>– Slide presentation for community coalition | Health department researchers, epidemiologists, and community nurse specialists | June 30 (start May 17) |

Community health nurses cultivate a network of relationships and partnerships in the community with individuals, groups, and organizations to promote health and address health inequities (Community Health Nurses of Canada [CHNC], 2011; Quad Council of Public Health Nursing Organizations, 2011). Community coalitions are a relatively common feature of these relationships. In preparation for practice, nursing students are expected to seek opportunities over the course of their undergraduate education to engage with partners and collaborate on strategies that improve the health of populations (Canadian Association of Schools of Nursing [CASN], 2014). The intent is to bring students face-to-face with particular populations, especially those facing inequities, and to experiences that expose them to essential skills, such as collaboration, advocacy, and capacity-building approaches, which take time to learn. Table 11.2 shows how community health nursing students might gain beginning competence in these areas as part of a community health project with coalitions, as described in this text.

For more than 30 years, coalitions have been a common feature of community-based health promotion initiatives, bringing together the resources of the community for mutual advantage and to achieve synergy. An introductory definition of **coalition**, on which this chapter builds, is "individuals representing diverse organizations, factions or constituencies, who agree to work together in order to achieve a common goal" (Feighery & Rogers, 1995, p. 1).

**Table 11.2: Adaptation of Community Health Nursing Process to Assess Coalitions**

| Steps of Process | Adaptation for Working with Coalitions |
| --- | --- |
| 1. Establish relationships and define project | – Review mandate, policy, and procedures of host agency and particular program(s).<br>– Determine policy and procedures of coalition, or if coalition is not yet established, those that would apply. |
| 2. Assess secondary data | Review literature, epidemiology, and sociodemographics related to health and social concerns to be addressed by the coalition.<br><br>Determine which sectors are relevant to the identified health and social concerns and explore their actual/potential involvement. |
| 3. Assess physical and social environment | Gain experience in coalition work by attending a coalition meeting, interviewing members, and observing coalition activities. Identify an assessment goal in relation to the stage of coalition building (e.g., during coalition formation, assess group/agency readiness to participate) and select an information-gathering approach. |
| 4. Assess primary data | Use selected assessment approach with stakeholders—program providers, partners, service recipients, and community members.<br><br>Initiate or adapt participant evaluation of meetings. |
| 5. Analyze assessment data | Determine action required to move coalition to next stage.<br><br>Provide a report in a format that is useful to the agency. |
| 6. Evaluate teamwork | Monitor formation of coalition building using structure and process indicators. |

Typically, coalitions involve long-term relationships, although community groups may participate at varying levels of intensity over the lifetime of a coalition. The term "consortium" is sometimes used interchangeably with "coalition"; however, Kreuter and Lezin (1998, p. 5) point out that a consortium tends to involve groups of the same type, such as universities or small business, whereas a coalition engages diverse community partners. The ability of the coalition to act in a unified way is crucial to its success. Although members may be more or less engaged in a coalition, there is an expectation that they will advocate on its behalf, which requires being able to put aside personal interests. This is quite different from the usual practice of community organizations, which is to concentrate deliberately on their own mandate and goals.

As you will recall from Chapter 1, collaboration with different sectors of society to promote health is consistent with the principles of primary health care, which recognize that the determinants of health and disease are embedded within the social, cultural, political, and economic fabric of a society (Commission on Social Determinants of Health, 2008) and cannot be addressed by the health sector alone. If you think about the issues that challenge communities today—families with young children are among the fastest growing group of the homeless; food banks are becoming a fixture in our cities; widespread substance use is contributing to injury rates in adolescents; the high prevalence of chronic illness in our aging populations is outstripping the availability of services—these issues are clearly health-related but they are also related to the social and economic environment. In order to have an impact on these pervasive and complex issues, it is necessary to address the underlying social conditions, which is beyond the capabilities of any one sector or organization. Coalitions are a way of bringing these diverse sectors together.

According to early reviews of the literature, coalitions provide a mechanism for intervening on multiple levels of society, consistent with a socioecological approach to health promotion, which makes them ideally suited to address complex health problems (Butterfoss, Goodman, & Wandersman, 1993; Wandersman et al., 1996). In keeping with socioecological theory, health promotion strategies need to target the determinants of health at different levels of the system: individuals and families, community and social policy (Green & Kreuter, 2005; Green, Richard, & Potvin, 1996; McLeroy, Kegler, Steckler, Burdine, & Wisotzky, 1994). This requires bringing together different sectors of the community—schools, businesses, and political groups—with health organizations to effectively harness resources and intervene with a range of health promotion strategies at different levels of society. Engaging all sectors of society promotes health equity by making sure that interventions reflect the needs and culture of the community (Brennan Ramirez, Baker, & Metzler, 2008; Butterfoss & Kegler, 2009; Center for Prevention Research and Development [CPRD], 2006).

A second and equally important goal of a coalition is to develop the capacity of the community (Butterfoss & Kegler, 2009; Goodman et al., 1998; Hawe, Noort, King, & Jordens, 1997). Generally, capacity is interpreted as competence or being able to change in a positive way. Drawing on earlier work by Cottrell (1976) and McKnight (1987), Robertson & Minkler (1994) equate capacity to the strengths, resources, and problem-solving abilities of individuals and collectives that will enable them to make a difference over time. With a view to understanding the construct as a base for measurement, Goodman and colleagues (1998, p. 259) define **community capacity** as "the characteristics of communities that affect their ability to identify, mobilize, and address social and public health problems." They identify 10 dimensions of capacity: leadership, citizen participation, skills, networks, resources, sense of community, community power, understanding community history, values, and critical reflection, but do not speculate on the processes by which capacity develops. One possibility is that bringing people together and strengthening social networks provides an opportunity for leadership to flourish and a forum for community problem solving. With the achievement of common goals, the sense of community is likely to increase, and the increased ability to solve community problems can then be applied to other issues and other situations (Moyer, Coristine, MacLean, & Meyer, 1999).

Given that improvements in health may be slow to materialize, several researchers have attempted to elucidate the theoretical basis of community capacity and develop indicators of community change to measure capacity-building efforts (e.g., Butterfoss & Kegler, 2009; Goodman et al., 1998; Laverack, 2003; MacLellan-Wright et al., 2007). The definition of **community capacity building** underpinning much of this effort is "an approach to the development of sustainable skills, organizational structures, resources and commitment to health improvement in health and other sectors, to prolong and multiply health gains many times over" (New South Wales Health Department, 2001).

The measurement approaches developed by Laverack (2003) and MacLellan-Wright and colleagues (2007) are examined here. While there are differences in terminology, the approaches have a similar focus and outcomes. For instance, Laverack (2003) identifies nine operational domains pertaining to the ability of the community: participation; leadership; community structures; asking why; resource mobilization; links with others; role of external supports; skills, knowledge, and learning; and sense of community. For example, "participation" is a measure of the extent that community members participate in small groups or organizations; "asking why" refers to the ability of a community to critically assess the social, political, economic, and other causes of inequality as a precursor to developing personal and social change strategies. MacLellan-Wright and colleagues (2007) use similar domains, chosen to show where capacity-building efforts would produce an observable or measureable impact within a relatively short time frame in the Community Capacity Building Tool (Public Health Agency of Canada [PHAC], Alberta/NWT Region, 2007, p. 12). For example, the tool measures "asking why" with the following questions:

- Have you explored the root causes of issues targeted by your project? Examples of root causes include lack of social support networks and barriers to accessing health services.
- Have you involved the target population in the process of asking why?
- Have you involved the target population in finding solutions to root causes of issues?
- Are there other activities you are doing to explore root causes or involve the target population in asking why? If yes, describe. (PHAC, Alberta/NWT Region, 2007, p. 12)

The potential responses are "just started," "on the road," "nearly there," and "we're there," with each statement briefly defined (PHAC, Alberta/NWT Region, 2007, p. 13). As you will probably notice, these practical tools can be used to support and guide coalition development as well as to measure progress in building community capacity.

## Formation and Development of Coalitions

Coalitions take a more formal approach to health promotion and capacity building than the community development approaches discussed in the previous chapter, but the ultimate goal, that the community will become healthier and better able to solve its own problems, is similar. Of the possible starting points for forming a community coalition, two approaches predominate. The first approach is professional led, where coalitions are formed deliberately as a first step toward developing a community-wide intervention to address a defined health issue, often in response to funding opportunities. The second approach is a volunteer- or grassroots-led initiative whereby community groups come together to address a common issue or concern (Butterfoss et al., 1993). As you might expect, there can also be a mix of the two approaches as coalitions evolve and change over time.

For many years, professional-led coalitions have been part of the funding require-ments of large-scale health promotion and prevention initiatives that seek to reduce the mortality and morbidity from chronic disease while fostering community involvement in health planning, and building community capacity (Butterfoss et al., 1993; CPRD, 2006; Wandersman et al., 1996). The intention of changing community norms is a com-mon feature of these initiatives, based on the understanding that the social environment greatly influences behavior. Typically, socioecological models of health (Green et al., 1996; Stokols, 1996) and social change theory (Thompson & Kinne, 1999) inform the interventions, delineating the most suitable points of intervention (what will be done, with whom, and where) and identify the most appropriate evidence-based interventions to address causal mechanisms. The complex interventions aim to bring about change at different levels of society and, consistent with a population health approach, are based on the understanding that the conditions that affect health are ubiquitous and that small changes will produce significant health gains for many people. Complementing these low-intensity interventions aimed at the population as a whole, community-wide interventions may include more intensive interventions tailored to subpopulations at high risk (Green & Kreuter, 2005).

When coalitions emerge from the grassroots, their exact starting point may be eas-ier to pinpoint in retrospect. For example, a critical event, such as the major employer in the area going out of business, or a fatal accident, might be the catalyst that brings everyone to a community meeting where the decision to take action is agreed upon. Or, the process may occur gradually as, over time, community groups have occasion to work with each other, develop partnerships, and broaden their focus to incorporate different issues and perspectives. Grassroots coalitions can be fostered deliberately by public or community health agencies with the intention of building community cap-acity. For example, Moyer and colleagues (1999) describe an intervention to reduce isolation in community living older adults, which led to partnerships with community groups providing programs and services to older adults, and eventually with commun-ity groups interested in developing friendly neighborhoods for persons of all ages. The model derived from the project describes how professionals marry the organizational mandate for health promotion and disease prevention with that of collaborating with community partners. Key features of the model are the staged and recursive process of engaging community groups in problem solving, the partnership between professionals and diverse sectors of the community, and the empowering agenda (Moyer et al., 1999).

McKnight (1997) offers a word of caution to health professionals engaged in community capacity building. He warns that there is a danger of extending the health system into the realm of community and supplanting the complex web of associations and informal links that underpin natural community functioning. Also challenging to health professionals are the ethical dilemmas posed by conflicting loyalties to the population, funders, and their organization in their role as community organizers (Minkler & Pies, 1997).

At this point, it is important to note that although coalitions are now seen as integral to current community health practice, evidence of their success in achieving health status change has not been demonstrated convincingly (CPRD, 2006; Kreuter & Lezin, 1998). On a positive note, process evaluation over the years has provided substantial evidence of best practices to guide the formation and development of coalitions. These can be found in an exhaustive review of coalitions addressing diverse issues such as substance abuse, HIV/AIDS, prenatal care, heart disease, cancer, and teen pregnancy (CPRD, 2006).

## Formation of a Coalition

There are many comprehensive, easy-to-use guides to coalition building grounded in decades of practical experience available online (e.g., Berkowitz & Wadud, 2014; Brennan Ramirez et al., 2008; Cohen, Baer, & Satterwhite, 2002; Centers for Disease Control and Prevention [CDC], 2012; Rabinowitz, 2014). See "Website Resources" at the end of this chapter for links.

These guides set out an orderly process of creating the conditions for success using a life-cycle approach (getting organized, maintenance, and ending the coalition) or organized by developmental stage (formation, implementation, and institutionalization). Coalitions tend to be long-term ventures and little is written about the final stages in the life of a coalition. Some dissolve once they feel their work is completed; others become institutionalized, which is what happens when the work of the coalition is subsumed in ongoing activities of the community (Wandersman et al., 1996). The important role community health nurses may play in creating community coalitions and carrying out the health action of coalitions is examined in more detail below.

## Creating the Conditions for Success—Advance Preparation

Much advance preparation is required to form a coalition and several factors have been identified as basic to success. Before agreeing to collaborate, community groups must recognize the existence of a common problem and acknowledge that they have a role in solving the problem but cannot do it alone. Usually, one organization, working alone, or through a small steering group, will take the lead. To be effective, the approach should be informed by a deep understanding of the community and its history, and should engage all those affected by the issue or problem (CPRD, 2006). Initial efforts aim to stimulate discussion and begin to articulate a vision prior to bringing groups together for more formal discussion. Community groups and organizations across different sectors will have various perspectives on an issue and can bring a wide range of knowledge, skills, and abilities to the table. By sharing resources, there is potential to achieve more

**Table 11.3: Potential Benefits to an Organization from Participation in a Coalition**

| Potential Benefits to Organization | |
|---|---|
| Shared responsibility | The organization can address new or broader community issues without having sole responsibility for managing or developing the response. |
| Leverage, political strength | Unified approaches demonstrate and develop widespread public support for taking action. |
| Synergy | Collaboration maximizes the power of groups through joint action. |
| Extended reach | Working together multiplies the response and minimizes duplication of effort and services. |
| Access to information and resources | Working collectively, organizations increase access to talents and can mobilize resources to influence an issue in more ways than any single organization could do alone. |
| Networking opportunities | There is increased potential for recruitment through connections to diverse constituencies, such as political, business, human service, social, and religious groups, and to less organized grassroots groups and individuals. |
| Skill enhancement | A coalition provides opportunity for individuals and organizations to develop skills and knowledge. |
| Recognition | Since coalition activities are carried out in a public forum, the abilities of participants can be recognized in the broader community. |
| Satisfaction | Individuals and organizations gain a sense of pride in making a contribution and helping to solve community problems. |

together than by working alone; however, each must see enough common ground before committing to work together toward a solution and see benefit in doing this.

Potential partners will likely weigh both the anticipated benefits and costs of participation in a coalition. The costs are mainly measured in time, effort, and money, but can include lost opportunities, such as not being able to expand services. Each organization and/or their individual representative will likely assess these costs and benefits differently, depending on their circumstances. For example, an organization might see an opportunity to expand its role in the community or the potential to gain access to resources and skill development for employees. Some potential benefits, identified in an early review of the emerging literature on coalitions (Butterfoss et al., 1993), and which continue to resonate in more recent reviews (McCLoskey et al., 2011), are described above in Table 11.3. Above all, participation has to be seen as meaningful; potential members need to be convinced that they will have a voice in decision making and that the benefits accruing to the organization are worth the costs. Otherwise, they may decline to participate (McCloskey et al., 2011). Negotiating the distribution of power and benefits against the cost of participation has to be handled with sensitivity so that everyone achieves a sense of "win-win," and this is likely to be a continuing challenge for coalitions.

The lead agency has a pivotal role in creating the conditions for success and must walk a fine line between leading and collaborating. Official community health agencies, particularly public health organizations, often assume this role because of their mandate and regional focus; however, the role should not to be undertaken lightly. Mittelmark (1996) argues that an organization should take stock of its capacity before taking on the task and recognize that coalition building requires a long-term commitment and sufficient resources if it is to succeed. An assessment of the capacity of public health

Mary meets with colleagues to identify potential community partners for the school-age physical activity coalition. She is delighted with the quality of information on program activities, identifies many community contacts, and summarizes the partnerships in a table with contact information.

Through conducting the interviews, Mary is able to form an opinion about cross-departmental collaboration and the level of interest in joining a community-wide coalition. She learns that people are proud of their work and want to share but fear losing control over the way their programs are offered. Some worry they will have less time for existing activities. Another cause for concern is that physical activity programs are used to draw people into other community-building activities, and this could be lost within a broader agenda.

Reflecting on the list, Mary and Jean identify that some partners are probably sending more than one representative to meet with health department programs. For example, a community health center might send one person to a diabetes prevention walking program meeting, another to an older adults' fall prevention meeting, and yet another to a meeting on bicycle safety. Thinking about the next step of bringing all the organizations to a common table, Jean identifies a possible selling point: community

partners can consolidate resources. She suggests that Mary reorganize the table to show the number and type of links with each agency or organization. This will allow them to flag the strongest partners and identify potential representatives for the coalition. Jean comments, "It is so important to have this information before you talk to outside agencies. You feel a little foolish if you discover that colleagues are partnering with an organization and you know nothing about it. It does not give a good impression; it makes us look disorganized and I worry that it might reduce my credibility also." Mary appreciates Jane's personal and political insight.

**Discussion Topics and Questions**

3. You are the nurse member of a steering group to build a coalition to improve services for developmentally disabled adults. List the types of agencies, groups, and organizations you would try to recruit.

4. A community asset can be a person—the stay-at-home mom or dad who organizes a playgroup; the policeman who helps with an afterschool club. Develop three questions to ask of potential community leaders to elicit information on how they might contribute to a program to reduce health disparities and increase youth physical activity.

agencies to work in partnership with communities identified four areas of relevance. The areas are: (1) the agency's skill in working with community groups and minority populations; (2) the agency workers' skill in working with community groups and minority populations; (3) the extent and frequency of community networking; and (4) community participation in health department planning (Parker, Margolis, Eng, & Henríquez-Roldán, 2003). Based on these findings, the authors recommend that public health organizations be held accountable for their capacity to be more community-based and foster community participation.

Canadian sources suggest that public and community health organizations have been building the capacity to support coalition development. Public health practitioners have shifted from working solely with individuals to working with groups and communities, and at the policy level (Edwards, Murphy, Moyer, & Wright, 1995). National studies show community health nurses are using a broader range of health promotion strategies, such as coalition building (Chambers et al., 1994; Schoenfeld & MacDonald, 2002). Furthermore, as noted earlier, community health nurses are expected to develop the requisite competencies and seek opportunities to participate in coalitions at entry to practice (CASN, 2014). In Canada and the United States, experienced community

**Table 11.4: Summary of Departmental Initiatives and Potential for Partnerships around School-Age Physical Activity**

| Adult Injury Prevention Initiatives | | | |
|---|---|---|---|
| **Community Partner** | **Initiatives** | **Potential for Involvement in School-Age Physical Activity Coalition** | **Contact Information** |
| – Heart Health Coalition<br>– Heart & Stroke Foundation<br>– Diabetes Association | – West End Mall walking program<br>– Walk Away from Diabetes program | Walking programs may be interested in expanding to include youth | Alex Logie, Coalition Chair, board member of Diabetes Association and local politician (222-8881) |
| YM-YWCA | YM-YWCA conduct training sessions with mall walkers | Offer many youth programs | Janet Bryzinscki, Director, Youth Programs (222-8882) |
| Community Health Centers (CHC) | Sunnyside CHC & Aboriginal HC are involved in Walk Away from Diabetes | – Sunnyside offers bicycle safety program<br>– Aboriginal HC runs a youth group | Kim Lee, Program Manager (222-8883) |
| Family Physicians network | Regular articles on injury prevention in quarterly newsletter distributed to all physicians in area | Health department fall prevention program distributes notepads with physical activity "prescription" for older adults, could repeat for youth | |
| City Recreation Department | Involved in Walk Away from Diabetes | Offer many youth programs in the community | Jim Brown (222-8884) |
| Shopping Mall<br>– management | Provide office space in six malls | | Glenna Sandre (222-8885) |
| Individual businesses | Support walking programs (e.g., offer discounts for coffee; donate prizes) | Car dealer sponsors afterschool youth center in West End | |
| Community Police West End | | Help to run the afterschool youth center | Sergeant Ravi Singh (222-8886) |

health nurses are expected to use strategies such as coalition building to overcome health inequities and to take on increasing responsibilities for coalitions as they assume managerial responsibilities (CHNC, 2011; Quad Council of Public Health Nursing Organizations, 2011).

## Getting Organized—Developing Organizational Structures

Whether formed from the bottom up or from the top down, all community coalitions have to function effectively. This entails making fundamental decisions about how the coalition will be organized and putting processes in place to carry out a plan of action (Butterfoss et al., 1993; McLeroy et al., 1994). To be effective, the coalition requires a critical mass of members, well-functioning organizational structures, collaborative relationships, and the ability to carry out the program of work for which the coalition is formed (Foster-Fishman, Shelby, Berkowitz, Lounsbury, & Allen, 2001).

Bringing groups together and getting organized takes considerable time and effort. Typically, the lead agency forms an ad hoc committee of community leaders to recruit members and organize (see diagram in Butterfoss et al., 1993, p. 320). In addition to health sector organizations, it is important to draw in business, education, social, and religious groups, as well as less organized grassroots groups and individuals (KU Work Group for Community Health and Development [KU Work Group], 2014a; McLeroy et al., 1994). Consideration should be given to those who would benefit from participation as well as those who can assist in meeting the goals of the coalition (KU Work Group, 2014b). The simplest approach is to generate a list of potential participants, and through informal discussion, explore interest, availability, and potential to contribute. This can be time-consuming and may require more than one contact to get agency participation.

Community health nurses are well qualified to assist with the formation of a coalition. They know the community, understand its diversity, and have access to hard-to-reach groups. They are likely to have connections with a wide range of community agencies and organizations, together with well-established links with practitioners from other disciplines. This brings an intimate understanding of the community: its culture and traditions, existing and emerging health issues, and the state of existing programs, services, and resources. Furthermore, community nurses are well regarded in the community and have skills in information gathering and organizing. All of these qualities can be put to good use in talking to groups and organizations to raise awareness and assess readiness to collaborate. More formal discussions may need to be conducted at the management level because of the need to commit organizational or group resources.

Kreuter and Lezin (1998, Appendix A) learned from experts in the field that realistic expectations for the first year of a coalition are as follows:

- Get organized
- Establish a clear vision and mission—a common purpose
- Clarify mode of operations
- Formalize process, procedures, and, as necessary, establish subcommittees around agreed-upon objectives
- Establish trust
- Develop an unambiguous plan of action
- Ascertain the group skills required to effectively manage the coalition

The evidence suggests that coalitions with a formal structure and clearly defined policies and procedures are more likely to succeed than ad hoc arrangements (CPRD, 2006; Nagy, 2014). Reaching agreement on a governance structure with rules to guide decision making helps to strengthen collaboration and may proceed at the same time as the development of the vision, mission, goals, and plan of work. Both structure and process are important, indeed necessary, for the coalition to run smoothly and secure the financial and human resources to carry out the work of the coalition. A comprehensive description of some of the different types of structure that may be put in place to guide decision making and oversee the work of the coalition can be found in the *Community Tool Box* (Nagy, 2014).

Strong leadership is vital to the success of a coalition. Recruiting an influential leader is one of the tasks of the lead agency or steering group. The person should command respect across the community and be able to draw into the coalition formal and informal leaders from the different sectors of the community (Butterfoss et al., 1993). Examples from the literature include: directors of a community organization, religious leaders, local politicians, and middle managers who can bridge the gap between employees and management (Wandersman et al., 1996). Many factors need to be taken into consideration. In addition to being acceptable to different constituencies, the leader should have energy, administrative experience, and interpersonal skills. Effective coalition leaders are characterized as being "open, task oriented and supportive to the group" (CPRD, 2006, p. 5). It takes a skilled communicator to conduct public meetings, lead discussions, problem solve, and resolve conflicts. Also, as the coalition spokesperson, the leader must be able to convey clearly where the coalition is going, both to coalition members and the broader community, possibly through the media. Finding such a person is an exacting task and sometimes the responsibilities have to be shared or the leadership rotated.

Employing skilled paid staff in a coalition is considered advantageous (Butterfoss & Kegler, 2009). For example, there is empirical evidence that paid staff lead to more highly rated strategic plans (Florin, Mitchell, Stevenson, & Klein, 2000). The authors do not speculate on why this happens but it may be because employees are able to dedicate time to the essential work of the coalition and have the necessary skills to ensure that the planned activities are carried out. On the other hand, it is important to be clear about staff-member roles to maintain volunteer involvement and avoid negative impact on the sustainability of the coalition activities when the project funding runs out.

## Relationships

Strong, collaborative relationships are fundamental to the success of a coalition (Foster-Fishman et al., 2001). The KU Work Group (2014a) identifies several factors that should be considered to foster participation and support:

- Recognition: People want to be recognized for their contributions.
- Respect: People want their values, culture, ideas, and time to be respected and considered in the organization's activities.
- Role: People want a clearly defined role in the coalition that makes them feel valuable and in which they can make a contribution.
- Relationships: People want the opportunity to establish and build networks both professionally and personally for greater influence and support.
- Reward: People expect the rewards of participating in a collaborative partnership to outweigh the costs and to benefit from the relationships established.

- Results: People respond to visible results that are clearly linked to outcomes that are important to them and that they can clearly link to their participation in the coalition.

In order to satisfy these requirements and maximize member input, organizers have to create a clear vision and quality management practices, such as "effective communication, conflict resolution, perception of fairness, and shared decision making" (CPRD, 2006, p. 5). Typically, coalition members bring a range of opinions on priorities and processes, and areas of disagreement can be anticipated from time to time, both on a personal and agency level. This will not necessarily threaten the partnership but will require continuing attention and, perhaps, delicate negotiation.

The challenge of bringing together diverse groups reinforces the need to understand the community context—the sociopolitical and socioeconomic conditions, community health status, and community infrastructure. Although inclusivity is essential (CPRD, 2006), in some situations it may be difficult to achieve. A study of 15 partnerships (Wandersman et al., 1996) found that greater ethnic and racial diversity in a community increased the difficulty of attaining a stable coalition. This was attributed to high levels of distrust and competition between groups and linguistic barriers. Other differences, such as social class, age, or political or religious orientation, can also be divisive. Guidelines suggest that it is advisable to anticipate some opposition or dissenting opinion from the outset and seek to achieve a compromise early on, rather than setting the stage for later confrontation. For example, coalitions lobbying for antismoking policies in public places were strongly opposed by restaurant and bar owners. Failing to provide a forum for open discussion can set back progress.

Integrating new members is an ongoing task for coalitions. Agencies and organizations are likely to be involved with a coalition over several years, but representatives change as people leave or take on new roles and responsibilities. As well, the coalition may determine it lacks certain skills or abilities and seek to recruit new members; maintaining the capacity to carry out its work is essential (CPRD, 2006). This means the coalition should plan ways to help new members fit into existing relationships and patterns of working and make a contribution. In addition to formally acknowledging new members and introducing them to others, orientation might include the provision of background material on the work of the coalition, and a meeting to discuss roles and issues. There are likely to be many sources of written information. For example, the work of the coalition is usually captured in the minutes of meetings. Other sources of information are operational documents, such as terms of reference, mission statements, goals, logic models, work plans, funding proposals, and reports. Attention to the socialization of new members will help to ensure the necessary ongoing commitment and enthusiasm required to sustain coalition activities. Being able to work with and support coalitions is a key role for community health nurses. The skills required to do this are essentially the same as those outlined in Chapter 2 on teamwork. The major difference is that the skills are being applied in larger and more diverse multidisciplinary teams, and that the team members come from many different work environments.

The injury prevention coalition is sponsoring a special meeting to bring together community groups with an interest in increasing physical activity in school-age children and youth. For some time, the coalition has wanted to address the needs of this population and extend the scope of the injury prevention coalition mandate. Several presentations are planned to educate members and to help them to explore the issues and determine common interests. Mary will present statistics on a local survey of physical activity in children and youth; the professor doing research in exercise physiology will provide an overview of the evidence of the benefits of exercise for children; and a school principal will talk about physical activity in the school curriculum. Presenters have been asked to keep their presentations to 10 minutes.

This is an important day for Mary, and she wants to do well. The assignment is timely because it fits with one of the tasks on her work plan. Also, she has found on more than one occasion that her knowledge and expertise in physical activity is being tested in subtle ways. She has had many questions about the type and amount of physical activity children need as part of a healthy lifestyle. Reviewing the literature will help to reacquaint her with the latest work and reassure her that she has mastery of the subject matter. It will also help her contribute to a draft action plan for the expected request for proposals to secure funds to carry out an intervention.

Preparing for the special meeting, Jean says, "Coalition meeting dates are set in September for the whole year and listed at the end of each set of minutes. Normally the agenda is distributed one week ahead of the meeting, but for a special meeting such as this, we have to give more lead time." Jean mentions that some agency representatives have only limited authority to speak for their organization. She adds, "We try

to make sure that participants know ahead of time when important decisions will be made. It allows the representative to seek guidance ahead of time, or to arrange for a more senior member of staff to participate.

"Another thing we have learned from experience is that our process has to be transparent. We used to meet ahead of time to try to move the meetings along more quickly but this was seen as too controlling. Now, we allow time for a full discussion of issues and make sure that all members have the opportunity to express their point of view and vote on the issues. Last month we began to evaluate each meeting using a brief checklist—people don't have to give their name (see Appendix to Chapter 11). This gives everyone a chance to give feedback on the meeting, right there. It helps to prevent concerns being aired outside the meeting, which gives the coalition a bad name in the community. It is working well."

**Discussion Topics and Questions**

5. You have been active in your community scout/guide group for several years and have been proposed as your organization's representative on a physical activity coalition. Identify three advantages for you and three for your organization in taking on this challenge.

6. As chair of a rural coalition on injury prevention of 20 health providers and community members, you have a loaded agenda with several important budget items to discuss. A representative from the Young Farmers' Association has just joined the coalition and, together with a family physician, is attending her first meeting. Your co-chair suggests that you leave the introductions until next time. Discuss the pros and cons of this option.

7. Identify three strategies a coalition chairperson might use to encourage regular attendance at meetings.

## Developing and Carrying Out a Plan of Action

Determining the mission and goals is a crucial step in the life of a coalition. Even with sufficient common interest to bring the coalition together, partners may have widely different priorities and expectations for what they would like to achieve. Ideally, the goal should be broad enough for everyone and yet sufficiently specific to guide planning. For example, Kreuter and Lezin (1998) describe the goal of the Harlem Hospital Injury Prevention Program: to reduce the childhood injury and death rate in central Harlem from a baseline rate of 1141/100,000 to the US rate of 656/100,000. The coalition had documented the significant need, which was addressed initially through injury surveillance and injury prevention education programs. Later on, smaller working groups or "sliding coalitions" initiated neighborhood projects to build safe playgrounds, which expanded across the country (Pressley et al., 2005). This approach exemplifies the principle that a good strategic plan is essential to the success of a coalition and should be based on a community needs assessment that clearly identifies the needs and concerns of the community (CPRD, 2006).

There are many guides to the planning process, especially now that coalitions are fundamental to many large-scale health promotion and prevention initiatives, such as the US Healthy Communities Program (see "Website Resources" in this chapter). Bracht, Kingsbury, and Rissel (1999) describe a five-stage planning model that has been success-fully used. The five stages are: (1) community analysis, (2) design initiation, (3) implementation, (4) maintenance and consolidation, and (5) dissemination and assessment. As you will recognize, these stages are similar to the phases of the community health nursing process. Since this chapter is focusing more on the formation of coalitions, only community analysis and design initiation are discussed below.

## Community Analysis and Design Initiation

A phrase often heard in the community health field is "start where the community is at" (Labonte & Robertson, 1996; Nyswander, 1956). For community health nurses, this requires marrying community and public health mandates with the concerns and needs of the community. A community analysis maps the community strengths and resources in relation to the issue at hand, and puts together what is known about the health issue. Gathering this information serves to raise awareness and focus the issue. You may want to review Chapter 3 and resources in the *Community Tool Box* (Heaven, 2014).

The PRECEDE-PROCEED model of health promotion planning and evaluation (Green & Kreuter, 2014) has long been used to guide the design of community health interventions. This ecological model conceptualizes health as "the product of the inter-dependence between the individual and subsystems of the ecosystem" (Green et al., 1996, p. 270). This implies that changes in the environment will have an impact on behavior and changes in human behavior have an impact on the environment.

In health promotion planning, the model uses a step-by-step investigative process to develop an understanding of community issues in stages (see Figure 11.1, below). Beginning with the felt needs, or quality-of-life concerns identified by the community, you work back to uncover the underlying health issues and their determinants. By draw-ing on theory and epidemiological studies, the multiple genetic, lifestyle (behavioral), and environmental factors and causal mechanisms that impact on health are identi-fied. Each factor is then examined in terms of its predisposing, enabling, and reinfor-cing antecedents (the PRECEDE component of the model). Any of these antecedents, defined in Box 11.1, may become the focus of intervention. This is another point where community input is crucial.

**Figure 11.1: The PRECEDE-PROCEED Model of Health Promotion Program Planning and Evaluation**

## PRECEDE-PROCEED Model

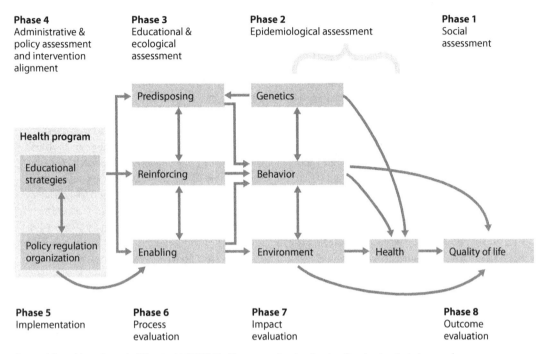

**Phase 4**
Administrative &
policy assessment
and intervention
alignment

**Phase 3**
Educational &
ecological
assessment

**Phase 2**
Epidemiological assessment

**Phase 1**
Social
assessment

**Phase 5**
Implementation

**Phase 6**
Process
evaluation

**Phase 7**
Impact
evaluation

**Phase 8**
Outcome
evaluation

*Source*: Adapted from Green, L., & Kreuter, M. (2005). *Health program planning: An educational and ecological approach* (4th ed., p. 10). New York, NY: McGraw-Hill.

Once the analysis is complete, evidence-based strategies are then identified to act on the modifiable conditions and bring about positive change in the lifestyle and the environment (the PROCEED component of the model). Further information on the model can be found in the "Website Resources" for this chapter.

The steps of the PRECEDE analytic process described above are illustrated here. The example identifies the predisposing, enabling, and reinforcing factors that affect physical activity in school-age children and youth. For a more in-depth understanding of the process, the reader is directed to the Green and Kreuter (2005) text.

BOX 11.1

**Example of PRECEDE Analysis—Promoting Physical Activity in Children and Youth**

**Quality-of-Life Issues**

People in your community tell you they value good health and fitness. Parents say they are concerned about how much time their children spend playing computer games. They want their children to play more outdoors with friends and to take part in sports, but they are worried about safety. Participation in organized sport is influenced by whether or not parents work outside the home. Some parents think involvement in local activities will make it less likely that their children will get involved in vandalism and petty crimes. Many think there should be more opportunities for physical activity at school to boost learning and help children grow up to be fit and healthy adults.

Recent social planning documents from your community show that the child population has been stable for several years. Social trends, however, such as the rising numbers of lone-parent families resulting from an increase in divorce rates and the breakup of partnerships, low minimum wages, the increasing number of working poor with children, and the lack of stability in the labor market contribute to increases in the number of children in need of health and social services.

**Health Issues**

There is compelling evidence that physical activity is an important determinant of health and quality of life in children, and that the effects extend into adulthood. The guidelines on recommended levels of activity for children and adolescents in Canada (Canadian Society for Exercise Physiology [CSEP], 2014) and the US (US Department of Health and Human Services [USDHHS], 2014), both of which provide "ready to use" resources and promotional material, are compared in Table 11.5. The Canadian guidelines include recommendations for limiting sedentary behavior. Otherwise, they are essentially the same and are consistent with international guidelines (World Health Organization, 2010).

In the US, childhood obesity has more than doubled in children and quadrupled in adolescents in the past 30 years (CDC, 2014b). Similarly, in Canada, measured obesity has increased 2.5 times in the last decade. A recent analysis of Canadian data reports the rate of measured obesity as 8.6 percent among children and youth ages 6 to 17, and that earlier estimates suggest

that 6.3 percent of children ages 2 to 5 are obese (Public Health Agency of Canada and Canadian Institute of Health Information, 2011). The rates of obesity are also high in Aboriginal children and youth, ranging from 16.9 percent among Métis, to 20 percent among off-reserve First Nations, to 25.6 among Inuit, based on self-reported data from children and youth, ages 6 to 14 years.

Like quitting smoking, effectively preventing obesity requires a multifaceted, long-term approach involving complementary interventions that operate at multiple levels: individual, community-wide, and public policy. Since the majority of children and youth spend a lot of their day at school, the school provides a channel for reaching them. A recent public health report identifies several community-based interventions with evidence of effectiveness: social marketing campaigns that emphasize physical activity, interventions to increase the frequency/duration of physical education classes, and school policies that increase access to healthier foods and beverages in vending machines and cafeterias (PHAC, Alberta/NWT Region, 2007). (As discussed by McLeroy, Norton, Kegler, Burdina, and Sumaya [2003], the term **community-based intervention** can have a wide range of meanings, such as "community as setting, community as target, community as agent, and community as resource.")

**Lifestyle (Behavioral) and Environmental Factors and Antecedents**

The physical activity guidelines provide a standard definition for comparison. The tenth annual report on physical activity in children and youth (Active Healthy Kids Canada, 2014) compares 10 countries, including Canada and the US, on 10 different indicators grouped into three categories: "Strategies and Investments; Settings & Sources of Influence (Family & Peers, School, Community & the Built Environment), and Behaviours that Contribute to Overall Physical Activity Levels (Organized Sport Participation, Active Play, Active Transportation, Sedentary Behaviours)." Despite some favorable results in other categories, overall physical activity levels for Canada and the US were rated at a D—"near the back of the pack." An important finding, based on 2009 data, is that only 7 percent of kids met the activity guidelines at ages 5 to 11, and only 4 percent for ages 12 to 17.

**Table 11.5: Physical Activity Guidelines for Children and Adolescents: Canada and US**

| | Canadian Physical Activity and Sedentary Behaviour Guidelines Handbook (CSEP, 2014) | Youth Physical Activity Guidelines Toolkit (USDHHS, 2014) |
|---|---|---|
| Age | Ages 5–11, 12–17 Accumulate at least 60 minutes of moderate- to vigorous-intensity physical activity daily. | Ages 6–17 years Children and adolescents should have 60 minutes or more of physical activity each day. |
| Type of Activity – at least 3 days per week | More activity provides better health. – vigorous intensity (activities that cause child to sweat and be out of breath, e.g., running, swimming) – muscle strengthening and bone strengthening | Most activity should be either moderate- or vigorous-intensity aerobic physical activity – vigorous intensity – muscle strengthening – bone strengthening |
| | Minimize sedentary behavior. – limit recreational screen time to no more than 2 hours per day; lower levels are associated with additional health benefits – limit sedentary (motorized) transport, extended sitting, and time spent indoors throughout the day More daily physical activity provides greater health benefits. | Replace inactivity with activity whenever possible. |
| Contextual Factors | Activity can take place at school, at play, inside or outside the home, and on the way to school and might involve family and friends. Physical activity should be fun. | It is important to encourage young people to participate in physical activities that are appropriate for their age, that are enjoyable, and that offer variety. |

The international and national guidelines and annual reports provide detailed information on an important health issue—physical activity in children and youth. In addition to generating information that can be used to design change, they provide standard measures, which can serve as a benchmark for measuring change once interventions are implemented to increase the level of activity in school children.

**Predisposing, Reinforcing, and Enabling Factors**
Systematic reviews identify several factors that determine lifestyle choices and environmental support for physical activity in young people (CDC, 2014b). These predisposing, reinforcing, and enabling factors, which suggest points of intervention that might be considered when promoting lifelong physical activity, are listed below.

Predisposing Factors:
- Enjoying different forms of physical activity and developing the skills to participate
- Understanding the relationship between physical activity and health
- Valuing physical activity

Reinforcing Factors:
- Parental support for participation in physical activity and support
- Parental role models and involvement of parents and guardians in physical activity instruction and programs for young people
- Promotion of lifelong physical activity by health providers

*continued on the following page*

continued from the previous page

Enabling Factors:
- Policies that promote enjoyable, lifelong physical activity
- Physical and social environments that encourage and enable physical activity
- Physical education curricula and instruction in schools
- Health education curricula and instruction in schools
- Extracurricular physical activity programs that meet the needs and interests of students
- Personnel training

- Health services for children and adolescents
- Developmentally appropriate community sports and recreation programs that are attractive to young people
- Regular evaluation of physical activity instruction, programs, and facilities

The preceding information is summarized in the following figure, based on the PRECEDE-PROCEED model (Green & Kreuter, 2005).

**Figure 11.2: Example of PRECEDE Analysis—Promoting Physical Activity in Children and Youth**

**Predisposing Factors**
*(Knowledge and Attitudes)*

Preferences influence the type of activity children engage in. Children (5–12 years) prefer to be active, or like active and quiet activities equally.
They also like equally well activities that are
- organized/unorganized,
- moderate/vigorous,
- competitive/non-competitive.[1]

**Reinforcing Factors**
*(Rewards and Feedback)*

Parental reinforcement and support increases their child's involvement in physical activity.
- 47% of parents believe their child gets enough Physical Education (PE) at school.[1]
- 82% of parents agree that the education system should place more importance on providing quality PE.[2]

**Enabling Factors**
*(Skills, Resources, Barriers)*

- Policies that promote enjoyable, lifelong physical activity
- Physical and social environments that encourage and enable physical activity
- Physical/Health Education curricula and instruction
- Personnel training
- Extracurricular physical activity programs that meet the needs and interests of students
- Health services for children and adolescents
- Developmentally appropriate community sports and recreation programs, attractive to young people
- Safe public spaces
- Regular evaluation of physical activity instruction, programs, and facilities

**Lifestyle Choices (Behavioral)**

- 54% of children and youth (5–19 years) are not active enough for optimal growth and development.
- 66% have Physical Education at school.
- 51% engage in other activity at school.
- 66% engage in activity elsewhere.[1]
- 7% of parents say they often played active games with their children in the past year.[2]
- 9% of parents support kids' physical activity financially (e.g., through fees, equipment).[2]
- 55% of Canadian school administrators report having a fully implemented policy for daily PE for all students.[2]

**Environment Supporting Engagement in Physical Activity**

- Over 94% of parents report local availability of parks/outdoor spaces and of public facilities and programs for physical activity, such as pools, arenas, and leagues.
- 59% of adults report living in a neighborhood that supports overall physical activity (e.g., has bike lanes, is walkable).
- A large majority of school administrators report students have access to gymnasiums (95%), playing fields (91%), bicycle racks (79%), and playground equipment (73%).
- Trained instruction and support is available.[2]

**Health**

*Notes:*
1. Canadian Fitness and Lifestyle Research Institute, 2014.
2. Active Healthy Kids Canada, 2014.

Developing and carrying out a plan of action is a complex undertaking, which benefits from broad involvement. Although communities and public health may appear to focus on different issues or look at issues from a different angle, they have many common concerns. The community understands health from lived experience and brings a vision of a community as a place to live well and raise families. Public and community health workers understand the science of causal mechanisms, modifiable risk, and protective factors, and the theoretical and research evidence for potential interventions. They know about health promotion. The two perspectives do not need to be at odds with each other. McKnight (1997) suggests that professionals can best contribute to community capacity building by respecting the wisdom of the community and working in partnership rather than trying to exert control; by providing access to information and resources and by using professional skills to strengthen the power of community associations. Community health workers should feel justly confident of their role in bringing professional knowledge and skills to the table, but they must listen to communities and, most important, act on the information that they hear and not disregard it (Kreuter, Lezin, Kreuter, & Green, 1998).

## Evaluating Coalitions

One of the main reasons given in support of coalitions is that they bring together the diverse resources required to change the health of populations. Yet, a critical review of the literature (Kreuter & Lezin, 1998) concludes that few coalitions can claim to have successfully achieved a long-term health impact. They offer three reasons: (1) most coalitions are inefficient and/or have insufficient mechanisms for planning and implementation; (2) achieving health status change through collaborative efforts is an unrealistic expectation, no matter how well the coalition performs; and (3) even if a change in health status was achieved it would be difficult to detect and attribute this to the efforts of a particular coalition because of the technical difficulties posed by evaluation. Despite the lack of evidence of success, Kreuter and Lezin (1998) argue that other perceived benefits, such as community capacity building, may be sufficient incentive to continue funding coalitions. They suggest the most appropriate action would be to provide more specific assistance and resources to support the formation of coalitions in settings where there is sufficient social capital. The authors define **social capital** as "the specific processes among people and organizations, working collaboratively in an atmosphere of trust, that lead to accomplishing a goal of *mutual social benefit*" (p. 34).

Given the difficulty in proving that coalitions have an impact on health, it becomes especially important to conduct a process evaluation to demonstrate that a coalition operates effectively and therefore contributes to community capacity (CPRD, 2006). A seminal article by Francisco, Paine, and Fawcett (1993) sets out a framework for evaluating the work of coalitions, which is still pertinent. The evaluation framework is based on the reasoning that a coalition must successfully complete successive stages of development—from formation through collaborative assessment, planning, and implementation—before it can effect more remote changes in health status. For each stage of development, the framework identifies indicators that can be used to monitor the formation of coalitions. More recent reviews narrow the focus of evaluation to the use of evidence-based practices to guide the formation of coalitions in key areas: community member competencies, relationships, intra-coalition operations, and the design and implementation of effective community-based programs (CPRD, 2006; Foster-Fishman et al., 2001).

Another important indicator is **coalition sustainability**, defined as "[a] community's ongoing capacity and resolve to work together to establish, advance, and maintain effective strategies that continuously improve health and quality of life for all" in a comprehensive planning guide (CDC, 2012). The guide recommends ongoing evaluation of sustainability in the following domains: strategic capacity, clear values or operating principles, core leadership with strong commitment, diverse membership, management capacity, community buy-in and support, and power and influence. More specifically, to be sustainable, coalitions require resources:

- Funding: Secure sources of multi-year funds, preferably from diverse sources, such as government, in kind, and donations.
- Leadership: This is exemplified in core members, strong commitment, clear governance, clear values and principles, sound financial and program management, capacity to carry out program activities, and credibility.
- Results: The outcomes show effectiveness and activities are seen to be addressing significant community needs.
- Community Support: Individual and organizations are champions of the coalition. (CDC, 2012; Foster-Fishman et al., 2001; Rabinowitz, 2014)

Many simple evaluation measures are now readily available to monitor the coalitions (e.g., Brown, 1997; MacLellan-Wright et al., 2007). Some examples of evaluation questions that might be asked in relation to the form and function of coalitions, and the type of data required to answer the questions, are provided in Box 11.2. The questions address how the coalition is structured; its policies and procedures for recruiting, retaining, and socializing members; and its achievements. (For a more comprehensive checklist, see Brown, 1997).

## Summary

Coalitions are integral to many health promotion interventions and are an important mechanism for supporting communities to create the conditions for health. It is essential that coalitions fairly represent the community of interest, that health issues are chosen carefully with the full cooperation of the community, and that specific and attainable goals are identified to guide the design of evidence-based, multi-level interventions.

Community health nurses are expected to gain the skills and knowledge to provide professional support to coalitions. This includes having the skills and knowledge to foster community participation, assist coalitions to complete key developmental tasks, and facilitate effective community health action. Monitoring and evaluating the coalition helps to ensure success, and this is another area where community health nurses can and do make a contribution. The scenarios in this chapter tell the story of how these skills can be developed by students and beginning practitioners to support physical activity in youth.

**Evaluating Coalitions—Questions and Evaluation Approaches**

*Question*: Is the membership of the coalition appropriate and are members committed?

*Evaluation Approach*: Document the number and type of coalition members.

- List members by the community sectors they represent and determine whether or not key sectors are represented.
- Ascertain what percentage of committee members attend meetings regularly, that is, are present for at least 50 percent of committee meetings.

*Question*: Does the coalition have adequate resources? Is there evidence that the community is willing to invest in the partnership?

*Evaluation Approach*: Document the resources obtained through the partnership.

- Money or in-kind donations, such as space or computers
- Number and type of trained volunteers who have been recruited and trained and are donating time to assist with implementation of the coalition plan

*Question*: Are members satisfied with the coalition?

*Evaluation Approach*: Questionnaire (See Appendix to Chapter 11 for an example of a questionnaire to evaluate the effectiveness of coalition meetings.)

- Is meeting time used effectively?

- Do you feel that, on the whole, members have an equal voice within the coalition? Please explain.
- How satisfied are you with the way decisions are made in the coalition? How is leadership exercised? Does one person, or a small group, make decisions for the coalition (Usually, Sometimes, Rarely)?

*Question*: Does the coalition conform to the standards of good partnership?

*Evaluation Approach*: Informal interview questions.

- How is decision making shared in the coalition?
- What resources does your organization contribute to the partnership? Do all coalition members make an equal contribution?
- Are the program and policy initiatives undertaken cooperatively?
- Has the coalition produced valued outcomes?
- Do the benefits of the partnership outweigh the costs?

*Question*: Is there tangible evidence of coalition planning?

*Evaluation Approach*: Document analysis.

- Documents on file: terms of reference; statement of mission and goals; action plan and logic models
- Meeting minutes of coalition and subcommittees
- Funding proposal—development and submission

A considerable body of research has identified that coalitions require stable funding and access to resources to reach their potential. They take sustained effort to set up and maintain and a long-term commitment to see the work to fruition. Given the reservations expressed by Kreuter and Lezin (1998) about the effectiveness of coalitions, it is important for health professionals to take these factors into account when using a coalition as part of a health promotion strategy. Government support and chronic disease prevention activities are evolving. To be effective, community health nurses need organizational support to engage with coalitions and support them in building communities' capacity for health action.

## Classroom and Seminar Exercises

1. Your health center is the lead agency of a coalition with new funding to prevent alcohol, tobacco, and other drug abuse in urban youth. List four or five points that you would address when seeking to engage the following community groups in the

Mary has completed a literature review and is collaborating with the national sport and recreation association survey team to develop the presentation on physical activity in school-age children and youth. Thanks to the foresight of the health department, who contributed additional funds to increase the size of the sample in the region, they are able to draw on local data.

The past four months have flown by. Mary now feels confident in her understanding of the issues around the promotion of physical activity in children and youth and has increased her understanding of coalition building. The pieces are starting to come together. The school-age physical activity team members have been named—she knows two of them quite well—and the team will start planning soon. Also, there will be an opportunity to participate in research: a professor who has a joint appointment with the health department is developing a research agenda around physical activity in school-age children. The best news is that Jean will be the team leader. Mary has enjoyed working with her over the past months and looks forward to continuing the relationship. Jean is equally happy with the arrangement and has already started to think about how they can improve the process of building a coalition.

When Jean asks her to put together a package of information for discussion at the first team meeting,

Mary knows exactly what she will include. She suggests to Jean that they use the meeting effectiveness questionnaire to evaluate their process (see Appendix to Chapter 11). "Yes," agrees Jean. "Let's set the standard and encourage open communication."

**Discussion Topics and Questions**

8.  Discuss how training workshops for members might benefit a coalition.
9.  Parents are constantly telling you that they want their children to be able to take advantage of the summer weather to play outdoors. Your city introduces guidelines to increase shade at outdoor facilities such as schoolyards, public pools, cottages, and backyards (for an example of Shade Guidelines, see www1.toronto.ca/city_of_toronto/toronto_public_health/healthy_public_policy/tcpc/files/pdf/shade_guidelines.pdf), and you find the below statement in the local newspaper. How would you build these ideas into a coalition action plan to increase physical activity in school children?

Dermatologist: Everyone is responsible for their own health, and one of our key mandates is to encourage people to adopt a healthy lifestyle by wearing adequate sunscreen, protective clothing, or finding a shady spot that safeguards them from the sun while allowing them to enjoy the outdoors.

coalition: (1) a sports club run by the community police, and (2) the local business group that includes restaurant and bar owners. Role-play with a partner on how you would deliver these points in an interview.

2.  Identify two community groups attended mainly by women, one health-related, one not health-related. Obtain a copy of their terms of reference, or attend a meeting. Identify how you might engage this organization in a community coalition on women's health.

3.  Attend a community coalition meeting, and evaluate the effectiveness of the meeting using the tools described in this chapter.

# References

Active Healthy Kids Canada. (2014). *2014 Active Healthy Kids Canada report card on physical activity for children and youth: Is Canada in the running?* Retrieved from www.activehealthykids.ca/ReportCard/2014ReportCard.aspx

Berkowitz, B., & Wadud, E. (2014). Identifying community assets and resources. *Community Tool Box* (Chapter 3, Section 8). Retrieved from http://ctb.ku.edu/en/table-of-contents/assessment/assessing-community-needs-and-resources/identify-community-assets/main

Bracht, N., Kingsbury, L., & Rissel, C. (1999). A five-stage community organization model for health promotion: Empowerment and partnership strategies. In N. Bracht (Ed.), *Health promotion at the community level: New advances* (2nd. ed., pp. 83–104). Thousand Oaks, CA: Sage.

Brennan Ramirez, L. K., Baker, E. A., & Metzler, M. (2008). *Promoting health equity: A resource to help communities address social determinants of health.* Atlanta, GA: US Department of Health and Human Services, Centers for Disease Control and Prevention. Retrieved from www.cdc.gov/nccdphp/dch/programs/healthycommunitiesprogram/tools/pdf/SDOH-workbook.pdf

Brown, C. R. (1997). Appendix 3: Coalition checklist. In M. Minkler (Ed.), *Community organizing and community building for health* (pp. 359–365). New Brunswick, NJ: Rutgers University Press.

Butterfoss, F. D., Goodman, R. M., & Wandersman, A. (1993). Community coalitions for prevention and health promotion. *Health Education Research, 8*(3), 315–330.

Butterfoss, F. D., & Kegler, M. C. (2009). The Community Coalition Action Theory (CCAT). In R. D. Clemente, R. A. Crosby, & M. C. Kegler (Eds.), *Emerging theories in health promotion practice and research* (2nd ed.). San Francisco, CA: Jossey-Bass.

Canadian Association of Schools of Nursing (CASN). (2014). *Entry-to-practice public health nursing competencies for undergraduate nursing education.* Retrieved from www.casn.ca/en/123/item/6

Canadian Society for Exercise Physiology (CSEP). (2014). *Canadian physical activity and sedentary behaviour guidelines handbook.* Retrieved from: www.csep.ca/CMFiles/Guidelines/CSEP_Guidelines_Handbook.pdf

Canadian Fitness and Lifestyle Research Institute. (2014). *2010–2011 physical activity monitor.* Retrieved from www.cflri.ca/pub_page/322

Centers for Disease Control and Prevention (CDC). (2014a). *A practitioner's guide for advancing health equity: Community strategies for preventing chronic disease.* Retrieved from www.cdc.gov/nccdphp/dch/pdfs/health-equity-guide/activeliving.pdf

Centers for Disease Control and Prevention (CDC). (2014b). *Youth physical activity guidelines toolkit.* Retrieved from www.cdc.gov/HealthyYouth/physicalactivity/guidelines.htm

Centers for Disease Control and Prevention, Healthy Communities Program & National Center for Chronic Disease Prevention and Health Promotion, Division of Adult and Community Health. (2012). *A sustainability planning guide for Healthy Communities.* Retrieved from http://stacks.cdc.gov/view/cdc/11700/

Center for Prevention Research and Development (CPRD). (2006). *Evidence-based practices for effective community coalitions.* Champaign, IL: Center for Prevention Research and Development, Institute of Government and Public Affairs, University of Illinois.

Chambers, L. W., Underwood, J., Halbert, T., Woodward, C. A., Heale, J., & Isaacs, S. (1994). 1992 Ontario survey of public health nurses: Perceptions of roles and activities. *Canadian Journal of Public Health, 85*(3), 175–179.

Cohen, L., Baer, N., & Satterwhite, P. (2002). Developing effective coalitions: An eight step guide. In M. E. Wurzbach (Ed.), *Community health education & promotion: A guide to program design and evaluation* (2nd ed., pp. 144–161). Gaithersburg, MD: Aspen Publishers Inc. Retrieved from http://thrive.preventioninstitute.org/pdf/eightstep.pdf

Commission on Social Determinants of Health. (2008). *Closing the gap in a generation: Health equity through action on the social determinants of health.* Final Report of the Commission on Social Determinants of Health. Geneva: World Health Organization. Retrieved from http://whqlibdoc.who.int/publications/2008/9789241563703_eng.pdf

Community Health Nurses of Canada (CHNC). (2011, March). *Canadian community health nursing professional practice model & standards of practice*. Retrieved from www.chnc.ca/nursing-standards-of-practice.cfm

Cottrell, L. S. (1976). The competent community. In B. H. Kaplan, R. N. Wilson, & A. H. Leighton (Eds.), *Further explorations in social psychiatry* (pp. 195–209). New York: Basic Books.

Edwards, N., Murphy, M., Moyer, A., & Wright, A. (1995). *Building and sustaining collective health action: A framework for community health practitioners* (No. DP95-1). Ottawa, ON: Community Health Research Unit.

Feighery, E., & Rogers, T. (1995). *Building and maintaining effective coalitions.* How-To Guides on Community Health Promotion, Health Promotion Resource Center. Retrieved from www.ttac.org/tcn/peers/pdfs/07.24.12/CA_BuildingAndMaintainingEffectiveCoalitions_Resource.pdf

Florin, P., Mitchell, R., Stevenson, J., & Klein, I. (2000). Predicting intermediate outcomes for prevention coalitions: A developmental perspective. *Evaluation and Program Planning, 23*(3), 341–346.

Foster-Fishman, P. G., Shelby, L., Berkowitz, D. W., Lounsbury, S. J., & Allen, N. A. (2001). Building collaborative capacity in community coalitions: A review and integrative framework. *American Journal of Community Psychology, 29*. Retrieved from http://systemexchange.msu.edu/upload/collab_capacity.pdf

Francisco, V. T., Paine, A. L., & Fawcett, S. B. (1993). A methodology for monitoring and evaluating community health coalitions. *Health Education Research, 8*(3), 403–416.

Goodman, R. M., Speers, M. A., McLeroy, K., Fawcett, S., Kegler, M., Parker, E., … & Wallerstein, N. (1998). Identifying and defining the dimensions of community capacity to provide a basis for measurement. *Health Education and Behaviour, 25*(3), 258–278.

Green, L., & Kreuter, M. (2005). *Health program planning: An educational and ecological approach* (4th ed.). New York: McGraw-Hill.

Green, L., & Kreuter, M. (2014). *The PRECEDE-PROCEED model of health program planning & evaluation.* Retrieved from www.lgreen.net/precede.htm

Green, L. W., Richard, L., & Potvin, L. (1996). Ecological foundations of health promotion. *American Journal of Health Promotion, 10*(4), 270–281.

Hawe, P., Noort, M., King, L., & Jordens, C. (1997). Multiplying health gains: The critical role of capacity-building within health promotion programs. *Health Policy, 39*, 29–42.

Heaven, C. (2014). Developing a plan for assessing local needs and resources. *Community Tool Box* (Chapter 3, Section 1). Retrieved from http://ctb.ku.edu/en/table-of-contents/assessment/assessing-community-needs-and-resources/develop-a-plan/main

Kreuter, M., & Lezin, N. (1998). Are consortia/collaboratives effective in changing health status and health systems? A critical review of the literature. Atlanta, GA: Health 2000 Inc., 2900 Chamblee Tucker Road, Building 8, Suite 3, 30341.

Kreuter, M., Lezin, N., Kreuter, M., & Green, L. (1998). *Community health promotion ideas that work: A field-book for practitioners.* Sudbury, MA: Jones and Bartlett.

KU Work Group for Community Health and Development. (2014a). Creating and maintaining partnerships. *Community Tool Box* (Chapter 1). Retrieved from http://ctb.ku.edu/en/creating-and-maintaining-partnerships

KU Work Group for Community Health and Development. (2014b). Increasing participation and membership. *Community Tool Box* (Chapter 8). Retrieved from http://ctb.ku.edu/en/increasing-participation-and-membership#node_toolkits_full_group_outline

Labonte, R., & Robertson, A. (1996). Delivering the goods, showing our stuff: The case for a constructivist paradigm for health promotion research and practice. *Health Education Quarterly, 23*(4), 431–447.

Laverack, G. (2003). Building capable communities: Experiences in a rural Fijian context. *Health Promotion International, 18*(2), 99–106.

MacLellan-Wright, M. F., Anderson, D., Barber, S., Smith, N., Cantin, B., Felix, R., & Raine, K. (2007). The development of measures of community capacity for community-based funding programs in Canada. *Health Promotion International, 22*(4), 299–306.

McCloskey, D. J., McDonald, M. A., Cook, J., Heurtin-Roberts, S., Updegrove, S., Sampson, D., ... & Eder, M. (2011). Community engagement: Definitions and organizing concepts from the literature. In Clinical and Translational Science Awards Consortium (CTSA) Community Engagement Key Function Committee Task Force on the Principles of Community Engagement (Ed.), *Principles of community engagement* (2nd ed.). Washington, DC: US Department of Health and Human Services. Available from www.atsdr.cdc.gov/communityengagement/

McKnight, J. L. (1987). Regenerating community. *Social Policy* (Winter), 54–58.

McKnight, J. L. (1997). Two tools for well-being: Health systems and communities. In M. Minkler (Ed.), *Community organizing and community building for health* (pp. 20–29). New Brunswick, NJ: Rutgers University Press.

McLeroy, K. R., Kegler, M., Steckler, A., Burdine, J. M., & Wisotzky, M. (1994). Community coalitions for health promotion: Summary and further reflections. *Health Education Research, 9*(1), 1–11.

McLeroy, K. R., Norton, B. L., Kegler, M. C., Burdina, J. B., & Sumaya, C. V. (2003). Community-based interventions. *American Journal of Public Health, 93*(4), 529–533.

Minkler, M., & Pies, C. (1997). Ethical issues in community organization and community participation. In M. Minkler (Ed.), *Community organizing and community building for health* (pp. 120–136). New Brunswick, NJ: Rutgers University Press.

Mittelmark, M. B. (1996). Centrally initiated health promotion: Getting on the agenda of a community and transforming a project to local ownership. Retrieved from http://iuhpe.org/rhpeo/ijhp-articles/1996/6/index.htm

Moyer, A., Coristine, M., MacLean, L., & Meyer, M. (1999). A model for building collective capacity in community-based programs: The Elderly in Need project. *Public Health Nursing, 16*(3), 205–214.

Nagy, J. (2014). Organizational structure: An overview. *Community Tool Box* (Chapter 9, Section 1). Retrieved from http://ctb.ku.edu/en/table-of-contents/structure/organizational-structure/overview/main

New South Wales Health Department. (2001). *A framework for building capacity to improve health* (No. SHPN: 990226). Sydney: New South Wales Health Department. Retrieved from www.thehealthcompass.org/sbcc-tools/framework-building-capacity-improve-health

Nyswander, D. (1956). Education for health: Some principles and their applications. *Health Education Monographs, 14*, 65–70.

Parker, E., Margolis, L. H., Eng, E., & Henríquez-Roldán, C. (2003). Assessing the capacity of health departments to engage in community-based participatory public health. *American Journal of Public Health, 93*(3), 472–476.

Pressley, J., Barlow, B., Durkin, M., Jacko, S. A., Dominguez, D. R., & Johnson, L. (2005). A national program for injury prevention for children and adolescents: The Injury Free Coalition for Kids. *Journal of Urban Health: Bulletin of New York Academy of Medicine, 82*, 389–402. Retrieved from www.injuryfree.org/resources/JournalOfUrbanHealth.pdf

Public Health Agency of Canada (PHAC), Alberta/NWT Region. (2007). Community capacity building tool. Retrieved from www.phac-aspc.gc.ca/canada/regions/ab-nwt-tno/documents/UserManual-January2007_e.pdf

Public Health Agency of Canada (PHAC) and Canadian Institute of Health Information (CIHI). (2011). *Obesity in Canada*. Ottawa, ON: Author.

Quad Council of Public Health Nursing Organizations. (2011). *Quad Council competencies for public health nurses*. Retrieved from www.achne.org/files/Quad%20Council/QuadCouncilCompetenciesforPublicHealthNurses.pdf

Rabinowitz, P. (2014). Coalition building I: Starting a coalition. *Community Tool Box* (Chapter 5, Section 5). Retrieved from http://ctb.ku.edu/en/table-of-contents/assessment/promotion-strategies/start-a-coalition/main

Robertson, A., & Minkler, M. (1994). New health promotion movement: A critical examination. *Health Education Quarterly, 21*(3), 295–312.

Schoenfeld, B. M., & MacDonald, M. B. (2002). Saskatchewan public health nursing survey: Perceptions of roles and activities. *Canadian Journal of Public Health, 93*(6), 452–456.

Stokols, D. (1996). Translating social ecological theory into guidelines for community health promotion. *American Journal of Health Promotion, 10*(4), 282–298.

Thompson, B., & Kinne, S. (1999). Social change theory: Application to community health. In N. Bracht (Ed.), *Health promotion at the community level: New advances* (2nd ed., pp. 29–46). Thousand Oaks, CA: Sage Publications.

US Department of Health and Human Services. (2014, March). *Youth physical activity guidelines toolkit.* Retrieved from www.cdc.gov/healthyyouth/physicalactivity/guidelines.htm

Wandersman, A., Valois, R., Ochs, L., de la Cruz, D. S., Adkins, E., & Goodman, R. M. (1996). Toward a social ecology of community coalitions. *American Journal of Health Promotion, 10*(4), 299–307.

World Health Organization (WHO). (2010). *Global recommendations on physical activity.* Retrieved from www.who.int/dietphysicalactivity/factsheet_recommendations/en/

## Website Resources

### Coalition Guides

Centers for Disease Control and Prevention (CDC), Division of Community Health: www.cdc.gov/nccdphp/dch/about/index.htm

This site provides access to the Healthy Communities Program at the National Center for Chronic Disease Prevention and Health Promotion. This program helps funded communities prevent chronic disease by building community capacity—commitment, resources, and skills. It also provides access to funded communities, success stories, and links to tools and guides, such as the Community Health Resources Database and CHANGE Tool and Action Guide.

Many of the websites listed in Chapter 10 also apply to Chapter 11. Search for specific coalitions by preceding the word "coalition" with an issue or population in your key word search, such as "tobacco," "poverty," "multicultural" or "youth," and you will find numerous examples.

Robert Wood Johnson Foundation and University of Wisconsin Population Health Institute, *County Health Rankings and Roadmaps*: www.countyhealthrankings.org/

The County Health Rankings measure the health of nearly all counties in the US and rank them within states. The indicators are informed by a model of population health that links social and environmental determinants—influencing factors—and health. County health rankings are linked to elements of the model. The Roadmaps section provides an action model, tools, and resources that communities can use to improve community health by taking action on selected health indicators.

# Appendix to Chapter 11

**Evaluation of Coalition Meeting**

Date:

Please circle the number that best represents your view on the way the coalition meetings are conducted.

| | Disagree | | | | Agree |
|---|---|---|---|---|---|
| 1. The objectives of the meeting were clear to me. | 1 | 2 | 3 | 4 | 5 |
| 2. The atmosphere created by the chairperson was conducive to exploring ideas. | 1 | 2 | 3 | 4 | 5 |
| 3. I was given opportunity to share my views and participate fully during the meeting. | 1 | 2 | 3 | 4 | 5 |
| 4. The number of participants was conducive to exploring and sharing ideas. | 1 | 2 | 3 | 4 | 5 |
| 5. The length of time allotted for discussion was appropriate. | 1 | 2 | 3 | 4 | 5 |
| 6. The decisions were made by the group as a whole, not just a few people. | 1 | 2 | 3 | 4 | 5 |
| 7. I was able to participate in decision making. | 1 | 2 | 3 | 4 | 5 |
| 8. Group members worked well with each other, and were not antagonistic. | 1 | 2 | 3 | 4 | 5 |
| 9. The group made good use of its time and accomplished objectives. | 1 | 2 | 3 | 4 | 5 |
| 10. The meeting was well organized and ran smoothly. | 1 | 2 | 3 | 4 | 5 |

Was there conflict present at this meeting?  ❑ No  ❑ Yes (please describe)

11. If there was conflict present, was it resolved?  ❑ No  ❑ Yes
If the conflict was not resolved, please indicate why:
❑ Conflict was avoided, not discussed
❑ Members argued with one another
❑ Other (specify)

Please circle the number that best represents your view on the relevance of the discussion at the coalition meetings.

| Choose: 1 = hardly ever; 2 = sometimes; 3 = half of the time; 4 = most of the time; 5 = always | 1 | 2 | 3 | 4 | 5 |
|---|---|---|---|---|---|
| 1. The discussions at meetings are relevant to: | | | | | |
|    a. the purpose of the meeting | 1 | 2 | 3 | 4 | 5 |
|    b. the focus of the coalition | 1 | 2 | 3 | 4 | 5 |
|    c. health and health care | 1 | 2 | 3 | 4 | 5 |
| 2. The ideas expressed are specific to the work of the coalition. | 1 | 2 | 3 | 4 | 5 |
| 3. The ideas expressed are relevant to my area of knowledge and skill. | 1 | 2 | 3 | 4 | 5 |

4. What could be done to make the meetings more effective?




Please add any additional comments about the meeting you would like to make:




Thank you for participating and completing this evaluation.

# Chapter 12

# Building Healthy Public Policy for Population Health

· · · · · · · · · · · · · · · · · · · · · · · · · · · · · · · · · · · · · · · · · · · · · · · · · · · · · · · · · · · · · · · · · · · · · · · · · · · · · · · · · · · · · · · · · · · ·

C
ommunity nurses practice within a policy framework and use policy to foster population health. This chapter provides an introduction to the role of nurses in developing policy to promote the health of communities. One of the five broad approaches to promoting the health of individuals, groups, and communities, healthy public policy works in synergy with other health promotion strategies to increase access to the determinants of health and create environments where the healthy choices are the easy choices.

The chapter differentiates between policy, health policy, and healthy public policy. It provides a guide to the policy change process, with emphasis on the knowledge and skills required by the beginning practitioner. These include identifying situations that require policy change, exploring evidence-based solutions, assessing community readiness, and engaging key decision makers to support the policy change process. Not least, building healthy public policy requires nurses to bring knowledge of community and community health, and to develop the leadership skills required, to work with nursing colleagues, community partners, and opinion leaders across the health spectrum.

Policy change requires a considerable investment in time and resources but works in synergy with other health promotion strategies to create long-term health benefits. Policy change draws together the community health nursing process and capacity-building approaches to increase the potential of communities to support health. The scenario features public health nurses contributing their expertise in developing healthy workplaces and support for breast-feeding to contribute to policy development in a coalition to create a Baby-Friendly Initiative in the city.

## Learning Objectives
· · · · · · · · · · · · · · · · · · · · · · · · · · · · · · · · · · · · · · · · · · · · · · · · · · · · · · · · · · · · · · · · · · · · · · · · · · · · · · · · · · · · ·

After reading this chapter and answering the questions throughout the chapter, you should be able to:

1. Discuss the use of policy as a health promotion strategy in community health nursing practice.
2. Describe the role of community nurses in creating healthy public policy.

3. Describe the policy change process.
4. Discuss strategies to assess community readiness for change.
5. Conduct a force field analysis and document the results.
6. Identify strategies to increase community involvement in policy initiatives.

## Policy and Community Health Nursing Practice

**Key Terms and Concepts**

force field analysis • healthy public policy • policy • sources of power: position, resources, expertise, personal qualities

**Policy** is a course or principle of action exemplified in the formal and informal rules and understandings that are adopted on a collective basis to guide individual and collective behavior (Schmid, Pratt, & Howze, 1995). Without doubt, unwritten rules and guidelines have a considerable influence on daily life, for example, the generally accepted policy of arriving for work on time, and treating others civilly. However, this chapter is concerned mainly with formal, written public policies, communicated in position papers, standards, guidelines, and policy statements, which have an impact on community health.

Community health nurses practice within a framework of national, provincial/territorial/state, and local (regional) policies that regulate health care. An important goal of health policy is an efficient and effective health care system (or, as some would say, illness care system). In common with other health providers, community nurses must understand the legislation, regulations, and policies that govern their professional practice with individuals, families, communities, and populations. In preparing for community health nursing practice, it is important for nurses to understand the economic, social, political, and environmental factors that inform health policy and guide the selection and delivery of community health programs and services. As well, the beginning practitioner must be competent in applying strategies that improve the health of populations across the life span (Canadian Association of Schools of Nursing, 2014; Quad Council of Public Health Nursing Organizations, 2011).

Of equal, or perhaps more, significance, community health nurses have a social and professional mandate to speak out on behalf of health in its broadest sense. Not only are they well placed to observe the impact of policy decisions on health, community health nurses have opportunities to raise issues and engage communities in policy discussions through their work with diverse client groups, disciplines, professional organizations, community groups, and intersectoral partners. Community nurses have a long history of concern with issues of equity and access (Canadian Nurses Association [CNA], 2000; Kang, 1995). Current initiatives, such as a report commissioned by CNA to analyze the impact of public policy and programming on the social determinants of health for the purpose of informing the evolution of nursing roles (Canadian Health Services Research Foundation, 2012), is just one example of how they continue to take this responsibility seriously. As policy change becomes an increasingly important part of community health practice (Chambers et al., 1994; Schoenfeld & MacDonald, 2002), community health nurses will need to continue to hone their skills in the policy arena.

Nurses usually undertake policy work as part of a multidisciplinary team or coalition that brings together different sectors of the community and community members. Some examples of how community health nurses become involved in policy change are shown in Table 12.2.

Janet is a public health nurse with the Workplace Health program. This program links with large and small businesses in the region to foster healthy workplaces and promote the health and well-being of employees. The program is meeting with two large employers in the area—an information technology (IT) firm and the new airport authority—to discuss ways of increasing support for women in the workplace. Both firms are concerned about absenteeism and retention of employees. The IT firm has always seen itself as a leader in promoting employee health and is a member of the Healthy Heart coalition. More than half of its employees are women, with the majority in the childbearing and child-rearing years. The IT firm laid off staff last year because of a downturn in the economy but is optimistic about the future and sees early signs of recovery. If this continues, the firm will begin rehiring in the coming months. The airport has just completed an expansion and is hiring new staff. In addition to improving conditions for employees, it wants to improve services for travelers with small children.

Both firms employ occupational health nurses, recreation staff, and counselors. Under discussion is the possibility of providing emergency day care, with a room for breast-feeding.

Janet seeks advice from a colleague on breast-feeding. Lillian, a public health nurse with the Healthy Children program, advocates for and assists in developing policies to support breast-feeding in the workplace, restaurants, shopping malls, and other public places. Her role includes enhancing knowledge and skills around breast-feeding. As a member of the coalition seeking Baby-Friendly status for the city, Lillian is excited at the thought of increasing support for breast-feeding in workplaces. Support for breast-feeding is an important element of this initiative of the World Health Organization (1998). Janet's idea also fits well with the Healthy Children program goal of increasing

the proportion of infants who are breast-fed up to six months to 50 percent by the year 2015. As an aside, Janet explains that she is supervising two nursing students in the community for the next 12 weeks and sees this as an opportunity for a student project.

After Janet leaves, Lillian thinks to herself, "This is an opportunity that can't be missed, but my plate is full already. Since joining the program last year after graduation, I have spent nearly two days a week at the well-baby clinics. Now that we have a new community nurse, maybe I can taper off. This would give me the time I need for breast-feeding projects. I will miss the contact with mothers and babies, but I would like to learn more about policy change. Thank goodness I have Jake as my supervisor. He has a lot of experience with policy development around tobacco and alcohol use and has many contacts in the business community. When I talk to him on Friday about my work plan for the next six months, I will propose that I drop the well-baby clinics for the next three months and take on this new project. I really want to increase my skills in policy development now that I see what is possible. Maybe I can negotiate some time with him. I will prepare another draft of my work plan (Table 12.1) to show how this new project will fit."

**Discussion Topics and Questions**
1. Identify public places in your community where mothers can, or might, choose to breast-feed their infants. Discuss what factors might support or detract from this practice.
2. Identify one or two policies pertaining to your clinical practice in the community, as a nursing student or community nurse, and discuss their potential impact on health.

For suggested responses, please see the Answer Key at the back of the book.

**Table 12.1: Draft Work Plan**

| Child Health Program<br>Lillian Smith    Draft Work Plan 2014–2015 | | (Revised: July 21, 2014) |
|---|---|---|
| **Activities** | **Timeline<br>(Responsibility)** | **Results and Comments** |
| 1. Revise departmental breast-feeding policy guidelines in line with the Baby-Friendly Initiative (BFI) | | |
| 1.1. Revise policies | Aug. 20, 2014<br>(Work group<br>[WG]) | Work group met three times and completed the revisions |
| 1.2. Submit revised policy to Policies & Procedures Committee for approval | Sept. 23, 2014<br>(LS) | Revised policy submitted |
| 1.3. Develop training resources | Dec. 16, 2014<br>(WG) | |
| 1.4. All staff training sessions | Jan.–March 2015<br>(WG) | |
| 2. Represent department on Baby-Friendly coalition—Project to get Baby-Friendly designation for city | | |
| 2.1. Attend monthly meetings | Sept. 1, 2014 | Ongoing |
| 2.2. Analyze breast-feeding policies submitted by members and prepare presentation on breast-feeding policies | Oct. 21, 2014<br>(LS, WG) | Completed |
| 2.3 Deliver slide presentation on findings | Nov. 21, 2014<br>(LS, Mary Myers) | |
| 3. Assist development of Workplace Health (WH) proposal for breast-feeding support project at two workplaces | | |
| 3.1 Prepare first draft of proposal | Oct. 12, 2014<br>(Jake Woods, LS) | First draft prepared |
| 3.2 Develop breast-feeding policies for selected workplaces | | |
| 3.3 Collaborate with WH to recruit businesses to the BFI coalition | Jan.1, 2015 | |

**Table 12.2: Community Health Nursing Roles in Policy Change**

| Community Health Issue | Nursing Action |
|---|---|
| Women living in an older adults' apartment building take part in an exercise group held in a common room where other residents smoke. One member leads the group with support from the community health nurse and the city recreation department. The women complain that the benefits of exercise are outweighed by their exposure to secondhand smoke. The room is exempt from city smoking bylaws, and the group wants this changed. | The nurse offers to provide information on the health impact of secondhand smoke and suggests approaches to use when talking to the tenants' association. |
| Several recent incidents of threats and physical assault have left nurses providing care in the home feeling vulnerable. Frequently, little information is available on new clients. | The nurses feel that their agency could do more to protect them and ask for a review of organizational policies around home visiting safety. |
| Women attending prenatal classes receive tokens for milk but cannot afford to buy winter clothing or equipment such as baby strollers. | The multidisciplinary team organizes a clothing exchange, and the program manager develops a partnership with a city-wide coalition on poverty that is advocating for increased maternal health benefits. |
| A community group running a drop-in center for young men living and working downtown offers bar workers a Smart Serve training program in support of municipal alcohol policies. The training course provides information and techniques on how to prevent alcohol-related incidents but lacks information on what to do when incidents occur. | Public health nurses support the alcohol policy indirectly by working with the community group to develop training on how to intervene when alcohol-related incidents do occur. |
| Following up on a missed appointment for TB monitoring, the public health nurse finds the family huddled in coats and blankets trying to keep warm. It is −20°C outside. In contravention of the law, the landlord turns down the heat in the apartment during the day. | The nurse advises the family on municipal housing policies and helps the parents file a report with housing authorities. |
| Community health nurses collaborated with the local school board to provide resources and workshops on increasing classroom physical activity. Their efforts are appreciated, but they realize that not all students will benefit because physical activity is not emphasized in the school curriculum. | The nurses develop a resolution directing their nursing association to lobby the government to introduce system-wide regulations on regular physical activity in schools. |

## Policy as a Health Promotion Strategy

Policy is one of several broad strategies used to promote population health by increasing access to the social and environmental determinants of health. (For a thoughtful discussion of how the concepts of public policy, the social determinants of health, and population health have been defined and continue to evolve, see Morrison, Gagnon, Morestin, & Keeling, 2014). As discussed in Chapter 6, in the context of health promotion, policy aims to achieve health goals in a society by creating environments where the "healthy choices are the easy choices" (Milio, 1989).

While policy change may overlap with other health promotion strategies, there are important differences. Traditional health education and awareness activities are rooted in the belief that failure to make healthy choices results from lack of information (Wallack, 1998). Within this model, education is designed to fill a knowledge gap that will lead to health-seeking behavior. Prenatal classes are examples of such educational activities aimed at preparing families for healthy pregnancy, childbirth, and parenting. Mass communication strategies use social marketing campaigns to increase public awareness of health risks, changing attitudes, and social norms to build support for policy change strategies (Public Health Nursing Section, 2001). As the name suggests, environmental change strategies may require policy support but are directed toward changing the physical and social climate, and providing resources to enable health. For example, public parks with climbing frames, trails, bicycle paths, and outdoor skating rinks enable year-round physical activity for all age groups (Stokols, 1996).

The policy formation model (Ontario Public Health Association [OPHA], 1996), a simplified version of the health cube (see Figure 6.1 in Chapter 6), depicts health promotion strategies to change policy, educate and raise awareness, and provide environmental support as being linked and nonhierarchical. In any given situation, one may be more appropriate than another. Choosing one, or any combination of the three, should be based on what is most likely to meet health goals.

## How Policies Affect Health

Significant health gains were made in the last century in developed countries through the introduction of legislation to provide food subsidies, safe drinking water, and better sanitation (McKeown, 1979). These policy measures, enacted through programs and services, and legislative, regulatory, or organizational mechanisms, were a key factor in reducing infectious diseases and improving community health (Schmid et al., 1995). More recently attention has been focused on using policy to influence healthy personal lifestyle choices—for example, around tobacco and seat belt use—implicated in the development of chronic disease, accidents, and injuries (Brownson, Newschaffer, & Ali-Abarghoui, 1997; Minkler, 1999; Schmid et al., 1995; Stokols, 1996). While individual health promotion strategies are effective, interventions employing multiple strategies at multiple levels are most effective (Jackson et al., 2006).

The Commission on Social Determinants of Health (2008) presents compelling evidence that personal life choices are strongly influenced by the socioeconomic environment. As our understanding of the central role of the social and environmental determinants of health has grown, so too has our appreciation of the role of policy in determining health. The determinants of health, as defined in Chapter 1, the circumstances in which people are born, grow up, and age, are shaped by the distribution of money, power, and resources at global, national, and local levels.

The term **healthy public policy** refers to the role of policy in promoting health of populations. Flynn (2000) identifies three levels of influence defined by which determinants of health are being addressed. The first level encompasses traditional health policy concerns involving health promotion, disease prevention, and the provision of health services. The second level comprises social, educational, and cultural policy. The third level is concerned with the broader economic and environmental policies that

**Table 12.3: Examples of Legislative/Regulatory and Organizational Policies for Different Levels of Healthy Public Policy**

| Healthy Public Policy Level | Policy Focus | |
| --- | --- | --- |
| | Legislative/Regulatory | Organizational |
| Health services | Regulation of Food Premises legislation | Policy requiring food-handler training prior to employment |
| Social, educational, cultural | Liquor License Act controlling the sale of alcohol | Workplace or school policy on use of alcohol on the premises |
| Economic and environmental | Maternity leave and benefits for pregnant women and new parents | Policies governing paid sick leave or extended leave allowances without penalty |

influence health, such as industrial development, transportation, and housing. This third level, also termed "health" in all policies, as described in the *Adelaide Statement on Health in All Policies* (WHO, 2010), advocates that all sectors of government—labor and business, justice, transportation, agriculture, and education—formulate policy with a view to its potential health impact (see examples in Table 12.3). A more recent qualitative research study to identify the essence of healthy public policy, and health impact assessment, identified healthy public policy as having four characteristics: concern with a broad definition of health, designing policy to improve people's health and reduce health inequities, intersectoral collaboration, and influencing the policy cycle from inception to completion (Harris, Kemp, & Sainsbury, 2012). Health impact assessment had the same number of characteristics: assessing policy proposal to predict population health and equity impacts, and a structured process for stakeholder dialogue, making recommendations, and flexibly adapting the policy process. In sum, the two were seen as different but mutually supporting.

Multi-level interventions to improve health and reduce inequities that include policy change have proven successful; however, the mechanisms of action are not fully understood (Sallis, Owen, & Fisher, 2008). Policy can change behavior by influencing the choices people make. For example, policies reduce exposure to health hazards by severely restricting opportunities to engage in unhealthy behavior, such as tobacco use, or by requiring people to follow proven, safe practices, such as using seat belts. With these so-called passive strategies, individuals do not have to take the initiative to choose healthy options. The required healthy behavior is maintained by monitoring and enforcing the legislation and by the pressure of public opinion. Policies also play a part in creating environments that foster certain behaviors and discourage others, as with bylaws that specify the use of green space in housing developments, limit pesticide use, or restrict smoking in public places to reduce exposure to secondhand tobacco smoke. More broadly, policies promote social justice or equitable access to the resources for health through measures such as a guaranteed minimum wage, welfare support, and entitlement to essential health care (Commission on Social Determinants of Health, 2008).

Building healthy public policy has an advantage over some of the other health promotion strategies. Not only is policy likely to have a broader reach than individual behavior change strategies, but unlike community capacity building, it can also be directed toward specific and tangible ends. Furthermore, policy is likely to have a long-lasting effect on the community. Once implemented, it is difficult to change, in contrast to program and service delivery, which can be withdrawn or pared down if funds dry up. On the other hand, evidence to support policy intervention is often lacking. Even in well-researched policy areas such as youth smoking, there has been limited evaluation of the effectiveness of policy in changing behavior (Multicultural Advocates for Social Change on Tobacco, 2004), and there are few well-controlled studies designed to assess the effects of policy interventions on health inequalities (Macintyre, Chalmers, Horton, & Smith, 2001). A possible reason for this is the complexity of conducting research and interventions based on ecological models (Sallis et al., 2008).

The most appropriate level for policy making is not always clear. Even though the lack of access to income and housing may be clearly visible in a community, some question whether policy change at this level can make a meaningful difference on the broad determinants of health. As Labonte (1997) points out, most economic and social policy is national and transnational in nature. This can leave communities vulnerable to shifts in national priorities and cuts in health care spending, unable to protect community programs or secure funding for local policy initiatives. Furthermore, there is apprehension within the health promotion field that policy interventions, such as the promotion of self-care, are viewed by government as a means of conserving health dollars through the withdrawal of costly individual services (Minkler, 1999). Choosing policy change as the most appropriate health promotion strategy needs careful consideration.

## Policy Change Process

There are several easy-to-follow guides to changing health-related policy. Some are written primarily for nurses; others are directed toward a broader audience of health care providers and community groups (Ewles & Simnett, 1999; Flynn, 2000; OPHA, 1996; Public Health Nursing Section, 2001). All the guides describe a systematic problem-solving approach that is similar to the community health nursing process and encompasses the four steps of assessment, planning, implementation, and evaluation. All advocate broad community involvement at all stages of policy development and recommend that decision making should be transparent, involve all the key stakeholders, and draw on evidence-based knowledge. Minor variation occurs in the number of steps, the terms used to describe them, and the level of policy change addressed—local or national. However, all are applicable to policy change at any level.

The following discussion follows a "road map" (Figure 12.1) based on an OPHA (1996) guide to policy change. The primary reason for choosing this guide is that it addresses policy change at the local level, which is likely to be the major focus for community nurses. As well, a workshop and useful tools have been developed from this resource and are available online (Public Health Ontario, 2012, 2013).

Lillian is now preparing a presentation for the Baby-Friendly coalition on breast-feeding policies. The coalition has representatives from all the major hospitals and community agencies, public and private, who provide breast-feeding support across the region. A sales representative, employed by a company selling baby formula, attends the bimonthly meetings, and there has been discussion about involving other businesses from different sectors of the community.

Since the last coalition meeting, Lillian's working group has gathered breast-feeding policies from member agencies and compared them with the World Health Organization's (WHO) Baby-Friendly Initiative (BFI) standards. This task proved to be much more onerous than anticipated. It took several weeks and many phone calls to collect information on the policies and practices, despite assurances they would be dispatched within one week of the previous meeting. The summer holidays further reduced the time available for meetings, leaving the team with only two weeks to complete the analysis. Lillian and her co-presenter worked late to complete the presentation. (For an example review, see the *Review of Breastfeeding Practices and Programs*, British Columbia Ministry of Health, 2012.)

Following a review of the Ten Steps to Successful Breast-Feeding, which underpin the BFI standards (see Box 12.1), Lillian presents the criteria for evaluating agency policies and a summary of the findings for discussion (see Box 12.2 and Box 12.3).

The chairperson thanks Lillian and her team for their hard work and invites questions. This is the first working group of the Baby-Friendly coalition to report back, and members are eager to discuss the findings. A few members say that they appreciate the team's sensitivity in presenting the findings, which shows there is much work to be done. One nurse comments, "Our agency was restructured last year, and we are employing more part-time staff—there is never any time to update policies. I am embarrassed to think when we last looked at them. This really gives us an incentive to do it." Another member says, "We know our policies

and practices are inconsistent across the hospital and have been meaning to tackle this for some time. Some units are more enthusiastic about the Baby-Friendly Initiative than others, and rooming-in seems to work more smoothly in those units." Members generally find the WHO evaluation criteria useful and acknowledge that policies are just the tip of the iceberg. More than one mentions that they expected to find considerable variation in the way the policies are implemented if they took a closer look. Everyone agrees there is no point in making excuses; it is time to make changes.

As a next step, the working group agrees to identify model policies on breast-feeding, rooming-in, and staff training for breast-feeding support, and a discharge policy around linking women to breast-feeding support groups.

Lillian recalls the meeting with Jake, when they had agreed that she assign one half day each week to this project for the remainder of the year. The time allocation appeared adequate then, allowing for some juggling of projects to meet deadlines, but it is no longer appropriate. "Life just gets more complicated," she thinks. "I will have to take another look at my commitments."

**Discussion Topics and Questions**

3. One Healthy People 2020 breast-feeding objective is to increase the proportion of employers providing an on-site lactation/mother's room from 25 percent in 2009 to 38 percent in 2020 (United States Breastfeeding Committee, 2013). Discuss how community nurses might support this objective, both as individuals and through their professional organization.

4. The WHO's "Ten Steps to Successful Breastfeeding" have implications for staff training. Discuss how a health service organization adopting a Baby-Friendly Initiative might comply with this requirement.

5. Discuss how you might respond to a colleague who says that if women want to feed their babies formula, that is their choice—we should let women decide what is best for their baby.

BOX 12.1
**Slide 1—Ten Steps to Successful Breast-Feeding**

Every facility providing maternity services and care for newborn infants should
1. have a written breast-feeding policy that is routinely communicated to all health care staff.
2. train all health care staff in skills necessary to implement this policy.
3. inform all pregnant women about the benefits and management of breast-feeding.
4. help mothers initiate breast-feeding within a half-hour of birth.
5. show mothers how to breast-feed and how to maintain lactation, even if they should be separated from their infants.
6. give newborn infants no food or drink other than breast milk, unless medically indicated.
7. practice rooming-in—allow mothers and infants to remain together—24 hours a day.
8. encourage breast-feeding on demand.
9. give no artificial teats or pacifiers (also called dummies or soothers) to breast-feeding infants.
10. foster the establishment of breast-feeding support groups and refer mothers to them on discharge from the hospital or clinic. (World Health Organization, 1998)

BOX 12.2
**Slide 2—Criteria for Evaluating Breast-Feeding Policies**

• There are appropriate policies on all practices concerning breast-feeding agreed between relevant authorities.
• Those policies are made explicit in a written document.
• All staff and patients are made aware of the policies. (World Health Organization, 1998)

BOX 12.3
**Slide 3—Summary of Findings**

• All agencies have some breast-feeding policies.
• The policies range from 2 to 22 pages; some agencies have a global policy, some are organized by themes.
• No two policies are the same on a particular topic—even within an organization.
• Close to two-thirds of hospitals are able to support rooming-in and all are moving toward that goal.
• There is significant variation in training plans and resources.
• Only two organizations have policies that contain a communication strategy.
• All the organizations have plans to update the policies.

**Figure 12.1: Policy Formation Model—THCU Road Map for Policy Development**

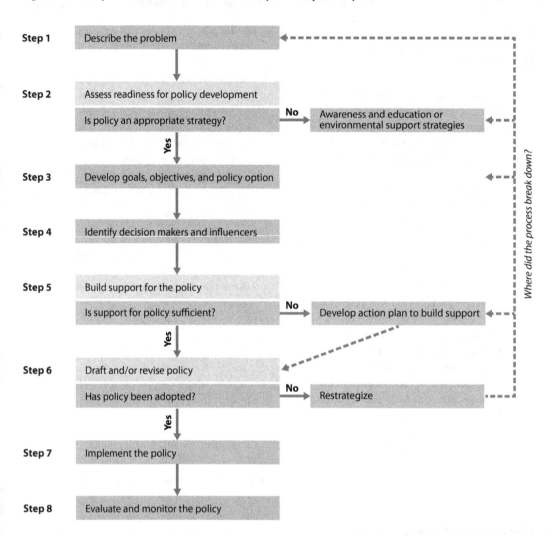

Source: Adapted from Ontario Agency for Health Protection and Promotion (Public Health Ontario). (2012). *Developing health promotion policies*. V3.18 [Internet]. Toronto, ON: Queen's Printer for Ontario. Cited 2014 Dec 22, Available from www.publichealthontario.ca/en/ eRepository/Developing_health_promotion_policies_2012.pdf.

The steps in the road map to policy change equate to phases in the community health nursing process. Table 11.1 from Chapter 11 can be modified slightly to fit the time scale and stage of a policy development community project. These phases, listed below, are used to structure the next section.

- Identify the problem and decide what to do.
- Develop an action plan for a policy change intervention.
- Implement the action plan.
- Evaluate the results.

## Identify the Problem and Decide What to Do (Road Map Steps 1–2)

The road to policy change starts with an identified issue or problem. This is where community nurses can play a key role in describing issues that might be addressed by policy change (see Table 12.2). It is important to gain a comprehensive understanding of the issue for the defined population and to determine that policy change is a viable solution to the problem. A preliminary analysis will document the nature and size of the problem; for instance, identifying who, and how many, are affected. A detailed analysis of the problem and a search for evidence will establish whether or not policy change offers a feasible solution. Policy change takes considerable time and effort; it should not be undertaken lightly.

Of equal importance is establishing that the issue is of concern to the community. This is fundamental; if the community does not recognize the problem, it is difficult to proceed. It is also necessary to determine whether or not the community has the capacity to address the problem. If the community is not aware or lacks capacity, then it would be more appropriate to use other strategies, such as awareness raising, or education or environmental support strategies.

Much of the foundation work of documenting community needs and strengths is carried out as part of ongoing surveillance of community health. As discussed in Chapters 3 to 5, this includes setting priorities and developing action statements to guide the choice of interventions for a particular issue. Before deciding on a policy change intervention, the following questions need to be answered:

- How likely is it that policy change will solve the problem?
- Is there evidence that policy change has worked before in similar situations?
- Are there other solutions that might be more appropriate?

To provide answers to these questions, look for evidence that has already been compiled in systematic reviews and position papers. For example, suppose the problem is tobacco use by youth. The National Institute for Health and Clinical Excellence (2007) provides evidence-based recommendations to prevent the uptake of smoking by children and young people. The recommendations address enforcing policies to prevent illegal sales to minors. Another focus of policy interventions is the price of cigarettes. When prices go down, the cost of cigarettes become less of a deterrent to smoking. As a best practice, Healthy People 2020 recommends increasing the excise tax on tobacco products to promote tobacco use cessation and reduce the initiation of tobacco use among youth (Centers for Disease Control and Prevention, 2014). Other promising strategies include aggressive media campaigns, teen smoking-cessation programs, social environment changes, and community interventions, especially if the strategies are coordinated to take advantage of potential synergies across interventions. Other credible sources of information may be found on websites such as the Public Health Agency of Canada's Canadian Best Practices Portal. This site provides a searchable list of health promotion policy interventions to address tobacco control. (See the Tar Wars example in Box 6.7 and "Website Resources" for this chapter.)

It takes time and effort to sift through the weight of information on health issues and assemble evidence to justify policy initiatives. Familiarity with the literature helps, and health practitioners can make an important contribution in this area. Before starting any policy change effort, it is important to determine that policy change is a realistic option associated with proven success and that there are sufficient resources to carry it out.

## Develop Goals, Objectives, and Policy Options (Action Plan) for a Policy Change Intervention (Road Map Steps 3–6)

The planning phase is concerned with clarifying the goals and objectives of the policy intervention, and critically reviewing policy options to provide clear direction for policy change. Key elements are tailoring the policy to the local situation, building a climate of acceptance and support, and crafting the policy statement and implementation guide. The aim is a scientifically sound and politically and socially acceptable policy that is economically feasible and administratively and technologically possible (Public Health Ontario, 2012). The planning process requires broad input, as well as a range of talents and abilities and commitment. It is crucial to have adequate resources, people, and funds to complete the many facets of the operation, all proceeding at the same time. A large team or coalition is probably best suited to undertake this work.

Several interlocking pieces have to be eased into place to make policy happen, and herein lies the challenge. It is important to remember that policies are an expression of people's values and beliefs. This means that in addition to being grounded in empirical evidence and research, a policy should reflect accumulated wisdom and public opinion. Public input has been likened to the second arm of a nutcracker, enabling the community to influence decision makers and take control of the process (Labonte, 1997).

### Identify Decision Makers and Build Support for Policy

In a democratic society it is very difficult to fully implement policies unless communities are ready for them. The statistics on tobacco support this. Smoking has been clearly identified as a risk factor for many chronic diseases and has been the primary cause of premature death in Canada for many years. Recent estimates predict that male smokers live to an average age of 71 years, whereas normal life expectancy is 78 years; female smokers live to an average age of 73 years compared to the normal life expectancy for women of 83 years (Health Canada, 2014). Yet despite widespread legislation to restrict the use of tobacco by young people and ban smoking in public places, in 2010–2011 the prevalence of smoking in school children, grades 6–9, ranged from a high of 4.4 percent in Quebec and Saskatchewan to a low of 2 percent in British Columbia (Reid, Hammond, Rynard, & Burholter, 2014).

While smoking rates have gradually decreased over the past 20 years, there have been significant differences in the adoption of smoking legislation across jurisdictions. For example, all Canadian provinces and territories have introduced comprehensive legislation to discourage tobacco use. However, 37 Ontario cities have more restrictive municipal bylaws than the province on smoking in buffer zones such as doorways, air intakes, and transit shelters, whereas only two cities in Quebec do (Non-Smokers Rights Association, 2014). This illustrates that the political will to implement policy controls varies from place to place.

## Conduct a Force Field Analysis

Ensuring sufficient support to drive change is an important part of laying the ground-work for policy implementation. **Force field analysis**, developed by psychologist and change theorist Kurt Lewin, is a process used to identify the driving and restraining forces associated with policy change. It entails identifying the key stakeholders, that is, all those who may be affected by the problem and the way it is resolved, both positively and negatively, and determining whether or not they are likely to support the policy.

One way to do this is to ask whether the individual or group will stand to gain or lose if the problem is resolved in a certain way. This may not be easy to determine. Positions on an issue are not always stated explicitly, and it is easy to fall into the trap of thinking that people share identical views just because they agree on some points. Stakeholders may be motivated by different and sometimes conflicting reasons or allegiances, some of which may be concealed. Silence does not necessarily signify consent (Ewles & Simnett, 1999). The information you require can be gathered through informal discussions with key informants, or more systematically through focus groups, surveys, or public meetings. As discussed in Chapter 4, all assessment methods have their advantages and disadvantages in terms of how representative they are of public opinion and the time required to gather the information. As with any assessment, it is useful to consult dif-ferent and complementary sources. For example, published material, such as council minutes, will tell you how councillors vote on a particular topic, which may or may not match what they say in private conversation.

The next step in the analysis is to describe each of the driving and restraining forces as completely as possible to show all potential influences on the policy process. For example, the tobacco manufacturers have been a powerful lobby against the introduc-tion of smoking bylaws; however, health promoters have mounted equally aggressive campaigns to counteract this influence. Conducting a force field analysis exercise will help you to understand the issue from many different viewpoints—those of the experts, the opinion leaders, and various subpopulations—and to understand the strength of feelings. Based on this understanding, strategies can be devised to increase the positive forces, decrease the restraining or negative forces, and formulate creative solutions that are acceptable to a wide range of people.

## Build Support and Engage Decision Makers

Securing broad public support as well as the support of key decision makers is important. This can be accomplished by talking to people (either one-on-one or at public meetings), giving media interviews, and writing newspaper articles; all provide an opportunity to raise awareness, generate discussion, and create support for policy options. If there is little interest in an issue, it may be necessary to conduct a social marketing campaign to influence public opinion before policy change can be attempted.

Early on, it is necessary to find out which agencies or departments are responsible for policy related to your issue, identify the key decision makers, and learn about their process for setting policy. For example, if the aim is to influence school policy, then you need to know how school policy is formed. Does each school have a policy committee or is there a regional committee? How often does the committee meet? What is the process for placing an item on the agenda? Who chairs the committee and who are its members?

The decision makers, both political and bureaucratic, steer the policy through the

The last hour of the December meeting of the Baby-Friendly community coalition is devoted to a consultant-led force field analysis. This starts with a brainstorming exercise to identify key stakeholders in the region. Moving quickly round the circle, each participant contributes information that is recorded on a flip chart. In 10 minutes, they have a long list of stakeholders. The list includes mothers, families in their childbearing and child-rearing years, health professionals (nurses, lactation consultants, dietitians, physicians, obstetricians), formula manufacturers and sales representatives, hospital administrators, and hospital and community health boards. Rather than waste meeting time, the consultant will develop a plan for gathering information from stakeholder groups to inform their work.

Using the same process, the group comes up with a list of barriers and facilitators for policy change. Lillian appreciates the wisdom of employing an external consultant to keep the group on track. Once or twice participants try to edit the list by saying things like "There's no point in listing the contacts with formula manufacturers because they are immovable," and "Why write that down? I don't think it is relevant to our community." The latter comment is in response to a remark from the airport manager, who has joined the group on Lillian's invitation. He draws attention to an article in *The Wall Street Journal* (Molla, 2014) entitled "5 reasons American women won't breastfeed." The article suggests that the convenience of the feeding method is a key driving force. After the consultant has discouraged debate, the group agrees it is better to simply record all the perspectives and analyze them later. A preliminary list of the forces appears in Table 12.4.

All the members are asked to review the driving and restraining forces and rank them in order of importance by an agreed-upon date. This will set the stage for the next meeting when they develop a strategy for influencing the forces and building community support.

In drawing the meeting to a close, the committee chair thanks the group for their efforts: "We are learning just how many angles there are to the issue. It will be a challenge to sort out the different points of view. Thank goodness the WHO has provided clear guidelines and some resources, because they have set high standards."

The next day, Lillian thinks about what she has agreed to do before the next meeting. The coalition executive has decided it is time to confirm management support for the BFI across the city. At the coalition chair's suggestion, she has agreed to prepare two slides on the results of the breast-feeding policies survey for an introductory presentation to senior management in the various agencies. While pleased that her work is valued, Lillian feels a little nervous at the prospect. Luckily, the focus of the next meeting with her program manager is about working with business leaders in the workplace health project.

At her program manager's suggestion, Lillian has started to keep a reflective journal on her work. Looking at her notes from the last meeting, she realizes she has learned a lot from working with the consultant and other disciplines and sectors. She appreciates that there are many priorities to consider. Seeing Janet at the coalition meeting with her students helped her to realize how far she has come in the last year. The students were compiling an inventory for the coalition of public places in the city where women could breast-feed. They were keen to learn more about policy development and had many questions for Lillian. With some satisfaction, Lillian realizes she is looking forward to the time when she will orient a student group to a policy development project. Closing the journal, Lillian makes a mental note to look back at these entries six months from now.

**Discussion Topics and Questions**

6. Read *The Wall Street Journal* article mentioned above. Rank the driving and restraining forces for breast-feeding mentioned in the article and discuss how the forces might facilitate or be a barrier to health policy change.

7. Legislation on the registration of firearms has had mixed success in Canada and is strongly opposed in the United States. Locate newspaper articles presenting different aspects of the issue and identify the driving and restraining forces to policy development.

**Table 12.4: Baby Friendly Initiative—Force Field Analysis**

| Driving Forces—Facilitators | Restraining Forces—Barriers |
|---|---|
| In 2011/2012, 89 percent of Canadian mothers breast-fed their infants; 26 percent breast-fed exclusively for six months or more (Glonet, 2013) | – Ease of bottle feeding; provision of formula samples in hospital<br>– Decreased revenue for hospitals and community boards from contracts with formula manufacturers |
| Increased media coverage of health benefits of breast-feeding (e.g., protects infants from many infectious diseases and may protect against obesity) | |
| Increased demand for Baby-Friendly settings by women with higher education | – Cost of restructuring in-patient settings to accommodate rooming-in<br>– Decreased support from formula companies for health provider educational activities and client teaching tools |
| BFI success well documented in many countries<br><br>– Easy-to-follow instructions<br>– Training programs<br>– Strong evidence base | – Reduced hospital stay and cuts to community-based programs offering breast-feeding support<br>– Opposition from staff who resist changes to work assignments |
| Social norms: increased media coverage of nurturing mother | Opposition from community members who believe that choices around breast-feeding should be left to women |
| Extended maternity benefits enable women to stay at home for one year | Social circumstances that deter breast-feeding, e.g., women who are not eligible for maternity benefits or who have to return to work when the benefits run out; women in low-income jobs who lack facilities for breast-feeding |

political process, so they need to be onside. Clearly, it is important to gain their support and work closely with them. Besides, there is good reason to think that bureaucratic decision making is influenced by many factors other than systematic empirical evidence. Macintyre and colleagues (2001, p. 223) list several factors that may have equal weight in swaying opinion:

- Cogent argument
- The scale of likely health benefits
- Likelihood that the policy will bring benefits other than health benefits
- Fit with existing or proposed government policy
- Possibility that the policy might do harm
- Ease and cost of implementation

In addition to weighing these rational arguments, decision makers may be motivated by personal values, a sense of duty, or needs, such as the desire to gain public approval and social status (Public Health Ontario, 2012). Hence the importance of balancing persuasive evidence with community campaigns to sway public opinion and influence key decision makers.

There are several ways to approach decision makers. With elected officials, the usual way is by letter, telephone call, or a face-to-face meeting; however email and social media may be a possibility. No one method is necessarily any better than another, and elected representatives often have a preferred approach that works best for them. Networking through professional associations, interest groups, and less formal channels offers another approach to gain access to opinion leaders. For those who wish to pursue this further, there are several guides with practical advice on how to make the first contact effectively (e.g., Nagy, 2014; Public Health Ontario, 2013).

Regardless of the initial approach, the aim is to build relationships and create alliances with decision makers and opinion leaders. To do this, community health nurses need to draw on the power they have to influence others. Ewles and Simnett (1999) describe four **sources of power: position, resources, expertise**, and **personal qualities**. As the name implies, position power is conferred through one's place in the hierarchy of an organization; resource power stems from being able to allocate resources. Both of these power sources are available to those in senior levels of management. Expert power comes from specialized knowledge or expertise and is a potential source of power for community health nurses. Personal power comes from personal attributes or leadership qualities such as intelligence, initiative, self-confidence, and charisma. Since persuading, negotiating, and making deals are a fundamental part of the process, community health nurses need to understand the different sources of power at their command and develop the appropriate influencing skills.

### Budget for Adequate Time and Resources

Planning policy change takes time, adequate resources, and endurance to achieve the goal. There are many strands to the work, and like any project, it will benefit from careful planning and coordination. Effective time management is essential to meet deadlines. Having said that, it is also important to be flexible to take advantage of opportunities and respond quickly when there is a change of plan. Policy change can be a slow process with many roadblocks; once underway, it is important to maintain the momentum and keep the process moving.

### Construct a Draft Policy

Clear goals and objectives help to focus the policy document. They should state which particular aspect of the problem is to be addressed and the expected health outcomes. For example, the policy might start with the following statement: "This policy aims to reduce smoking among young girls by increasing the price of cigarettes." Specific, measurable objectives further define the content of the policy.

A policy is likely to go through several iterations before it is approved. The draft policy serves a number of purposes:

- The ideas, expressed in writing, are available for discussion and debate.
- The succinct statement of intent can be used to inform others and negotiate support.
- The draft document reduces later effort because it is easier to modify something that is already written than to construct a policy from scratch.

The approach to developing a policy is no different than designing any intervention. There should be evidence to show that the policy, when implemented, will bring about the desired changes. (You may find it helpful to refer to Chapters 5 and 6.)

It is at the draft stage that the proposed policy may undergo a health impact assessment (HIA). As discussed in earlier chapters, this is a structured process to help decision makers examine the population health and equity impacts of a policy. Many tools are available to guide the process, for example, identifying what should be assessed, who to involve, and providing a framework for assessment. The report of an HIA makes recommendations for improving the policy to mitigate negative impacts and strengthen positive impacts, and sets out a plan for monitoring and evaluating the policy. In many ways, HIA mirrors the policy development process itself. (See Canadian Nurses Association in "Website Resources" for this chapter.)

Health impact assessment provides an opportunity for broad community involvement in the policy process. Community health nurses can play a part in engaging community members so that policies are relevant to community needs. With policies originating in sectors other than health, community health providers may be called on to contribute their expertise in assessing the health and equity impact of the policies. Harris and colleagues (2012) acknowledge that the process is not without difficulty. Participants may not have sufficient expertise to properly assess impact and, in many cases, the evidence is just not available. Decision makers may have failed to evaluate the impact of previous health policy initiatives (Macintyre, 2003), and sensitive measures to evaluate the impact of policy change on key target groups may not be readily available (Davidoff, 2004). Another factor is that health policy, as with health promotion in general, may take years to achieve its impact on health determinants (Leon, Walt, & Gilson, 2001). Assembling the strongest evidence possible and a plausible argument for why one option is preferred over another offers a way forward.

## Formal Policy and Its Parts

Formal policy has several parts: the rationale or preamble, which explains why the policy is needed; definitions; the components, which explain how the policy is implemented; the communication strategy; and the plan for enforcement and monitoring (Public Health Ontario, 2012). A sample municipal alcohol policy is provided in the Appendix to Chapter 12. The parts of the policy are explained below.

### Rationale
The rationale is summarized in a succinct statement that explains the reason for the policy and what it is trying to achieve. Sometimes the reasons are contained in statements beginning with "Whereas...."

### Definitions
A definition of key terms using clear language helps to prevent ambiguity. For example, the following definition makes it clear that merely holding a lit cigarette qualifies as smoking: "Smoking includes carrying a lighted cigar, cigarette, pipe or any other lighted smoking instrument and smoke has a corresponding meaning." It is often necessary to

define the setting where a specific policy is in force. For example, in the smoking policy below, "Enclosed Public Place" requires definition.

### Components of the Policy

The components of the policy explain where, when, and how the policy will be implemented. For example, a smoking policy might give the following directions:

- No person shall smoke in any Enclosed Public Place within the city whether or not a No Smoking sign is posted.
- Every proprietor of an Enclosed Public Place shall post signs at every entrance to the Enclosed Public Place in accordance with Section 4.1 of this by law.

The municipal alcohol policy example in the Appendix to Chapter 12 is much more complex and requires careful reading because it has many components.

### Communication Strategy

The purpose of the communication strategy is to explain how the policy will be made known to those who are likely to be affected by it. An important consideration is that everyone touched by the policy understands what it is about, knows when it will come into effect, and can determine how it will affect daily life. It also flags where there is a need for advance preparation, such as training. For example, the sample municipal alcohol policy (see Appendix to Chapter 12) contains training implications. The policy dictates that bartenders, or alcohol servers, must undergo special training in order to meet their new responsibilities. When planning the implementation, sufficient time should be allowed to spread the key messages. This allows the necessary supports to be put in place so that the implementation will run smoothly.

Another aim of the communication strategy is to prepare the public and create acceptance of the policy before it is introduced so that most people will comply. Policy that is likely to affect the whole population, for instance, car seat belt legislation, is often introduced through a media campaign, with television and radio advertisements, talk show discussion, and informational websites. Public officials and managers will likely be responsible for policy implementation, including the preparatory work, but these aspects need to be considered at the planning stage. Community health nurses have a role to play in creating awareness of policy change, for example, by advising clients, participating in talk shows, and writing letters to the editor in support of the policy.

### Plan for Enforcement and Monitoring

This section of the policy states how it will be enforced and lays out the consequences of failure to comply. The penalties need to be sufficient to act as a deterrent but may start with a warning and escalate for repeated offenses. The municipal alcohol policy (see Appendix to Chapter 12) provides an example. The advantages of compliance can be used as an incentive. For example, by promoting moderate alcohol use and protecting patrons from intoxication, alcohol servers may avoid brawls and liability in case of an accident.

As with evaluation, the plan for monitoring should be in place before the policy comes into effect. Monitoring helps to identify situations where the policy is unclear or difficult to apply. It can also provide information on whether the policy is being applied as intended and applied consistently. Such feedback can be used to improve implementation and thereby help to attain the long-term goals. Keep in mind that no policy will be completely flawless, especially when it is being implemented for the first time.

## Implement the Action Plan (Road Map Step 7)

Community health nurses may or may not have a direct role to play in the implementation of policy, depending on where the responsibility for implementation lies and the nature of the policy. They may, however, play a valuable role in providing education to support policy change. For example, they may offer smoking cessation programs, provide telephone advice and resources to help smokers quit, organize support for car seat installation at well-baby clinics, and provide training on breast-feeding support. Another possible area of involvement is informal monitoring in places where nurses practice. In the case of smoking, this could be in community settings such as schools and day care facilities.

## Evaluate the Results (Road Map Step 8)

As discussed earlier, evaluation is a step in policy work that is often neglected. The question of ultimate importance is "Did the policy achieve the desired impact on health?" This is a difficult question to answer for many reasons. Baseline data before the policy change may be unavailable or nonexistent; it is difficult to distinguish the impact of policy change from the many other factors influencing health behavior; and there is often a time lag between innovation and change in health status. As a result, evaluation often looks for clues that policy change is moving in the right direction: Was the policy implemented as planned? How well is the policy being accepted? Are there measurable effects on attitudes, if not behavior? Are there beneficial effects that were not anticipated?

It is also useful to reflect on the process of policy development: Did it go as planned? What tips can be shared with others starting on a similar journey? What lessons were learned about the issue? About the policy change process? This learning from process evaluation can guide future policy initiatives or be applied in other situations. The Policy Implementation Checklist, in the Appendix to Chapter 12, provides a tool for evaluating the policy change process (The Health Communication Unit, 2004).

## Summary

Healthy public policy is an important strategy for influencing the health of populations. Although the process takes considerable time and resources, the impact of healthy public policy is long term. Health policies are used to create supportive environments that increase access for all to the social determinants of health and enable healthy choices. Community health nurses may contribute to the development of healthy public policy in many ways: by collaborating with community members to identify issues that lend themselves to a policy solution, providing evidence that policy change is effective, participating in the policy development process, and monitoring the impact of policy change.

The scenarios in this chapter illustrate the application of concepts and principles of policy development to support breast-feeding in the workplace and Baby-Friendly communities. Understanding the practicalities of developing healthy public policy and acquiring the skills to support the policy development process are essential learning for community health nurses.

## Classroom and Seminar Exercises

1. Accidents and injuries are major contributors to present-day mortality and morbidity in youth. Identify key stakeholders in developing policies around water safety in a waterfront community, and describe possible driving and restraining forces.
2. Increased rates of smoking among girls and women are described as a national priority, and policies around tobacco prices have shown promise (CDC, 2014). Discuss how you might influence the driving and restraining forces for such policies in Aboriginal/Native American communities.
3. Legislation on the registration of firearms has had mixed success in Canada and is strongly opposed in the United States. Locate newspaper articles presenting different aspects of the issue and suggest how the approach to policy development might be influenced.
4. Assess the support in your community for a municipal alcohol policy, as shown in the Appendix to Chapter 12.
5. Develop a model organizational policy pertaining to employee safety in a neighborhood with high crime rates for (a) a new health clinic, or (b) community health agencies visiting clients in the home.

## References

British Columbia Ministry of Health. (2012). *Review of breastfeeding practices and programs: British Columbia and pan-Canadian jurisdictional scan*. Retrieved from www.health.gov. bc.ca/library/publications/year/2012/breastfeeding-jurisdictional-scan.pdf

Brownson, R. C., Newschaffer, C. J., & Ali-Abarghoui, F. (1997). Policy research for disease prevention: Challenges and practical recommendations. *American Journal of Public Health, 87*(5), 735–739.

Canadian Association of Schools of Nursing. (2014, May). *Entry-to-practice public health nursing competencies for undergraduate nursing education*. Retrieved from www.casn.ca/en/123/item/6

Canadian Health Services Research Foundation. (2012). *Better health: An analysis of public policy and programming focusing on the determinants of health and health outcomes that are effective in achieving the healthiest populations*. Retrieved from www.cfhi-fcass.ca/sf-docs/default-source/commissioned-research-reports/Muntaner-BetterCare-EN.pdf?sfvrsn=0

Canadian Nurses Association. (2000). Nursing is a political act—the bigger picture. *Nursing Now: Issues and Trends in Canadian Nursing, 8*, 1–5.

Centers for Disease Control and Prevention (CDC). (2014). *Best practices for comprehensive tobacco control programs—2014, appendix B: Program and policy recommendations for comprehensive tobacco control programs*. Retrieved from www.cdc.gov/tobacco/stateandcommunity/best_practices/pdfs/2014/comprehensive.pdf

Chambers, L. W., Underwood, J., Halbert, T., Woodward, C. A., Heale, J., & Isaacs, S. (1994). 1992 Ontario survey of public health nurses: Perceptions of roles and activities. *Canadian Journal of Public Health, 85*(3), 175–179.

Commission on Social Determinants of Health. (2008). *Closing the gap in a generation: Health equity through action on the social determinants of health*. Final Report of the Commission on Social Determinants of Health. Geneva: World Health Organization. Retrieved from http://whqlibdoc.who.int/publications/2008/9789241563703_eng.pdf

Davidoff, A. (2004). Identifying children with special health care needs in the National Health Interview Survey: A new resource for policy analysis. *Health Services Research, 39*(1), 53–71.

Ewles, L., & Simnett, I. (1999). *Promoting health: A practical guide* (4th ed.). Edinburgh: Baillière Tindall.

Flynn, B. C. (2000). Health policy for healthy cities and communities. In E. T. Anderson & J. McFarlane (Eds.), *Community as partner: Theory and practice in nursing* (3rd ed., pp. 137–149). Philadelphia, PA: Lippincott Williams & Wilkins.

Glonet, L. (2013) *Breastfeeding trends in Canada* (Catalogue no. 82-624-X). Ottawa, ON: Statistics Canada. Retrieved from www.statcan.gc.ca/pub/82-624-x/2013001/article/11879-eng.htm

Harris, P. J., Kemp, L. A., & Sainsbury, P. (2012). The essential elements of health impact assessment and healthy public policy: A qualitative study of practitioner perspectives. *British Medical Journal Open, 2*(e001245). doi:10.1136/bmjopen-2012-001245

Health Canada. (2014). *Smoking and mortality*. Retrieved from www.hc-sc.gc.ca/hc-ps/tobac-tabac/legislation/label-etiquette/mortal-eng.php

Jackson, S. F., Perkins, F., Khandor, E., Cordwell, L., Hamann, S., & Busai, S. (2006). Integrated health promotion strategies: A contribution to tackling current and future health challenges. *Health Promotion International, 21*(Suppl. 1), 75–83.

Kang, R. (1995). Building community capacity for health promotion: A challenge for public health nurses. *Public Health Nursing, 12*(5), 312–318.

Labonte, R. (1997). Community, community development and the forming of authentic partnerships: Some critical reflections. In M. Minkler (Ed.), *Community organizing and community building for health* (pp. 88–102). New Brunswick, NJ: Rutgers University Press.

Leon, D. A., Walt, G., & Gilson, L. (2001). International perspectives on health inequalities and policy. *British Medical Journal, 322*, 591–594.

Macintyre, S. (2003). Evidence based policy making. *British Medical Journal, 326*, 5–6.

Macintyre, S., Chalmers, I., Horton, R., & Smith, R. (2001). Using evidence to inform health policy: Case study. *British Medical Journal, 322*, 222–225.

McKeown, T. (1979). *The role of medicine: Dream, mirage, or nemesis*. Princeton, NJ: Princeton University Press.

Milio, N. (1989). Making healthy public policy; developing the science by learning the art: An ecological framework for policy studies. In B. Badura & I. Kickbusch (Eds.), *Health promotion research: Towards a new social epidemiology* (pp. 7–27). Copenhagen: World Health Organization Regional Office for Europe.

Minkler, M. (1999). Personal responsibility for health? A review of the arguments and the evidence at century's end. *Health Education Quarterly, 26*(1), 121–140.

Molla, R. (2014, April 14). 5 reasons American women won't breastfeed. *The Wall Street Journal*. Retrieved from http://blogs.wsj.com/briefly/2014/04/14/5

Morrison, V., Gagnon, F., Morestin, F., & Keeling, M. (2014). *Keywords in healthy public policy.* Montreal, QC: National Collaborating Centre for Healthy Public Policy. Retrieved from www.ncchpp.ca/41/What_s_New_.ccnpps?id_article=1206

Multicultural Advocates for Social Change on Tobacco. (2004). *Smoking prevention and control strategies for youth.* Retrieved from www.mascotcoalition.org/education/youth_smoking.html

Nagy, J. (2014). Writing letters to elected officials. *Community Tool Box* (Chapter 33, Section 1). Retrieved from http://ctb.ku.edu/en/table-of-contents/advocacy/direct-action/letters-to-elected-officials/main

National Institute for Health and Clinical Excellence (NICE). (2007). *Preventing the uptake of smoking by children and young people* (NICE guidelines PH14). Retrieved from www.nice.org.uk/guidance/ph14

Non-Smokers Rights Association (NSRA). (2014). *Compendium of 100% smoke-free municipal bylaws* (Spring 2012 update). Retrieved from www.nsra-adnf.ca/cms/file/files/Summary_table_Spring_2012.pdf

Ontario Agency for Health Protection and Promotion (Public Health Ontario). (2012). *Developing health promotion policies.* V3.18 [Internet]. Toronto, ON: Queen's Printer for Ontario. Cited 2014 Dec 22, Available from www.publichealthontario.ca/en/eRepository/Developing_health_promotion_policies_2012.pdf

Ontario Public Health Association (OPHA). (1996). *Making a difference in your community: A guide for policy change* (2nd ed.). Toronto: OPHA. Retrieved from http://opha.on.ca/OPHA/media/Resources/Resource%20Documents/Making_a_Difference-PolicyChange.pdf?ext=.pdf

Public Health Nursing Section. (2001). *Public health interventions: Applications for public health nursing practice.* St. Paul, MN: Minnesota Department of Health.

Public Health Ontario. (2012). *Developing health promotion policies.* Retrieved from www.publichealthontario.ca

Public Health Ontario. (2013). *At a glance: The eight steps to developing a healthy public policy* (Version 4). Retrieved from www.publichealthontario.ca

Quad Council of Public Health Nursing Organizations. (2011). *Quad Council competencies for public health nurses.* Retrieved from www.phf.org/resourcestools/Pages/Public_Health_Nursing_Competencies.aspx.

Reid, J. L., Hammond, D., Rynard, V. L., & Burholter, R. (2014). *Tobacco use in Canada: Patterns and trends.* Policy Supplement. Waterloo, ON: Propel Centre for Population Health Impact, University of Waterloo. Retrieved from www.tobaccoreport.ca/2014/index.cfm

Sallis, J. F., Owen, N., & Fisher, E. B. (2008). Ecological models of health behavior. In K. Glanz, B. K. Rimer, & Viswanath, K. (Eds.), *Health behavior and health education: Theory, research, and practice* (4th ed., pp. 465–485). San Francisco, CA: Jossey-Bass.

Schmid, T. L., Pratt, M., & Howze, E. (1995). Policy as intervention: Environmental and policy approaches to the prevention of cardiovascular disease. *American Journal of Public Health, 85*(9), 1207–1211.

Schoenfeld, B. M., & MacDonald, M. B. (2002). Saskatchewan public health nursing survey: Perceptions of roles and activities. *Canadian Journal of Public Health, 93*(6), 452–456.

Stokols, D. (1996). Translating social ecological theory into guidelines for community health promotion. *American Journal of Health Promotion, 10*(4), 282–298.

The Health Communication Unit (THCU) at the Centre for Health Promotion University of Toronto. (2004). Developing health promotion policies. Version 1. Toronto ON: THCU.

United States Breastfeeding Committee. (2013). *Healthy People 2020: Breastfeeding objectives.* Retrieved from www.usbreastfeeding.org/LegislationPolicy/FederalPoliciesInitiatives/HealthyPeople2020BreastfeedingObjectives/tabid/120/Default.aspx

Wallack, L. (1998). Media advocacy: A strategy for empowering people and communities. In M. Minkler (Ed.), *Community organizing and community building for health* (pp. 339–352). New Brunswick, NJ: Rutgers University Press.

World Health Organization. (1998). *Evidence for the ten steps to successful breastfeeding.* Retrieved from www.who.int/child-adolescent-health/publications/NUTRITION/WHO_CHD_98.9.htm

World Health Organization (WHO). (2010). *Adelaide Statement on Health in All Policies.* Adelaide: Government of South Australia. Retrieved from www.who.int/social_determinants/hiap_statement_who_sa_final.pdf

## Website Resources

### Policy Resources

National Collaborating Centre for Healthy Public Policy: www.ncchpp.ca/en/
   This website for the Quebec collaborating center for public health (one of six in Canada) promotes the use of scientific research and other knowledge to strengthen public health practice. The site provides a graphic link to its projects on the home page, each of which leads to resources.

Canadian Nurses Association: https://nurseone.ca/en
   This site provides links to sample health impact assessments (HIA). First, select "Tools." Under the "Tools" sidebar, select "Health in All Policies Toolkit." Click on "Assessment Tools/Health Impact Assessment."

KU Work Group for Community Health and Development, *Community Tool Box: Changing Policies*: http://ctb.ku.edu/en/table-of-contents/implement/changing-policies
   This entry page to Chapter 25, "Changing Policies," provides direct links to Tool Box resources on influencing policy development.

### Topic-Specific Policy

National and international sites, such as WHO, CDC, and PHAC (see "Website Resources" for Chapter 3), provide links to policy implication under specific health topics. The Baby-Friendly Initiative below provides an example.

World Health Organization (WHO), *Baby-Friendly Hospital Initiative*: www.who.int/nutrition/topics/bfhi/en/
   This site describes the success of the initiative and planned expansion to communities and other settings, and provides a link to a comprehensive resource package. See "Website Resources" for Chapter 3 for links to national sites where information on breast-feeding (or nutrition) can be found under "Health Topics."

# Appendix to Chapter 12

## Example of a Municipal Alcohol Policy

**Municipal Alcohol Policy**

*Rationale (Why the policy is needed)*

It is the intention of the Municipality of Summerland to provide for the safe and responsible use of alcohol in municipally owned properties, to minimize the legal responsibility for users as well as the Municipality's broad legal liability, and to foster awareness of the responsibilities of the Special Occasion Permits to the Users so that they in turn may encourage the responsible consumption of alcohol.

*Components (Explains how the policy is implemented)*

A special permit is required for special occasion events where alcohol will be sold. Events can be held only in designated locations.

Responsibility for the event is assigned to a designated person or "event User." The Liquor Licence Act of Ontario clearly states that the event User has a "duty of control," that is, to protect participants from foreseeable harm to themselves and others. The Act also states that the server of alcohol is responsible for intoxicated individuals until they regain sobriety, not only until they arrive home safely. Be aware that you and your group can be held liable for injuries and damages arising from failure to adhere to the Liquor Licence Act of (Province/Territory/State). Infractions to the Act include:

- serving someone to intoxication
- serving someone who is already intoxicated
- serving minors
- failing to prevent impaired individuals from driving

The User must provide proof of insurance (at least 1 million dollars) for alcohol-related events (e.g., carnival, rock concert, or any event with attendance over 500 people) and indemnify the municipality.

Minors are prohibited from attending unless accompanied by a responsible adult; it is forbidden to serve alcohol to those who do attend.

The User must follow sensible alcohol marketing practices (no oversized drinks, double shots of spirits, drinking contests, volume discounts, and unlimited free alcohol, which encourage increased immoderate consumption).

An appropriate number of properly educated servers should be present. Bar, floor, and door supervisors must be 19 years of age or over; numbers based on estimated attendance on permit. They must be certified by a recognized alcohol server training course such as Smart Serve (a 4-hour training course that provides the event workers with information and techniques on how to prevent alcohol-related problems from occurring and how to intervene when they do occur). Monthly training sessions are held at City Hall. [Contact person named]. A Smart Serve Resource Bank has been created for persons wishing to hire the services of certified Smart Serve event workers. A list is available at the Parks and Recreation Department.

**Enforcement** (*The penalties for failing to comply with the policy*)

If Users fail to adhere to the policy guidelines and controls, the following enforcement procedures will be taken:

First infraction:
The User will be sent a Registered letter outlining the consequences of further infractions.

Second infraction:
The User will be sent a Registered letter stating that they will lose all scheduled privileges for a three (3) month period including all monies related to their rental and are suspended from all functions at any municipal property for the same period of time.

Third infraction:
The User will be sent a Registered letter stating that they will lose all rental privileges for one (1) year and are suspended from all functions at any municipal property for the same length of time. Prior to the end of the suspension period, the User must meet personally with a municipal representative to discuss how they will ensure that all rules will be followed in the future so that similar incidents do not occur.

The municipality will report any infraction of this policy to legal authorities, including the Liquor License Board, whenever it believes such action is required.

**Policy Monitoring and Revision**

Municipal staff will monitor the events where alcohol is served in municipal facilities.

Minor variations to the policy can be approved, on an event-by-event basis, by the Commissioner having jurisdiction over the facility/location, for events requiring exception to the policy.

The Municipal Alcohol Policy will be reviewed annually and updated to reflect any subsequent legislative changes.

**Guidelines and Controls**

The User must

- acknowledge intent to observe and comply with the controls of the policy, specified below, by initialing the facility permit or rental agreement.
- obtain and display the necessary permit, provide evidence that event workers are properly trained, and purchase liability insurance.
- be present at the event, support staff, refrain from using alcohol, and be in charge of decision making.
- employ appropriate numbers of trained staff, advise them of their legal responsibilities, ensure they are present at all times, and refrain from alcohol; ensure adequate security staff.
- observe that alcohol is sold under safe conditions and consumed on premises.
- restrict sale of alcohol to reasonable amounts—4 tickets at a time, not to underage youth, and check identification (unmask if participating in masquerade events).
- provide non-alcohol drinks and low-alcohol beverages at lower cost than alcohol.
- serve sufficient, appropriate food; avoid salty snacks.
- take steps to discourage excessive drinking; e.g., if tickets are used, allow them to be cashed at any time; do not flag closing time to avoid stocking up; stop on time, clear up, and remove liquor from premises swiftly.
- provide a safe physical setting, monitor exits, safe transportation options. Take immediate action to prevent the outbreak of disturbances.

**Policy Implementation Checklist**

1. Have you identified and analyzed the issues your policy needs to address?
2. Do you have sufficient information about these issues to support and justify the implementation of your policy?
3. Are your policy goals reasonable, and your policy objectives measurable?
4. Do you have the required support and approval of key decision makers? If not, how will this be obtained?
5. Have you selected your policy components and prepared a written policy that describes these components and a strategy for implementation?
6. Do you have an accurate estimate of the resources (time, money, person power, and expertise) needed to implement and monitor your policy?
7. Is the timeline for implementation realistic?
8. Does your policy specify who is responsible for doing what?
9. Have you identified the barriers to implementation you are likely to encounter?
10. Do you have a plan for dealing with these barriers?
11. Have you shared your draft policy with other key stakeholders who will be responsible for implementation?
12. Is this the appropriate time to start implementing your policy? (THCU, 2004, p. 63)

Chapter 13

# Evaluating Community Health Programs

I n previous chapters we discussed how the community health nursing process is applied systematically to assess, plan, implement, and evaluate short-term health projects in the community. Such projects provide an opportunity for students and new practitioners to apply the principles of primary health care, perfect problem-solving skills, and hone communication techniques while addressing a community health issue of significance. It is also important, however, to view the projects in perspective: each project is conducted over a relatively short period of time in the life of a community and is embedded in a complex web of community health programs and services. It is important to understand and appreciate how such projects fit with, and contribute to, community health. Program evaluation is key to that understanding. The evaluation of program effectiveness is a critical skill for community health nurses.

The significant health issue chosen to illustrate the application of the concepts and principles of program evaluation is the risk of infection in two population groups: foreign-born students attending English-as-a-Second-Language classes, at risk for tuberculosis (TB); and older adults at risk for influenza. The scenarios illustrate how community health nurses evaluate the impact of the programs they deliver in order to modify programs to the health needs of the population.

## Learning Objectives

After reading this chapter and answering the questions throughout the chapter, you should be able to:

1. Adapt the concepts and principles of the community health nursing process for an evaluation project.
2. Discuss the importance of community involvement in program evaluation.
3. Discuss the program logic model used to guide program evaluation.
4. Create a program logic model to describe a community program.
5. Develop an observation checklist for the purpose of evaluation.
6. Document and communicate observations.

### Key Terms and Concepts

cold chain • directly observed therapy, short course (DOTS) • drug-resistant TB • evaluability assessment • program • program evaluation • program logic model • service delivery outcomes

A poster catches Mai's eye as she enters the public health department building: "Get your flu shot now." Mai exchanges a smile with her fellow student, Fadma. On their way to the first meeting with the project team, they have been chatting about the scramble it has been to complete their immunizations to obtain proof of their up-to-date immunization status before the start of the clinical course.

The program manager welcomes them to the team meeting and makes introductions. Millie, a public health nurse and the team leader, asks, "Why did you choose to join the communicable disease team?" Laughing, she adds, "Most students think that communicable disease is boring." Fadma explains that she volunteers at a community health center, well attended by women from the Somali community, and she finds it surprising that many of the women are fearful of immunization. She gives two examples. One day she overheard women at the food bank agreeing that it was better for children to catch measles and develop natural immunity. Another day she heard a woman angrily say that she did not need TB testing because she came from a region where there was none and her family had always been healthy. This has made Fadma realize that she needs to better understand how to talk to people about immunization and communicable disease control.

Mai says she wants to learn how to organize a mass immunization campaign and that she is also attracted by the opportunity to learn more about program evaluation, which she understands will be a major focus of the assignment.

At this first meeting, the students learn that planning for influenza (flu) usually starts in June so the annual campaign will be ready to launch at the end of September. "Just in time for the flu season," says Millie. She provides them with a pack of material on the influenza program, including a program logic model, and suggests they read this through to become familiar with the program.

Moving on to the student project, Millie explains that the health unit promotes a community-wide influenza campaign each year to ensure that residents who need it have access to free vaccination. Several organizations take part, including community health centers, resource centers, home health organizations, pharmacies, and multicultural associations. After explaining how the campaign is organized, she zeroes in on their project. Last year, the community health centers (CHCs) were dissatisfied with the low uptake of immunization over previous years. Although they had increased the number of clinics, they did not reach as many older adults as expected. The turnout at sessions held in conjunction with programs for older adults was particularly disappointing. This year, the team wants to conduct a stronger evaluation of the flu clinics, with the help of the students, to understand what factors influence attendance.

**Discussion Topics and Questions**

1. Discuss whether the basis for an evaluation should be the "program as delivered" or the "program as planned."
2. Discuss the advantages and disadvantages of community involvement in program evaluation.

For suggested responses, please see the Answer Key at the back of the book.

## Program Evaluation

A project that deals only with evaluation may make you feel that you can skip earlier steps in the community health nursing process. That is not the case. Some adaptations are necessary; however, your team will still progress through all the steps of the process to ensure that the evaluation is appropriate to the situation. Table 13.1 shows how the process is adapted for an evaluation project.

**Table 13.1: Adaptation of Community Health Nursing Project for Program Evaluation**

| Steps of Community Health Nursing Project | Adaptation for Evaluation of a Community Program |
|---|---|
| Orient to project | Review mandate, policy, and procedures of agency and particular program. Orient to issue and population and community. |
| Assess secondary data | Review program needs assessment, including sociodemographic data, epidemiology and evidence base, and program plan. |
| Assess primary data | Interview key informants—program providers, partners, and recipients. Determine availability of similar or related programs and services. Observe program delivery at two or more sites. |
| Analyze assessment data | Review program description and program logic model to identify program goals and activities. |
| Plan | Plan the evaluation:<br>– describe the program as it is being delivered<br>– clarify the purpose of the evaluation and define the questions to be answered<br>– develop the evaluation plan<br>– develop evaluation measures or tools |
| Act | Conduct pilot of evaluation measures.<br>Carry out the evaluation. |
| Evaluate | Determine results/impact and provide report in format useful to agency. Reflect on teamwork. |

## Community Health Programs and Program Evaluation

A **program** is an organized public health action (Centers for Disease Control and Prevention, Program Performance and Evaluation Office, 2012) consisting of closely related activities intended to achieve specific outcomes or results with specific individuals, groups, or communities (Porteous, Sheldrick, & Stewart, 1997). The questions that follow provide a framework for understanding the dimensions of a specific program.

1. What is the goal of the program? (What specific outcomes or results are expected?)
2. What population group does the program address?
3. What resources (e.g., people, money) are required to deliver the program?
4. What activities are carried out to achieve the program goal?

An example is provided by state, provincial, and territorial health department programs that seek to control and manage infectious diseases. The overarching goal of these broad programs is to reduce or eliminate specific infectious diseases, such as TB and certain vaccine-preventable diseases, within a given population and to prevent epidemics. Typically, they provide guidelines for the management of reportable and communicable diseases, and explain the emergency response structures required to manage outbreaks. Other goals are the prevention of food- and water-borne disease and infection control in public institutions, day care centers, and personal service settings. At the local level, public health departments are responsible for the infectious disease control budget and employ program staff to perform activities that include surveillance, case finding, contact tracing, immunization, infection control, and risk assessment. Together, these programs assure effective control of infectious diseases in a region (see "Website Resources" for links to regional, national, and international infection control sites and infection control program standards and protocols).

Even though the infrastructure for infectious disease control has been in place for a long time in developed countries and the programs usually run smoothly, they must constantly adapt to changing conditions. For instance, new and improved vaccines entail changes in immunization schedules, and internationally orchestrated strategies to eliminate common diseases such as polio and measles periodically demand a shift in resources. The situation is further complicated with outbreaks of disease such as Ebola, H1N1, or Severe Acute Respiratory Syndrome (SARS), which can encircle the globe with breathtaking rapidity through international travel. As a result, the control of infectious disease is under continuous scrutiny, and program managers and community boards must routinely evaluate local programs to make sure they are effective and synchronous with national and international standards.

The changing patterns of an infectious disease such as tuberculosis present an ongoing challenge. Although TB rates are declining in North America, there is a significant burden of disease concentrated in foreign-born individuals and certain racial and ethnic groups. Furthermore, high levels of poverty, poor nutrition, and lack of adequate housing are creating vulnerable populations with low levels of protection against infection in some parts of Canada (MacDonald, Hébert, & Stanbrook, 2011) and the US (Alami et al., 2014). For example, TB is more prevalent in Aboriginals in Canada than in the general population. Another troubling issue is that drug-resistant strains of TB are becoming a serious threat. A person is said to have **drug-resistant TB** if the strain of *Mycobacterium tuberculosis* causing the disease is resistant to one or more of the four first-line drugs (Public Health Agency of Canada, 2012). Drug resistance occurs when people do not complete the full course of treatment; when health care providers prescribe the wrong drug, dose, or length of treatment; when supply is not available; or when the drugs are of poor quality (Centers for Disease Control and Prevention [CDC], 2014a; Chang, Wheeler, & Farrell, 2002; Uppaluri et al., 2002). As might be expected, the burden of drug-resistant TB is concentrated more and more in countries with a high incidence of TB and low resources (Ormerod, 2005).

Many national tuberculosis programs are based on the **DOTS** (directly observed therapy, short course) strategy. DOTS is central to the "Stop TB Strategy," the goal of which is "to dramatically reduce the global burden of TB by 2015 in line with the Millennium Development Goals" (WHO, 2014, p. 18). The DOTS strategy has five elements: (1) political commitment with increased and sustained financing; (2) case detection through quality-assured bacteriology; (3) standardized treatment, with supervision and patient support; (4) an effective drug supply and management system, and monitoring and evaluation system; and (5) impact measurement. The third element—standardized treatment—is elaborated on in the description of an innovative TB prevention program below.

# Program Logic Model for a TB Prevention Program

A **program logic model** synthesizes program elements into a picture of how a program is supposed to work (Milstein, Wetterhall, & CDC Evaluation Working Group, 2014). Applicable to almost any program, a logic model provides a visual representation of program activities, in a flow chart or table, and links them to the stated program goals. The main value of the program logic model, as the name implies, is that it illuminates the underlying logic or causal reasoning that connects program activities to the expected results. Box 13.1 describes an innovative TB prevention program offered in conjunction with English-as-a-Second-Language (ESL) classes for new immigrants (Moyer, Verhovsek, & Wilson, 1997). The program is first described and then used to illustrate a program logic model.

---

BOX 13.1
**Example TB Prevention Program**

A public health nurse administers the tuberculin skin test to participating students attending English-as-a-Second-Language (ESL) classes. After 48 to 72 hours have passed, the nurse returns to assess the results and provide counseling. If the results are positive, the nurse refers the student to a community health clinic for treatment, traces and screens contacts, and provides case management until treatment is completed. In order to be available to as many students as possible, the program is offered at a variety of times and places throughout the week in ESL classrooms across the region.

The public health nurse undertakes a range of activities to increase awareness, knowledge, and referrals to the program, such as the following:
- Placing advertisements in grocery stores, shopping centers, pharmacies, and so forth
- Writing articles for community newspapers
- Sending letters to physicians to let them know about the program

In order to create support for treatment, the public health nurse works with the ESL teachers, school boards, and immigrant organizations to make available educational materials on TB prevention and control and healthy lifestyles, information on community resources, and to develop strategies to help students build informal support networks with other students and community groups.

These activities are expected to
- increase students' knowledge of the risk of TB and the benefits of treatment.
- increase knowledge of community resources.
- increase links with other students undergoing treatment.

As a result, the program is expected to increase the number of students who present themselves for TB testing and complete the screening process. In turn, this should increase the number of persons with active TB who are accurately identified; who initiate and complete treatment; and whose contacts are traced, screened, and, if necessary, treated. Ultimately, the program will decrease the number of persons with active TB and increase the number of persons who have successfully completed treatment for TB. Not least, the program will help to build the capacity of the community to provide a supportive environment for its immigrant population.

## Elements of Program Logic Model

The program logic model has three main elements: (1) program activities, (2) short-term outcomes, and (3) long-term outcomes. As discussed in Chapter 6, the program activities are expected to bring about the short-term and long-term outcomes. The next section explains the program elements and discusses how they are assembled into a program and depicted in a program logic model. The example of the TB prevention program in Box 13.1 is used to illustrate the elements. To make it easier to follow, the elements are discussed in reverse order: long-term outcomes, short-term outcomes, and program activities.

### Long-Term and Short-Term Outcomes

The outcomes describe what the program is trying to accomplish. The long-term outcomes of a program are the final endpoint of what the program was designed to achieve. In health promotion programs, this might be an improvement in health status, or an increase in community capacity, and so on. The short-term or more immediate outcomes, such as changes in knowledge, skills, attitudes, and intentions, act as stepping stones to the long-term outcome of improved health (see the discussion on objectives in Chapter 6). For example, intending to register for a smoking-cessation program is a precursor to registering, which is a precursor to learning techniques to help stop smoking, which is a precursor to smoking cessation. When the causative relationship is confirmed by research, then it is reasonable to believe that a short-term outcome will lead to the long-term outcome, and this assumption is often made (Israel et al., 1995). Thanks to years of research, there are well-established links between smoking and lung cancer. Therefore, it is assumed that successful smoking-cessation programs will contribute to lower rates of lung cancer, though it would probably be more accurate to say that they reduce the risk that the disease will develop.

In the TB prevention program described earlier, the identification of TB in ESL students (a potentially high-risk group) represents a short-term or immediate outcome of screening activities. The long-term outcome of reduced incidence of TB is dependent on many interrelated factors, including the prescription of the right medication and the completion of a full course of treatment, both of which can be more or less successful. From these examples, it can be seen that "long-term" and "short-term" represent points on a continuum rather than a defined period of time.

### Program Activities

The program activities are informed by health promotion strategies (health education and creation of supportive environments) with case management. These activities are chosen based on evidence that they will produce the desired outcomes with the population of interest. As with the process of linking interventions and outcomes discussed in Chapter 6, this involves tailoring the intervention to community needs and resources.

To continue with the previous example, it is well known that new immigrants encounter many barriers to TB diagnosis and treatment. For example, fear that the discovery of disease will result in deportation, or lack of medical insurance to cover immediate health care costs, may deter new immigrants from seeking treatment (Uppaluri et al., 2002). A case management approach using directly observed therapy (DOT) has been successful in ensuring that persons with active tuberculosis complete the full course of

**Figure 13.1: Program Logic Model of TB Prevention Program**

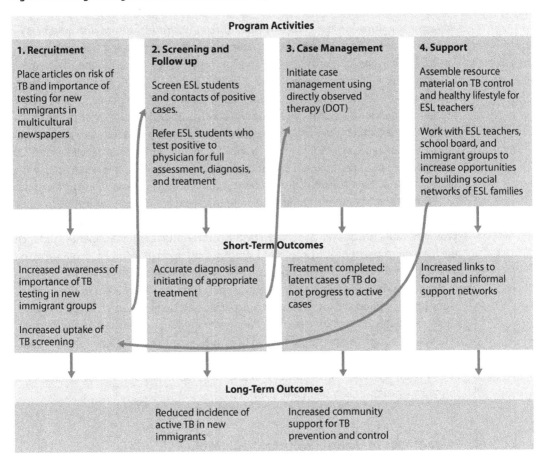

anti-tuberculosis drugs required to bring the disease under control. With DOT, health and community workers and trained volunteers observe and record that patients have swallowed the drugs over the duration of the treatment (for a fuller description of DOT, see British Columbia Centre for Disease Control, 2011).

The currently recommended course of treatment for drug-susceptible TB is a six-month regimen of four first-line drugs: isoniazad, rifampicin, ethambutol, and pyrazinamide (Tiemersma, van der Werf, Borgdorff, Williams, & Nagelkerke, 2011). Incomplete treatment brings the risk of secondary drug resistance. Close contacts of a person with active TB are at high risk for developing the disease. Therefore, it is important to trace and assess contacts and, if necessary, provide prophylactic treatment to prevent the progression of latent TB to active TB. The two steps together contribute to the ultimate program goal of decreased incidence of TB.

These program elements—activities, short-term outcomes, and long-term outcomes—and the links between them are summarized graphically in the program logic model shown in Figure 13.1.

## Service Delivery Outcomes

Program activities can be further defined in the logic model to provide measures of service delivery. The **service delivery outcomes** specify the types and frequency of service to be delivered for each activity. In other words, they prescribe the "dose" to be administered. For example, one of the activities described in the TB program plan is that program staff will submit articles to community newspapers for different ethnic groups on the importance of TB testing and control. A service delivery outcome might be: "submission of a 1000-word article to three local English-language newspapers and one foreign-language newspaper read by specified community groups, each month." Of course there are many practical considerations to take into account when setting the targets, such as the readership, distribution, and daily/weekly status of the newspapers.

Ideally, the program logic model is developed as part of program planning to guide program delivery. As described in Chapter 6, the program goals are defined—what the program wants to achieve, as indicated by the community needs assessment—and then the most appropriate health promotion strategies are selected to inform program activities to meet short- and long-term goals. Macaskill and colleagues (2000) use the term **evaluability assessment** to describe extensive stakeholder collaboration in the development phase to increase the success of a program and determine that it can be evaluated in a reliable and credible fashion. Poor program design is one reason for program evaluation failures. When the program logic model is constructed after implementation, evaluators have to consult program documentation, such as program proposals, annual reports, and operating data, and talk to knowledgeable program staff to gain insight into how a program is actually being offered.

## Advantages of Using a Program Logic Model

Program logic models take time to complete but are worth the effort because of the advantages described below.

- Drawing the model requires that you show the connections between program elements. This clarifies the program logic and identifies which program activities are crucial for attaining the long-term goals.
- The model can help to identify duplication of activities or weak links before the program is implemented.
- The model promotes a common understanding among program staff and can be used to describe the program to stakeholders, thereby facilitating involvement.
- The definition of activities assists the program manager to calculate the resources that will be required at different stages of the program.
- When the logic model is constructed during program planning, it helps to ensure that the program is evaluable and that evaluation is a focus up front. The program outputs and outcome indicators are explicit from the outset, which makes it easier to set up systems to gather critical operational data.

# Evaluation of Community Health Programs

**Program evaluation** is defined as a systematic investigation of three interrelated program domains: merit (or quality); worth (or value, i.e., cost-effectiveness); and significance (or importance) of the program (CDC, Program Performance and Evaluation Office, 2012). Evaluation shares some common features with research, such as the careful framing of questions and the methodical approach to seeking answers. However, rather than seeking to create new knowledge—which is the hallmark of research—program evaluation has a more practical orientation. Program evaluation generates information that will be used to guide decision making and program development (Porteous et al., 1997). It addresses the following questions:

1. Did we do what we said we would do?
2. What did we learn about what worked and what did not work?
3. What difference did we make?
4. What could we do differently?
5. How do we plan to use evaluation findings for continuous learning? (Health Canada, 2002)

As a general rule, the evaluation of health promotion programs should take into account their complexity and be consistent with the way the programs are carried out (Rootman, Goodstadt, Potvin, & Springett, 2001). Programs are offered in a range of settings, from health clinics to schools, shopping malls, and homes, where health care delivery is just one of many activities being carried out. Program activities are often combined in a way that makes sense for the participants. For example, a resource center might offer a well-baby clinic and include a session on parenting (family health program), immunization (infection control program), free milk, and access to a food bank (food security program), all at the same time. It goes without saying that natural settings are more complex and difficult to control than laboratories, which makes it difficult to isolate cause and effect. Therefore experts in the field advise against imposing evaluation strategies and methods suitable for quantitative sciences on community situations (Nutbeam, 1998; Pirie, Stone, Assaf, Flora, & Maschewsky-Schneider, 1994; Rootman et al., 2001).

Also consistent with the way that health promotion programs operate, more attention is being paid to their collaborative nature, and evaluation is approached as a participatory endeavor and capacity-building opportunity. This means involving stakeholders, adopting empowering processes, and considering the multiple dimensions and time frame of program activities (Rootman et al., 2001). Rather than being seen as a specialist activity carried out by program evaluators and researchers, following strict scientific methods, stakeholders may be directly involved in all phases of the evaluation, including the design, conduct, and writing of the report. All of this adds to the complexity of program evaluation. On the other hand, the more participatory the approach, the more likely it is that the evaluation will meet the information needs of all stakeholders.

Mai and Fadma are dismayed when they see the pile of the documents for review: public health program guidelines, several articles on influenza immunization, a report on best practices, regional statistics for the previous year, and, not least, the program report. This will not be easy reading! "We are never going to get through this in one morning," says Mai. After a few minutes of griping, Fadma says, "What we need is a plan. Let's make a list of what we need to know to get started." They quickly generate the following questions:

1. What is the public health mandate regarding influenza immunization?
2. How does the influenza program operate?
3. When was the last needs assessment carried out?
4. What are the key facts on influenza and influenza prevention?
5. Who should be immunized—what is the schedule?
6. Are there side effects to immunization?
7. What proportion of the population is immunized; who does not get immunized but should?
8. Are there other health measures that help to prevent influenza?
9. What are the statistics on the number of cases of influenza?
10. Where were the outbreaks of influenza last year?

Fadma elects to quickly read through the program documents to answer these questions and get a better sense of the influenza program. Mai will find out more about influenza and its prevention. They write key findings on a white board as they go along. At the end of two hours they review the findings:

- The previous year's influenza campaign was directed to three groups: adults 65 years of age and over, adults with chronic disease, and formal and informal caregivers. This is consistent with the regional mandate.
- The program maintains effective working relationships with community health centers, school boards, ESL teachers, and family practitioners through an annual community consultation plus individual meetings. This year, the ethno-cultural community resource centers will participate so that their needs can be addressed.

- Influenza prevention resource materials are disseminated through the media (TV, radio, newspapers) and community organizations, including those serving multicultural groups.
- Educational material is disseminated to family practice/medical centers; for example, last year influenza fact sheets in eight languages were distributed in the community, and 1794 prescription notepads, with a message to get the flu vaccine, went to doctors' offices.

Mai starts to put the information in a logic model (see Table 13.2). She says, "The arrows indicate that the program activities lead to the short-term objectives but I am not certain how this actually happens."

Millie explains how the various activities contribute to the outcomes: "The community consultation fulfills several functions. It brings together the key provider groups for an update on this year's campaign. We review changes to the vaccines and the immunization protocol, reinforce the importance of maintaining the cold chain, and discuss reporting and documentation. This helps to ensure a consistent approach and good records. Also, we have to make sure that everyone in the region has access to the government-funded vaccine, so the meeting provides an opportunity to talk about the clinics."

"What is the cold chain?" asks Fadma. Millie explains that "the vaccine **cold chain** is a temperature-controlled environment used to maintain and distribute vaccines in optimal condition" (CDC, 2014b). It is vitally important to store vaccines at the correct temperature to maintain potency—they should not be too hot or too cold. In their area, the health department is responsible for ensuring that proper conditions are maintained, wherever vaccines are stored.

Millie continues: "Many people go to their family doctor, pharmacy, or flu clinic for the flu shot, but this year the health centers will offer clinics in community locations to try to increase the uptake. Last year, we conducted a needs assessment in the Italian and Chinese communities and found many older adults did not attend the flu clinics because they did not speak English. This year a health center is offering a clinic at a residence for older adults, in the Italian community, which has interpreters.

**Table 13.2: Draft Influenza Program Logic Model**

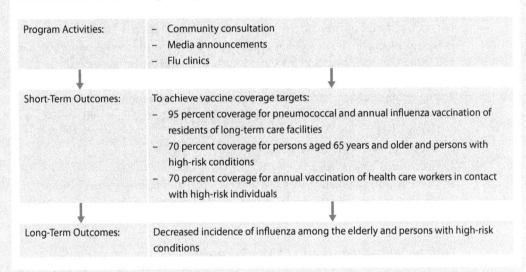

| Program Activities: | – Community consultation<br>– Media announcements<br>– Flu clinics |
|---|---|
| Short-Term Outcomes: | To achieve vaccine coverage targets:<br>– 95 percent coverage for pneumococcal and annual influenza vaccination of residents of long-term care facilities<br>– 70 percent coverage for persons aged 65 years and older and persons with high-risk conditions<br>– 70 percent coverage for annual vaccination of health care workers in contact with high-risk individuals |
| Long-Term Outcomes: | Decreased incidence of influenza among the elderly and persons with high-risk conditions |

"The fact sheets, newspaper articles, and public announcements promote immunization in two ways. First, we use articles, fact sheets, and local television shows to disseminate factual information on influenza and explain why it is important to prevent the flu in older adults and others whose health is compromised. The general public hears the message, not just the at-risk group, and we know that informal support networks are an important influence on health behavior. Second, throughout the campaign we advertise where and when the clinics are being held each week."

The students begin to see how the program activities contribute to the short-term outcome of increasing uptake of flu vaccine and expand the description of program activities in the logic model drawing. They identify some service delivery outcomes, such as the number of clinics to be held at each site.

Millie helps the students to interpret the previous year's clinic statistics and shows Mai how to log on to FluWatch—on the Public Health Agency of Canada website—to compare them with provincial and national statistics. They find the incidence was lower than in the previous year. Mai follows the links to the World Health Organization (WHO) FluLine and is excited to find so much information with so little effort. The

FluLine tabulates weekly influenza statistics from around the world, identifies the causal agents, and plots the outbreaks on a world map. This allows a comparison of rates between regions and countries and against the rates for previous years (see "Website Resources" for links).

At the end of their second day in the program, the students agree they have completed the first steps of the community health nursing project and are ready to start thinking about program evaluation for the planning meeting next week. Before the meeting, they want to see a flu clinic in action. Millie suggests they visit the Sunnyside health clinic—"I told the nurses to expect you any time." They decide to visit together. Mai will then attend another community clinic and Fadma will go to the Italian residence.

**Discussion Topics and Questions**

3. Discuss how you might evaluate the success of activities to build the support networks of students attending ESL classes.
4. Discuss the resources required to carry out the TB prevention program described in Box 13.1.

# Conducting a Program Evaluation

Program evaluation can be broken down into several steps. The steps, listed below, serve to organize the following discussion. It is worth noting that steps 2 to 3 are not entirely independent and do not proceed in a lock-step fashion. Usually there is movement back and forward as the evaluation design, methods, and tools are being decided.

1. Engage stakeholders and clarify the purpose of the evaluation.
2. Describe the program, design the evaluation approach, and determine questions to be answered.
3. Decide on the methods and tools.
4. Gather credible evidence.
5. Document the evaluation in an evaluation report and justify the conclusions.
6. Ensure use and share lessons learned.

## Engage Stakeholders and Clarify Purpose

It is important to involve multiple stakeholders in all phases of program development, including program evaluation (Israel et al., 1995; Rootman et al., 2001). A participatory approach helps to bring together all those with an investment in the program, including community partners and those served by the program. Evaluation is increasingly considered an integral part of program delivery and is carried out by operational staff rather than external evaluators. Depending on the scope and complexity of the evaluation, persons with specialist knowledge, such as health planners, epidemiologists, and measurement experts, may also be included in the evaluation team or used as consultants. As with all teamwork, it is important to agree on the roles and responsibilities of team members at the outset.

Bear in mind that evaluation is rooted in values, and members of the evaluation team may have different priorities regarding what should be evaluated. For example, health providers may want to show the value of their work and let other health providers know which health promotion strategies work best with particular communities; managers at different levels of the health system require information to make informed decisions about the use of resources; community leaders look for guidance on policy development; academics are interested in developing the body of knowledge of health promotion theory; funding agencies want to know what has been accomplished with project funds; and community members want to know that community health programs are improving health and offer value for money.

Fundamentally, program evaluation is about making program decisions, so it is helpful to clarify at the outset the general nature of the decisions to be made and to establish a time frame for when the results are expected. This may seem obvious, but it is easy to assume that everyone has the same agenda when they do not. The initial, broad direction will probably come from the program manager or a program steering group. Reaching agreement on whether the main purpose of the evaluation is to improve program delivery, provide evidence of cost-effectiveness, or determine whether or not to continue to offer a program provides a context for the inquiry and helps to establish the scope of

**Table 13.3: Evaluation Plan**

| Task | By Whom | By When |
|---|---|---|
| Assemble evaluation team, clarify purpose of evaluation (including budget) | Evaluation team leader | September 10 |
| Prepare the evaluation plan | Evaluation team leader, with team input | September 10 |
| Describe the program | Team members | September 16 |
| Determine what questions the evaluation will answer | Team | September 30 |
| Identify key stakeholders | Team | September 30 |
| Interview stakeholders | Delegated team members | October |
| Define the methods and tools | Team | October |
| Conduct the evaluation | Delegated team members | November |
| Write the report | Delegated team members | December 1–14 |
| Present results | Team leader/team | December 18 |

the evaluation. An explicit agenda, even if it holds the prospect of program closure, can be used to build cooperation. As well, it is helpful to confirm the level of management support for conducting the evaluation and what resources will be committed. Bear in mind that as planning proceeds, some of the parameters may change.

Once the evaluation team is assembled, and the broad purpose and scope of the evaluation is agreed upon, the next step is to develop a work plan. The work plan lays out the main tasks, sets timelines, and allocates resources, the details of which can be elaborated. A simple format is shown in Table 13.3. As you can see, the process is similar to that provided in the timeline and Gantt chart in Chapters 6 and 7.

## Describe Program, Design Evaluation Approach, and Determine Questions

A complete and accurate description of the program to be evaluated is an essential starting point. As discussed earlier, a program logic model may have been developed when the program was planned, but programs can drift away from their original form. Besides, some program elements are planned but never implemented for various reasons. Lack of funds, a change in priorities, a change in work responsibilities, and timing conflicts are among the possible explanations. Given that community programs operate in a natural setting, variations from the plan are not unexpected. Before starting an evaluation it is important to make sure the program logic model reflects the program being delivered and describes what is really happening, rather than what the program should ideally look like. This is where it helps to have someone who is not intimately involved in the program to ask questions and seek clarification on the program description. If necessary, the program logic model can be redrawn until there is consensus that it accurately captures the reality of the program.

The program logic model provides a framework for designing the evaluation approach and determining the specific questions to be answered. Keep in mind that evaluation serves a different purpose at different stages of program development. In the early stages

**Table 13.4: Types of Evaluation**

| Type of Evaluation/ Alternative Terms | Questions Guiding Evaluation |
|---|---|
| Process Evaluation/ Formative Evaluation | How did the program address issues of continuity, coordination, and sequencing? |
| | What activities were provided: where, under what conditions, by whom, to what audience, and with what level of effort? |
| | What were the differences between program sites? |
| | Who participated—is the program reaching the specified audience? Who does it fail to reach and why? |
| | What was the nature of staff-client interaction? |
| | What did participants experience—were they satisfied with the experience? |
| | Which activities worked and which did not? |
| | What are the strengths and weaknesses of the program? |
| Short-Term (Immediate) Outcome Evaluation/Short-Term Impact Evaluation/ Summative Evaluation | What changes occurred in knowledge, attitudes, beliefs and behavior of participants, programs, and policies of organizations and governments as a result of the program? |
| Long-Term (Ultimate) Outcome Evaluation/Long-Term Impact Evaluation/ Summative Evaluation | What changes occurred in health status, morbidity, and mortality as a result of the program? |

of program implementation, evaluation is concerned with how the program is being delivered. Later on the focus of evaluation turns to whether the program is achieving the desired results. These types of evaluation are termed process evaluation and outcome evaluation, respectively (see also Chapter 7).

Process evaluation provides information of progress toward the achievement of the short- and long-term outcomes, and permits mid-course adjustments (Israel et al., 1995). Broadly speaking, it answers the question "Are we doing what we said we were going to do?" For example, in the TB prevention program described earlier, suppose that after six weeks of a twelve-week series of ESL classes, the number of students screened at each site ranges from a low of four at site A to a high of 60 students at site Z. Process evaluation might ask "Why is there such a difference? Is the program being offered the same way across the ESL sites? What factors explain the difference in attendance?"

Process evaluation is particularly important in community programs where the health outcomes are not likely to be observed for many years. Process evaluation helps to distill learning: What is working and why? Such information can be used to improve the way the program is delivered by identifying which aspects of the program can be improved and which aspects can be continued without change (Pirie et al., 1994).

Outcome evaluation is concerned with the change brought about as a result of the program. It answers the question "What difference has the program made?" Both the more immediate effects, such as changes in knowledge, attitudes, or behavior, and the longer-term effects, such as changes in health status, are of interest. The findings from a process evaluation can contribute to outcome evaluation by helping to interpret why the outcomes were or were not achieved and by providing clues to what might be done differently.

Adapted from the work of Israel and colleagues (1995, p. 368), Table 13.4 compares the different types of evaluation, identifies alternative terms used to describe them, and provides sample questions pertinent to the type of evaluation.

For an evaluation to be useful, it should respond to the needs of key users. A key question to ask is "What information is needed to aid decision making now?" At the same time, program evaluation, especially of mandated programs, tends to be dominated by professional interests, and evaluators are well advised to remember that program decisions are best taken in collaboration with the community (Nutbeam, 1998; Rootman et al., 2001). Stakeholder input can be obtained equally well through key informant interviews, surveys, or possibly a group meeting. Keep in mind that participatory approaches tend to take a long time because of the high level of interaction required. It is important to consider the time and resources required, as well as the strengths and weaknesses of the various approaches. (It may be useful to review the section on key informant interviewing in Chapter 4.) As with any data, the input from stakeholders must be collated and summarized for analysis. One way to do this is to use the program logic model as a guide and organize the feedback in relation to the elements of the model, that is, by specific program activities and short-term and long-term outcomes. Evaluation questions can then be drawn out for each element.

For example, the following feedback on the TB prevention program, discussed earlier, relates to the way the program is being offered across the sites:

- Program manager, program staff, volunteers, and ESL students say many clinics are being cancelled at two sites because the clinic space is needed for other activities.
- Stakeholders say there are insufficient nurses for the number of ESL students attending the clinic. The ESL students say there is not enough time to complete TB testing before class or during breaks.
- Two female students tell the interviewer it is not considered appropriate for women to receive health care from men in their culture. They say women will not attend clinics run by a male nurse.
- Many participants tell you that "some clinics are very busy, others are empty."

The final selection of the evaluation questions rests with the evaluation team and may involve some negotiation. Explicit criteria can be used to decide which questions have the highest priority. For example, one approach would be to set priorities based on the relevance of the information to immediate decision-making needs and the importance of the question to more than one stakeholder. Inevitably, other considerations such as time and resources will play a part in the final selection. Once the questions have been decided, then they can be reformulated so that they are specific and measurable (see discussion on SMART objectives in Chapter 6).

## Determine the Evaluation Methods and Tools

Ask yourself what data is required to answer the questions and where the data can be obtained—who has the information. Then determine the most appropriate method for data collection and identify specific data collection instruments. Using the worksheet in Table 13.5 as an example, you can see that the first question to be answered is "Were the clinics implemented as planned across the city?" This question relates to one of the project activities from the program described earlier: holding scheduled TB screening clinics in ESL classes. The evaluators will consider this activity to have been carried out successfully if 90 percent of the clinics are held as scheduled. The question will be answered by auditing clinic site records to determine which scheduled clinics were held and which were cancelled. The clinic nurse holds the records. The percentage of cancelled clinics can then be calculated for each site and the sites compared.

## Determine Tools: Observation as a Means of Collecting Evaluation Data

Between-site variation in program delivery can have a bearing on overall program success. One way of gathering information about possible site differences is to observe and compare activities across sites. Observational data can be used to complement data gathered using other data collection methods, but it can also provide unique insights. For example, through observation, you can identify key differences in the physical and social environment and in the clinical context. The value of the approach is that it does not disturb the natural order of things; life can go on just as it does every day. As a result, the observer has access to what people say and do, which may be different from what they say, or think, they do. Also, some activities become so ritualized that people perform them without thinking or questioning why they are doing them; these habitual activities may be difficult to recall as significant. Without being obtrusive, a trained observer can

**Table 13.5: Evaluation Questions for Selected Program Activities—Indicators of Success, Evaluation Approach, and Source of Information**

| Evaluation Question | Program Activity | Indicator of Success | Evaluation Approach | Potential Source of Data |
|---|---|---|---|---|
| Were the clinics implemented as planned across the city? | Scheduled clinics held across the city in ESL classes | 90 percent of clinics held as scheduled | Audit of clinic records | Program staff |
| | TB screening carried out | 75 percent of students screened | Audit of clinic records | Program staff |
| How were barriers to access addressed? | Barriers to clinic access identified and, where possible, removed | List of barriers, and efforts to eliminate them described, with estimated degree of success | Audit of "barriers list" / Observation checklist to identify barriers | Program staff / Independent observer |

view experiences in context, learn what is typical and what is not, and gain insight into what the experience means to people in the place where it happens (Hammersley & Atkinson, 2007; Patton, 1990).

Observation and description is the first step to understanding a phenomenon. Things have to be described before they can be measured. Gathering observational data is integral to nursing practice, and the same skills can be applied in collecting observational data for the purpose of evaluating community programs. The approach to observation can be more or less structured, depending on how much is known about the subject of interest. Less structure is an advantage if little is known. However, it is impossible to observe everything when in a natural setting, so it is helpful to have an organizing framework in mind. Patton (1990) identifies some options for organizing an observation session:

- Chronology: Describe events as they happen in time. For example, document all interactions with staff from the time a person enters a clinic setting to the time he or she leaves.
- Key events: Record critical events (for example, unusual or unexpected events, or events that exceed or do not meet expectations).
- Setting: Describe the physical and social aspects of the environment.
- People: Choose a location, for example, the registration desk. Describe the people in the setting, what they say and do, including the non-verbal.
- Processes: Make note of the key processes that happen in a setting, for example, at the flu clinic: registration, waiting for immunization, booking appointments.
- Issues: Questions arising from reflection on the observations. (p. 377)

Another approach to observation is to start with sensitizing concepts. These are concepts known to be fundamental to the issue of concern. For example, the previous discussion on the TB prevention logic model identified the crucial role of screening. This sensitizes the observer to look for factors that support or prevent screening at the sites. The factors can be specified in more detail once their salience is confirmed. As you will probably observe, this flexibility in approach is an advantage when using observation as a data collection technique in the early stages of an inquiry (Patton, 1990).

A more structured approach to observation entails the use of an observation checklist. The checklist helps to keep track of observations and promotes a consistent approach, thereby enabling comparison. Items on the checklist can be pre-coded to indicate what response is expected, for example, a yes or no. This is particularly useful when the key variables are already well known. An advantage of using a checklist is that it helps to minimize the degree of inference required by the observer. A disadvantage is the lack of flexibility. Combining a checklist and unstructured observations can remedy this and allow the observer to add items to the list for systematic observation.

A sample checklist, developed to assess the barriers to clinic access, is shown in the Appendix to Chapter 13. The checklist is structured to record observations from the perspective of a clinic participant, starting with the approach to the clinic. Attached to the checklist is a list of tips to help you obtain reliable information.

The students eagerly discuss their experience at the flu clinics. Since the first clinic was quiet, they were able to observe several immunizations and had time to talk to the clients and the clinic nurse. Mai had a similar experience at the second community clinic. In contrast, only two older women attended the clinic at the Italian residence; neither was Italian. The clinic nurse told Fadma this low attendance was the norm.

The students meet with the program manager about their project. She explains that the flu program has stable funding but it is not sufficient to cover the anticipated increase in the older adult population served by the program. She would like the evaluation to identify how the program can make better use of resources. An evaluation group, which has already been set up, is meeting next week. The students will assist Millie to prepare the program logic model for the meeting, conduct the stakeholder interviews, and report back to the evaluation team. Depending on progress, they may have time to conduct a small part of the evaluation—their exact focus will be decided in collaboration with the evaluation team once the evaluation questions are agreed upon.

Millie provides a list of the main stakeholders for the influenza prevention program: community health centers, the multicultural resource center, and three specific population groups—older adults, persons with chronic disease, and health providers. As Millie points out, all are represented on the steering group. Fadma and Mai decide to randomly choose one person from each category of stakeholder. Millie provides the contact information to set up interviews. The students ask interviewees what questions they have about the flu clinics that the evaluation might address and tabulate the answers (see Table 13.6).

### Table 13.6: Inventory of Stakeholder Input to the Evaluation

| Interviewee | Interviewee Input: Questions and Observations |
| --- | --- |
| Program Manager | "According to program staff, the Monday evening clinics are always quiet. I am wondering if we should eliminate that clinic altogether and increase staff at other clinics." |
| | "I would like to know who is attending the clinics. Are we reaching the specified group?" |
| Program Staff | "The health center clinics are working well. We get a lot of people we have never seen before. I wish there was more time to talk. The other day, an older man came in. He was very quiet and had soup stains on his shirt. I intended to talk to him but the clinic was full, and he left before I had a chance to speak to him." |
| | "How many clinics at the resource center are cancelled because of other activities going on?" |
| | "Is clinic staffing based on attendance?" |
| | "Some clinics are combined with a drop-in clinic. This is not usually a problem, but it is difficult to keep track of people when there are many drop-in patients." |
| Community Partner | "There is limited parking at the center, and it is expensive. We get a lot of complaints about this." |
| Volunteer | "Some clinics are very quiet—no one there—others are so busy you feel exhausted when you get home." |
| | "The handout does not say anything about side effects. A lot of people ask me if they are likely to get mild flu symptoms with the injection. What should I say?" |
| Participants | The clinic is easy to get to by public transit but several women said the waiting times are too long. The clinic hours, 5:00–7:30 p.m., conflict with dinner. |
| | "The parking is too far from the center. My mother-in-law uses a walker, and it is tiring for her to walk so far. No one would help me get a wheelchair." |

The evaluation team reviews the input, and there is consensus that the priority for the evaluation is to determine whether the flu clinics are being implemented as planned across the sites and whether they are reaching the specified group. Four specific questions are composed, indicators of success are defined, and evaluation tools are specified, together with information on the sources of data required to answer the questions (see Table 13.7).

The evaluation team decides, in consultation with Mai and Fadma, that the students will complete an observation study of the screening clinics to identify barriers and facilitators. With input from Millie, the students develop a work plan to guide their study. The main items are listed below:

1. Adapt the clinic checklist (see Appendix to Chapter 13) for observation at flu clinics (by week 6).
2. Select 25 percent of clinics (10 clinics) and schedule two observation periods at each, as agreed with the evaluation team (by week 6).
3. Check agreement between observers: two observers conduct four parallel sets of observations, compare results and resolve differences, aiming for 80 percent agreement between observers. (Millie, program volunteer on the evaluation team, Mai, and Fadma). Compare observations and discuss and resolve differences (weeks 6–7).

4. Conduct observations (weeks 7–9).
5. Summarize all observations on an enlarged observation sheet (weeks 9–10).
6. Identify barriers to access and cluster by themes, for example, transportation and parking, hours of operation, language of service (by week 11).
7. Prepare three overheads (methods, overview of clinic sample, results) for a 5- to 10-minute presentation at evaluation meeting (week 11).
8. Write section of evaluation report, incorporating comments from evaluation team (week 11–12).
9. Attend debriefing of evaluation team, program team, and project team (week 12).

**Discussion Topics and Questions**

5. Identify factors that might interfere with gathering observational data on access issues at a flu clinic (see Appendix to Chapter 13), or have an impact on the quality of the data.
6. How might the mix of health promotion activities at a clinic—combinations of well-baby assessment, immunization, parenting sessions, free milk, and access to a food bank—have an impact on immunization rates in babies and toddlers?
7. Identify potential short-term and long-term outcomes for a program promoting alcohol-free high-school graduation ceremonies.

**Table 13.7: Worksheet for Flu Clinic Evaluation**

| Evaluation Question | Activity | Indicator of Success | Evaluation Tool | Information Source |
|---|---|---|---|---|
| Were activities implemented as planned? (How many clinics were held and where?) | Document scheduled flu clinics held across the city in CHCs, older adult residences, and resource centers | 90 percent of clinics are held as scheduled | Audit clinic records | Program staff |
| What are the barriers and facilitators of accessibility? | Observation study at 10 clinics | Barriers and facilitators identified | Clinic observation checklist | Evaluator |
| Are participants satisfied with the program? | Random administration of short questionnaire | At least 60 percent of participants are satisfied with the service | Client satisfaction questionnaire | Evaluator |
| What percentage of those immunized are in a specified group? | Extract information from random sample of immunization records | More than 60 percent of those immunized are in the specified group | Audit of clinic records | Program staff |

## Conduct Evaluation, Analyze Data, and Summarize Findings for Inclusion in an Evaluation Report

Gathering evaluation data and the analytic process is as described in Chapters 6, 7, and 8. For example, if you are collecting observation data with the observation checklist found in the Appendix to Chapter 13, use a blank copy to summarize observations and make comparisons across the settings. Highlight barriers and facilitators, and note their frequency, for example, all clinics offer free parking; only one clinic offers services in French. Another analytical strategy might be to develop a profile of a barrier-free clinic and compare other clinics to this profile. Whatever the analytical approach, it is important to remember that each set of data collected—observations, audits, interviews—must be analyzed and synthesized in the final report.

## Summary

It is difficult to grasp all the ramifications of a community health program. Participating in a program evaluation challenges all those involved with a program to pool their wits and work together to provide the information that is necessary to guide decision making. A program logic model is a useful evaluation tool. The logic model helps evaluators to comprehend the program activities and understand how the various elements of a community program work together in order to determine whether or not they are successful in bringing about changes that are likely to have an impact on health. Developing skills and using program evaluation tools is an important part of community health nursing practice. As exemplified in the scenarios for this chapter, the technical challenge of evaluating community programs has to be placed in context in order to appreciate its complexity.

## Classroom and Seminar Exercises

1. Debate whether the decision to immunize children against measles should be left up to parents.
2. Many agencies offer prenatal programs. Working in groups of three, use the following questions to interview program staff about the program. Use the information to draw a program logic model. Compare similarities and differences between the programs.
   a. What is the goal of the program? (What specific outcomes or results are expected?)
   b. What population group does the program address?
   c. What resources (e.g., people, money) are required to deliver the program?
   d. What activities are carried out to achieve the program goal?
3. Discuss how you would use a program logic model to tell program volunteers about the program.

4. Develop an observation checklist to evaluate parents' ability to install their car seat after a workshop demonstration.

5. Identify three short-term outcomes that might be used to evaluate the success of a TV commercial in conveying the importance to older adults of getting a flu shot.

## References

Alami, N. N., Yuen, C., M., Miramontes, R., Pratt, R., Price, S. F., & Navin, T. R. (2014). Trends in tuberculosis—United States, 2013. *Morbidity & Mortality Weekly Report (MMWR)*, *63*(11), 229–233.

British Columbia Centre for Disease Control. (2011). *Tuberculosis manual, Appendix K: Directly observed therapy.* Retrieved from www.bccdc.ca/NR/rdonlyres/57623012-34A9-4886-9B6D-00D8576BA190/0/TB_Manual_BCCDC_June2010.pdf

Butterfoss, F., & Francisco, V. (2004). Evaluating community partnerships and coalitions with practitioners in mind. *Health Promotion Practice, 5*(2), 108–114.

Centers for Disease Control and Prevention (CDC). (2014a). *Drug-resistant TB.* Retrieved from www.cdc.gov/tb/topic/drtb/default.htm

Centers for Disease Control and Prevention (CDC). (2014b). *Vaccine storage and handling toolkit.* Retrieved from www.cdc.gov/vaccines/recs/default.htm

Centers for Disease Control and Prevention, Program Performance and Evaluation Office. (2012). *A framework for program evaluation.* Retrieved from www.cdc.gov/eval/framework/

Chang, S., Wheeler, L. S. M., & Farrell, K. P. (2002). Public health impact of targeted tuberculosis screening in public schools. *American Journal of Public Health, 92*(12), 1942–1945.

Hammersley, M., & Atkinson, P. (2007). *Ethnography: Principles in practice* (3rd ed.). New York: Routledge.

Health Canada. (2002). *Guide to project evaluation: A participatory approach.* Retrieved from www.collectionscanada.gc.ca/webarchives/20071225031208/http://www.phac-aspc.gc.ca/ph-sp/phdd/resources/guide/framwork.htm

Israel, B. A., Cummings, K. M., Dignan, M. B., Heaney, C. A., Perales, D. P., Simons-Morton, B. G., & Zimmerman, M. A. (1995). Evaluation of health education programs: Current assessment and future direction. *Health Education Quarterly, 22*, 364–389.

Macaskill, L., Dwyer, J. J. M., Uetrecht, C., Dombrow, C., Crompton, R., Wilck, B., & Stone, J. (2000). An evaluability assessment to develop a restaurant health promotion program in Canada. *Health Promotion International, 15*, 57–69. doi:10.1093/heapro/15.1.57

MacDonald, N., Hébert, P. C., & Stanbrook, M. B. (2011). Tuberculosis in Nunavut: A century of failure [Editorial]. *Canadian Medical Association Journal, 183*. doi:10.1503/cmaj.110160

Milstein, B., Wetherhall, S., & CDC Evaluation Working Group. (2014). A framework for program evaluation: A gateway to tools. *Community Tool Box* (Chapter 36, Section 1). Retrieved from http://ctb.ku.edu/en/table-of-contents/evaluate/evaluation/framework-for-evaluation/main

Moyer, A., Verhovsek, H., & Wilson, V. (1997). Facilitating the shift to population-based public health programs: Innovation through the use of framework and logic models. *Canadian Journal of Public Health, 88*(95), 95–98.

Nutbeam, D. (1998). Evaluating health promotion-progress, problems and solutions. *Health Promotion International, 13*(1), 27–44.

Ormerod, L. (2005). Multidrug-resistant tuberculosis (MDR-TB): Epidemiology, prevention and treatment. *British Medical Bulletin, 73–74*(1), 17–24. doi:10.1093/bmb/ldh047

Patton, M. Q. (1990). Qualitative evaluation and research methods (4th ed.). Newbury Park, CA: Sage Publications.

Pirie, P. L., Stone, E. J., Assaf, A. R., Flora, J. A., & Maschewsky-Schneider, U. (1994). Program evaluation strategies for community-based health promotion programs: Perspectives from the cardiovascular disease community research and demonstration studies. *Health Education Research, 9*(1), 23–26.

Porteous, N. L., Sheldrick, B. J., & Stewart, P. J. (1997). The logic model: A blueprint for describing programs. Retrieved from http://research.familymed.ubc.ca/files/2012/03/logic_model_e.pdf

Public Health Agency of Canada. (2012). *Tuberculosis: Drug resistance in Canada—2012.* Retrieved from www.phac-aspc.gc.ca/tbpc-latb/pubs/tb-dr2012/index-eng.php#methods

Rootman, I., Goodstadt, M., Potvin, L., & Springett, J. (2001). A framework for health promotion evaluation. In I. Rootman, M. Goodstadt, B. Hyndman, D. V. McQueen, L. Potvin, J. Springett, & E. Ziglio (Eds.), *Evaluation in health promotion: Principles and perspectives.* Geneva: World Health Organization.

Tiemersma, E. W., van der Werf, M. J., Borgdorff, M. W., Williams, B. G., & Nagelkerke, N. J. (2011). Natural history of tuberculosis: Duration and fatality of untreated pulmonary tuberculosis in HIV negative patients: A systematic review. *Plos ONE, 6*, e17601. Retrieved from http://journals.plos.org/plosone/article?id=10.1371/journal.pone.0017601

Uppaluri, A., Naus, M., Heywood, N., Brunton, J., Kerbel, D., & Wobeser, W. (2002). Effectiveness of the immigration medical surveillance program for tuberculosis in Ontario. *Canadian Journal of Public Health, 93*(2), 88–91.

World Health Organization (WHO). (2014). *Global Tuberculosis Report 2014.* Retrieved from www.who.int/tb/publications/global_report/en/

## Website Resources

### International, National, State/Provincial, and Territorial Infection Control Sites

Centers for Disease Control and Prevention: www.cdc.gov/
Follow the links on the main menu: "Diseases and Conditions"/Flu (Influenza); and "Healthy Living"/Vaccines and Immunizations. The Influenza (Flu) page provides detailed information on flu basics, treatment and resources, information for health professionals, and approved vaccines for the current year, together with a map of flu activity and surveillance across the US. It also provides links to other influenza websites and international flu activities supported by CDC.

Under "About CDC" on the main page, you will find a link to "Morbidity and Mortality Weekly Report (MMWR)" at www.cdc.gov/mmwr/. The MMWR home page provides links to surveillance summaries and specific topical reports. Under "Other Resources," there is a link to State Health Departments.

Public Health Agency of Canada: www.phac-aspc.gc.ca/id-mi/index-eng.php
The main menu provides links to pages on "Infectious Diseases," "Immunizations and Vaccines," and other relevant topics, such as "Food Safety" and "Travel Health." The "Infectious Diseases" page provides links, arranged alphabetically, to "Influenza" and particular strains of influenza such as "H1N1." The "Immunizations and Vaccines" page provides links to provincial and territorial websites and immunization schedules.

**Infectious Diseases and Environmental Health Program Standards and Protocols**

Ontario Ministry of Health and Long-Term Care, *Ontario Public Health Standards*: www.
health.gov.on.ca/en/pro/programs/publichealth/oph_standards/ophsprotocols.aspx
   This site provides a link to Infectious Disease and Environmental Health program standards
and protocols.

World Health Organization Fact Sheet on Influenza: www.who.int/topics/influenza/en/
   This site provides links to fact sheets on influenza, reports and statistics from different parts
of the world, and links to the WHO surveillance systems and to related topics such as vaccines.

World Health Organization FluNet: www.who.int/influenza/gisrs_laboratory/flunet/en/
   Follow the links to national and international influenza pages.


**Program Evaluation Resources**

Centers for Disease Control and Prevention, Program Performance and Evaluation Office
(PPEO)—Program Evaluation, *A Framework for Program Evaluation*: www.cdc.gov/eval/frame-
work/index.htm
   The CDC framework for evaluation describes steps and standards for program evaluation
and is used to organize links to numerous other evaluation resources.

KU Work Group for Community Health and Development, *Community Tool Box: A
Framework for Program Evaluation*: http://ctb.ku.edu/en/table-of-contents/evaluate/evaluation/
framework-for-evaluation/main
   This web page offers "a gateway to tools" for program evalution, and includes numerous
references and links to Web resources.

Public Health Ontario: www.publichealthontario.ca/EN/Pages/default.aspx
   The site provides links to a variety of professional development resources, such as seminars
and workshops. Under "Services and Tools," you will find an interactive program planner, and
other resources can be located using the site search feature.

# Appendix to Chapter 13

## Clinic—Observational Assessment

### Tips on Making Reliable Observations

1. Try to minimize your impact on the setting. Let people get used to your presence before the observation starts. Remember, the presence of an observer may have an impact on behavior. Think about what happens when a police is car parked on the side of the road—people slow down. When you know someone is watching you, you may do things "by the book" or try to show yourself in the best light.

2. Spend enough time in the setting to differentiate the typical from the atypical.

3. Vary observations with regard to people, place, and time; try to capture the full range of possibilities, for example, do not always observe the same person at the same time each day.

4. Weigh the advantages and disadvantages of staying in one location or moving around. With the former, you can blend into the background; with the latter, you can choose to focus on particular events.

5. Schedule observations for manageable periods of time to avoid fatigue (e.g., 10 minutes on and 10 minutes off). What we see and what we attend to is influenced by our expectations, by our emotions, and by our physical state.

6. Pair up with another observer to avoid selectivity and bias; check that your observations are in agreement.

7. Clarify the need for ethical clearance. Generally speaking, conducting observations at clinical sites does not present ethical issues any different to those that might arise in the course of clinical practice. However, health provider–client interactions are considered confidential, and observations for the purpose of evaluation may require informed consent.

8. Think about how you will respond during your observation if you are asked to help out at the clinic when it gets busy.

Observation Date/Time (dd/mm/yyyy/start and stop time): _____ Observer _____

| Clinic Name | Sunnyside CHC Clinic #1 | Sunnyside CHC Golden Age Club Clinic #2 | William Street Community Center | Family Medicine Center |
|---|---|---|---|---|
| Location | 212 42nd Street East | Corner of 5th Avenue & Market Street | 9 William Street | Corner of Main & 2nd Avenue |
| Accessibility | | | | |
| Parking available<br>– Yes/No | | | | |
| – cost/hour | | | | |
| Transport nearby<br>– bus stop | | | | |
| – subway stop | | | | |
| Building signs<br>– Yes/No | | | | |
| Wheelchair access<br>– Yes/No | | | | |
| Waiting Area | | | | |
| Seating available<br>– Yes/No | | | | |
| – average wait time | | | | |

| Clinic Name | Sunnyside CHC Clinic #1 | Sunnyside CHC Golden Age Club Clinic #2 | William Street Community Center | Family Medicine Center |
|---|---|---|---|---|
| Educational matter on display related to clinic focus, e.g., flu posters/pamphlets<br>– Yes/No | | | | |
| Languages spoken<br>– English<br>– French<br>– Other | | | | |
| Staffing numbers<br>– nurses<br>– volunteers | | | | |
| Observations | | | | |
| Clinic Operations | | | | |
| Days/hours of week | | | | |
| Appointment system<br>– Yes/No | | | | |
| Attendance Record (previous month) | | | | |
| – average per clinic<br>– largest attendance<br>– smallest attendance<br>– total clients | | | | |
| Number of clinics cancelled per month | | | | |

# Chapter 14

# Community Health Nursing Roles in Disaster and Emergency Management

$\mathsf{C}$ommunity health nurses have an important role in addressing all aspects of natural and man-made disasters. This chapter explains and illustrates those roles by examining the four components of emergency management—prevention and mitigation, preparation, response, and recovery—used by the Federal Emergency Management Agency (FEMA) in the US and Public Safety Canada. The four components are the basis of the all-hazard approach to emergency management used by governments.

In this chapter, the four components are also used to feature the fundamental concepts and procedures used throughout this text: community health nursing values, beliefs, standards, and competencies; teamwork; approaches used to engage community members and organizations; and following a systematic process. For example, the chapter and scenarios identify the processes needed to provide appropriate support and services to people who are vulnerable and therefore at greater risk than others during a disaster, thereby involving the social determinants of health and social justice.

Two of the three scenarios in the chapter deal with initiating partnerships with organizations who have the expertise to serve vulnerable populations during a disaster. One scenario relates to identifying relevant partners during prevention and mitigation, and the second with emergency shelter management during response. The third scenario indicates how a student team or new practitioner could be involved in determining ways to recruit and train additional nurses for a flu pandemic. Each of the three scenarios outlines community nursing experiences for an approximate six-week period.

## Learning Objectives

After reading this chapter and answering the questions throughout the chapter, you should be able to:

1. Apply what you have learned about working on a team and in the community to disaster and emergency management.
2. Identify the four components of disaster and emergency management.
3. Apply community health nursing concepts, procedures, research, and standards/ competencies during disaster and emergency management.

4. Develop an approach to recruit partners during prevention and mitigation, and for emergency shelters during response.
5. Develop an approach to plan for surge capacity for an influenza pandemic.
6. Promote the management of social media during emergencies.

**Key Terms and Concepts**

all-hazard approach • CMIST (Communication, Medical needs, Independence, Supervision, and Transport) • continuity of operation plans (COOPs) • disaster • emergency management: prevention and mitigation, preparedness, response, recovery • emergency shelter • hazard • incident management system • pandemic • resilience • risk • risk-based • social media • surge capacity • triage

## Building on Work with Groups and Communities to Learning to Practice during Emergencies

This text has provided you with fundamental community health nursing knowledge and skills to prepare you to work in a range of situations. In this final chapter on emergency management, you can challenge yourself to use the skills and knowledge gained from community health nursing values and concepts, teamwork, short-term group projects, and work at the community level. Understanding the role of community health nurses during emergency management will assist you in being able to stay calm and contribute to the care of community members when needed.

**SCENARIO: Preparing for Emergencies in Public Health**

The public health department of North Columbia, with a population of about 600,000, determined that it needed to review the procedures it had in place to deal with emergencies and was also required to submit updated plans to the city. The public health nursing section was tasked with reviewing its role. Since preparation for emergencies would involve all their staff, the public health nurses also decided to use the preparation for dealing with disasters and emergencies as a way to illustrate the use of the community health nursing standards in practice.

A nursing manager was assigned to form a task group to coordinate the review for nursing and drew nursing representatives from all the nursing programs. After a preliminary scan at the first meeting, the task group decided that they would likely need more members to update their plans in three areas: mass immunizations, shelters, and preparing the community to deal with disasters. The manager requested and received approval for three community health nursing student teams to work with the task force on the review. The teams will provide examples of incorporating the community/public health nursing standards or competencies in their report.

**Discussion Topics and Questions**
1. What are examples of infectious diseases that often require mass immunizations in North America?
2. What knowledge and skills could community health nurses contribute in an emergency situation?

For suggested responses, please see the Answer Key at the back of the book.

# Disaster and Emergency Management

An important component of community health nursing education is being prepared to promote health during disaster and emergency (Association of Community Health Nursing Educators [ACHNE], 2008). An emergency occurs when a hazard overwhelms a population and creates a disaster. An emergency occurs when normal procedures are overwhelmed and extraordinary measures are initiated to quickly coordinate actions to protect the health, safety, or welfare of people, or to limit damage to property or the environment. A **hazard** is a potentially damaging natural or man-made event that may cause the loss of life or injury, property damage, social and economic disruption, or environmental damage. A **disaster** is a natural or man-made event that results when a hazard impacts a vulnerable community in a way that overwhelms the community's ability to cope and may cause serious harm to the safety, health, welfare, property, or environment.

Hazards and the resulting disasters and emergencies are difficult to manage because they are unpredictable. Here is an example of an emergency that could occur anywhere. A hazard is caused by a stalled vehicle on a busy major highway when visibility is poor and the road is slippery. The hazard becomes a disaster when more and more vehicles crash into each other, resulting in injured people, damaged vehicles, and a blocked highway. The multiple vehicle crashes overwhelm the local police and ambulance services, and require immediate emergency response measures to control the situation, evacuate the injured, and remove the damaged vehicles. When the injured are taken to hospital and the damaged vehicles removed from the highway, recovery begins with repairs to the highway to allow the regular flow of traffic. Recovery also involves investigating areas that should or could have prevented the emergency, such as policing and highway conditions, signage, and speed, to identify action that could prevent or mitigate the hazard in this and similar situations.

Emergency management is based on principles of risk management. **Risk** is the combination of the likelihood and the consequence of a specified hazard being realized. It refers to the vulnerability, proximity, or exposure to hazards, which affects the likelihood of adverse impact (Public Safety Canada, 2014a). **Risk-based** is the concept that sound emergency management decision making requires an understanding and evaluation of hazards, risks, and vulnerabilities. Vulnerability is measured in emergency management according to how well prepared and equipped a community is in terms of physical, social, and environmental factors and processes to minimize the impact of, or cope with, hazards.

Two broad types of hazards cause disasters: natural hazards and disasters, and human-induced disasters (Public Safety Canada, 2014b). Natural hazards are outbreaks of disease, floods, hurricanes, storm surges, tsunamis, avalanches, landslides, tornadoes, forest fires near houses, and earthquakes. Human-induced disasters include intentional events, such as terrorist or cyber attacks, human or technological accidents or failures, including electrical power outages, or other disruptions, such as loss of water supply and telecommunications. With most if not all hazards, the concern is for the impact on people, the life of communities, and the environment.

Rather than working out plans to deal with each type of disaster, the US and Canadian governments have taken an all-hazard approach to managing disasters and emergencies

**Four Components of Disaster and Emergency Management**

**Prevention and mitigation** actions eliminate or reduce the risks of disasters in order to protect lives, property, and the environment, and reduce economic disruption. Prevention and mitigation measures include hazard and vulnerability assessment, and structural and nonstructural methods, such as the construction of floodways and dikes, anti-skid surfacing, use of speed restrictions on roads, seat belt requirements, building codes, and land-use planning. Compared to the other three components, prevention and mitigation to minimize illness and injury continues throughout all components of emergency management.

**Preparedness** involves actions taken prior to an emergency or disaster to ensure an effective response, for example, emergency response plans, mutual assistance agreements, resource inventories, and training, equipment, and exercise programs.

**Response** occurs during or immediately before or after a disaster to manage its consequences through, for example, emergency public communication, search and rescue, emergency medical assistance, shelter, and evacuation to minimize suffering and losses associated with disasters.

**Recovery** involves repairing or restoring conditions to an acceptable level through measures taken after a disaster, for example, return of evacuees, trauma counseling, reconstruction, economic impact studies, and financial assistance. There is a strong relationship between long-term sustainable recovery and prevention and mitigation of future disasters. Recovery efforts should be conducted with a view toward disaster risk reduction.

*Sources*: Emergency Management Ontario, 2010; Public Safety Canada, 2014b.

(Public Health Emergency, 2009; Public Safety Canada, 2014b). An **all-hazard approach** means that common components that apply to all disasters and emergencies are used in preparation and management (Public Safety Canada, 2014b; US Department of Education, 2010). **Emergency management** is the organization of all activities and risk management measures related to prevention and mitigation, preparedness, response, and recovery. When the disaster is identified, the preparations are adjusted as needed. The ultimate purpose of emergency management is to save lives, preserve the environment, and protect property and the economy (Public Safety Canada, 2014a). Box 14.1 describes the four components.

The following illustration (Figure 14.1) indicates how the four emergency management components are interrelated. For example, long-term prevention/mitigation and preparedness are pre-disaster measures that are expected to reduce the risk and effect of disasters. However, prevention and mitigation of illness and injury must be considered throughout the whole cycle. The response and relief provided during emergency management is followed by short- and long-term recovery, which cycles into prevention and mitigation. When the four components are strengthened, and prevention and mitigation of illness and injury are continued through the full cycle, the number and impact of disasters and emergencies can be reduced.

## Public Health Responsibilities during Disasters and Emergencies

Public health plays a critical role in most emergency situations. According to the British Columbia Ministry of Health (2013), public health responsibilities include those that are directly health-related, such as influenza pandemics, as well as other emergencies/

**Figure 14.1: Disaster and Emergency Management**

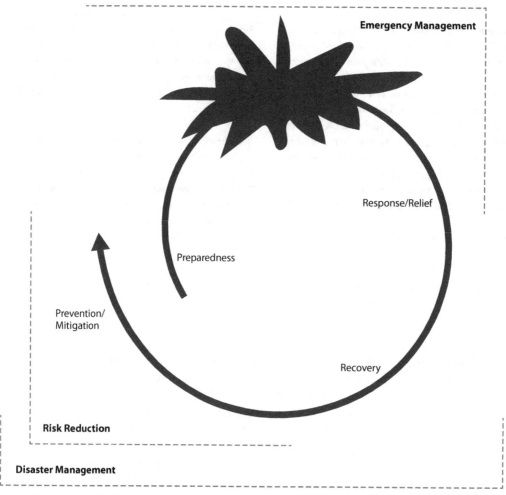

*Source*: Adapted from Public Safety Canada. (2014). *An emergency management framework for Canada* (2nd ed.). Retrieved from www.publicsafety.gc.ca/cnt/rsrcs/pblctns/mrgnc-mngmnt-frmwrk/index-eng.aspx; and World Health Organization (WHO). (2002). *Disasters and emergencies training package*. Retrieved from http://apps.who.int/disasters/repo/7656.pdf

disasters that have health consequences, such as floods, earthquakes, or forest fires. Within the health system, public health plays a key role in coordination and collaboration across several areas, including acute care, long-term care, pre-hospital, mental health, and home and community care (British Columbia Ministry of Health, 2013).

During prevention and mitigation, preparation, response, and recovery efforts, public health is responsible for fostering a population that is resilient to emergencies (British Columbia Ministry of Health, 2013). This means that public health is the local government organization responsible for preparing the population by informing them about the different types of emergencies, how to prepare their family for emergencies, and, during an actual emergency, where to obtain reliable information, maintain themselves without municipal services, and obtain assistance. **Resilience** during emergencies minimizes vulnerability, dependence, and susceptibility by strengthening the capacity to cope with, respond to, recover from, and learn from emergencies (British Columbia Ministry of Health, 2013). According to the Federal Emergency Management Agency (FEMA, 2011), incorporating the whole community approach in emergency management contributes to community security and resiliency. The three core principles of the whole community approach are: (1) understanding and meeting the actual needs of the whole community, (2) engaging and empowering all segments of the community, and (3) strengthening what usually works well in communities.

Coordination and collaboration require fast and accurate communication. If properly managed, social media can provide that service. During a disaster, **social media**, if properly managed, can assist with monitoring, communicating, and evaluation. Box 14.2 provides information and instructions for using and managing social media.

## Community Health Nursing in Disaster and Emergency Management

Research articles and reviews on nursing in disaster and emergency management consistently identify that nurses, as the largest health care workforce, have a major role as first responders/receivers, caregivers, and leaders (Baack & Alfred, 2013; Littleton-Kearney & Slepski, 2008; Stangeland, 2010; Weiner, Irwin, Trangenstein, & Gordon, 2005). Studies also identify that the limited nursing research and training in emergency management does not provide sufficient knowledge and skills for nurses to respond in a disaster with confidence and authority (Jacobson et al., 2010; Stangeland, 2010; Veenema, 2006). For example, a three-year survey of schools of nursing in the US, begun immediately following September 11, 2001, showed that the amount of disaster preparedness in the curriculum remained at four hours and that 75 percent of nursing faculty felt inadequately prepared to teach the content (Weiner et al., 2005).

Recommendations for training include the principles of disaster preparedness, mass casualty care and disaster management skills (Littleton-Kearney & Slepski, 2008), and the ethical and legal issues that arise during a disaster (Aliakbari, Hammad, Bahrami, & Aein, 2014). Preferred training methods include small group workshops with instructor-led and Internet-based training (Jacobson et al., 2010). (See "Website Resources" in this chapter for relevant links.)

---

BOX 14.2
**Social Media in Disasters**

During the Oregon wildfires in 2011, *Emergency Management* reported that a Virtual Operations Support Team (VOST) was activated to keep emergency communications and response updated for 19 days (Katims, 2013). The magazine article explains that each VOST contains a leader and a team of individuals trained to use social media to support affected organizations and jurisdictions during a disaster. The article concludes by stating that every emergency management organization should build a VOST to be prepared to keep up with the constant and overwhelming flow of information during a disaster.

As an indication of the widespread use of mobile phones, a survey conducted with 495 Medical Reserve Corps coordinators and volunteers identified that 99 percent owned a mobile phone (Scheller, Peck, & Olson, 2014). However, only 23 percent used them during a response to browse the Internet for emergency response information. The study found that 80 percent preferred to use email to send or receive response instructions.

The DelValle Institute for Emergency Preparedness (2014) in Boston provides the following guidance for effectively using social media for emergency management:
1. Develop social media policies related to monitoring, communicating, and evaluation.
2. Use Twitter to communicate with the public, TweetDeck to manage information, and Twitter Alerts to receive emergency updates from specific organizations.
3. Explore geographical data before, during, and after emergency.
4. Cross-train staff to become part of a VOST.

The focus of community health nursing during emergency management is promoting community resilience and mitigating the potential for physical or psychological illness and injury during the stress of emergency situations. The following sections expand on the principles of disaster preparedness by describing the community health nursing responsibilities in the four components of disaster and emergency management: prevention and mitigation, preparedness, response, and recovery.

## Emergency Prevention and Mitigation

The three broad roles for community health nurses in prevention and mitigation are: (1) using their knowledge of the community to identify and report potential risks or hazards, (2) working on community and organizational emergency management committees, and (3) specific involvement in identifying and planning support for vulnerable populations.

The broad perspective of community health nurses is particularly important in preventing and mitigating disasters because they are aware of concerns and vulnerabilities from their work in the community. Concerns such as substandard housing and isolated elderly become major issues in an emergency.

An example of concerns escalating into a series of disasters involves Attawapiskat, a First Nations community on the shore of Hudson Bay in Northern Ontario. Attawapiskat first made the news in 2011 with the announcement that the community was experiencing a severe housing crisis. The Chiefs of Ontario (2011) identified that 128 families were living in condemned buildings, 19 families were living in makeshift sheds without water or electricity, and 5 families were living in uninsulated tents. Some improvements were made by the federal government, but the basic infrastructure still remains substandard. In 2013, parts of the village were evacuated because of a fire in a trailer park, and in 2013 and 2014, parts were again evacuated due to flooding (Tahirali, 2014).

Knowledge of the physical structures of the community helps community health nurses to identify potential hazards, such as a sudden flow of water down a street, vehicle congestion following a special event, or limited security around road or building sites. They also know where to report such hazards. They know the location of resources, such as the fire station, and how the resources are used, such as the numerous activities that take place at the elementary school.

In this and all components of disaster and community management, community health nurses become members of organizational and municipal disaster planning groups. Community health nurses not only contribute their expertise but also gain information and assistance in recognizing and addressing community health issues. They are also in a position to ask about plans to use social media to keep the community informed and to provide a quick means of communication among emergency workers.

Part of the prevention and mitigation component is informing the community about potential emergencies. Government and other organizations provide very useful resources on their websites to help people prepare for emergencies. For example, a Federal Emergency Management Agency (2014a) website assists kids, parents, and educators in planning for a disaster. The educators' section has material on a variety of disaster topics, such as emergency preparedness, structured in three groupings that encompass

The team assigned to the assessment of vulnerability has some help in getting started. The public health nurse advisor serves on the city emergency management committee dealing with vulnerable populations and provides an initial list of 10 organizations with contact names and phone numbers from the committee.

After the team has familiarized themselves with the sociodemographics of the city, and the city and national websites on emergencies and disasters, they meet with the advisor to discuss how to use the list of organizations. They could just start at the top of the list and call them all or could call a few who could help them work out an approach to use with the others. The advisor likes the idea of starting with a few people who would collaborate with them. She indicates four people on the list who would be helpful and provide different perspectives. The team decides that the purpose is to identify key community organizations serving vulnerable people and to develop a common approach with them that the organizations can use in informing their clients about potential disasters.

The team then explains that all the websites dealing with disasters have detailed information about preparing an emergency kit. Although the information about the emergency kits is quite consistent across websites, the team wonders if the information is provided anywhere else and if people are given any assistance in preparing the kit. Considering the

vulnerability of the people they are assessing, the team feels that the emergency kit, with supplies like extra water and medication, is very important. The advisor says that the issue was raised at the committee meeting, but has not been addressed. She thinks it would be a good issue to raise during the assessment.

With advice from the initial key informants from the Meals on Wheels program, a church with a homeless shelter, a social worker from the city low-cost housing, and a home care manager, the team organizes short Internet teleconferences with groups of three to five key informants and the advisor. At each teleconference, they discuss various options to identify vulnerable people and ways to inform them of how to prepare for an emergency, including preparing an emergency kit. The team analyzes the responses and provides a report that includes useful options for providing disaster information and support for preparing an emergency kit that the advisor will give to the city management committee.

**Discussion Topics and Questions**

3. What community health nursing values, processes, and beliefs (Chapter 1) were involved in emergency planning with organizations serving vulnerable people?

4. Which nursing standards and competencies apply to the work the team is doing for the city emergency management committee?

grades 1 to 12. (Links are provided in "Website Resources" at the end of the chapter.)

Another responsibility of community health nursing in this first component is assessing the vulnerabilities of community members (ACHNE, 2008). People who are vulnerable in normal circumstances because of lack of income, education, social supports, age, or disability become even more vulnerable during an emergency. For example, if a storm were threatening an area, vulnerable people might not hear about it because they are less connected to others and may not listen or have access to news reports. This would mean that they would likely not have extra food, flashlights, medications, or water on hand to weather the storm. Vulnerable people would also be less likely to know about or attend immunization clinics unless special efforts were made to make the clinics accessible to them.

Assessing the community to identify vulnerable people requires teamwork, engagement of community organizations and services, and following a process. Teamwork allows you to cover a larger area using a consistent and efficient process. The assessment process detailed in Chapters 3 and 4—orientation, review of secondary data, mapping of the community, and interviewing key informants—can help you identify the organizations and programs serving vulnerable people. During prevention and mitigation, the process would likely involve partnering with the different community organizations, such as homeless shelters, drop-in programs for women and single mothers, churches, home care services, social services, and low-income housing managers, to tailor an approach for each organization to identify, inform, and refer vulnerable people in the case of a disaster.

## Emergency Preparedness

Preparedness is closer in time to a potential or actual emergency than prevention and mitigation. During preparedness, actual plans are put in place to deal with a disaster and team training occurs. Preparation occurs throughout the community and country with individuals and families, organizations, communities, municipalities, and regional and national governments. The activities involved in preparedness focus community planning and training on individual and family emergency planning, and pandemic planning.

### Preparing Plans and Training

Preparation emphasizes the updating of local disaster and emergency plans and conducting training, and community health nurses have important roles to play in both areas (ACHNE, 2008). In preparation, community health nurses continue to contribute their knowledge of the community in planning but the plans become more specific. Plans are developed to manage command and control functions during an emergency, organize mass immunization clinics, or arrange an emergency shelter.

These planning activities, whether at the state/provincial/territorial or local municipal level, follow a format determined at the national level. In Canada, most municipalities, provinces, and territories have their own Emergency Measures Organization (Government of Canada, 2013b). US emergency organizations can be found on the Public Health Emergency (2014) website.

Community health nurses need to be aware of the universal incident management system, called the IMS, so they can effectively assist with local planning and understand reporting structures once a disaster occurs (ACHNE, 2008). The **incident management system** (IMS) provides a standardized approach to emergency management at the international, national, and local levels in five areas: command, operations, planning, logistics, and finance/administration (Federal Emergency Management Agency [FEMA], 2014b). During an emergency, community health nurses usually work in the area of operations but a few may be assigned to the command or planning sections.

Community health nurses are involved in disaster training both at the organization and community levels. Organizational training includes education, and exercises could focus on mass immunization clinics or home assessments during an emergency. Community disaster training can involve a few or multiple community organizations participating in some aspect of a mock disaster situation. Mock disasters could mimic a plane or train crash, a bomb threat in a building, or contamination of the municipal drinking water.

Disaster and emergency training are necessary for people to prepare mentally for working during a disaster and to learn the necessary knowledge and skills. Governments at all levels in the US (FEMA, 2013) and Canada (Emergency Management Ontario, 2009) provide detailed information on planning, conducting, and evaluating emergency training exercises. Both sources emphasize the importance of an established emergency training program over unevaluated occasional exercises that are relatively unconnected to emergency management. A training program is a risk-based process for programming exercises that tests elements of your emergency plan, including equipment and the functions of personnel. It enables you to plan the best series of exercises for your organization, conduct the exercises, evaluate each exercise to see if it tested what you planned to test, and analyze the results so that you are able to make any needed changes and report the results to your emergency management committee (Emergency Management Ontario, 2009). Since this programming is similar to the community health nursing process, community health nurses are a valuable asset in preparing and conducing training programs in their organization and the community.

Two basic types of exercises are used in training programs (Emergency Management Ontario, 2009): discussion-based and operations-based. Discussion-based exercises familiarize participants with current, or develop new, plans, policies, agreements, and procedures. In community health nursing, a discussion-based exercise might be used to develop policy on the elements and timing of emergency training. Operations-based exercises validate plans, policies, agreements, and procedures; clarify roles and responsibilities; and identify resource gaps in an operational environment, either within an organization or in a community. In community health nursing, an operations-based exercise might be conducted with municipal housing services to identify people who would need assistance if a disaster resulted in a power outage.

## Individual and Family Preparedness

Community health nurses have an important role in helping to inform families and the community about how to prepare for an emergency, including preparing their own emergency kit (ACHNE, 2008). Community health nurses are role models for health in the community, and their descriptions of preparing their emergency kits help to emphasize the importance of preparation. Individuals and families need to be prepared to keep informed of the disaster developments and be able to take care of their most important needs for 72 hours following a disaster. Seventy-two hours is the longest time they would expect to wait before rescue services could reach them in most types of disasters. Both the US government (FEMA, 2014a) and the Canadian government (Government of Canada, 2013a) provide extensive information on their websites to encourage individuals, families with children and pets, and people with disabilities to plan for emergencies, keep informed, and prepare an emergency kit. Canada designates the first full week in May as Emergency Preparedness Week, and the US designates September as National Preparedness Month. Community health nurses can work with other community groups to raise awareness about the need for families to learn about disasters and how to prepare. They can help organize or promote events associated with emergency preparedness.

## Pandemic Preparedness

Preparedness for a pandemic outbreak is a paramount concern for public and community health nursing. No one can predict specifics, but everyone can keep up to date on the general approach to dealing with a pandemic and skills such as infection control and immunization. A **pandemic** is a global disease outbreak whose status as such is determined by how the disease spreads, and not how many deaths it causes (Department of Health and Human Services, 2014). When a new or novel influenza A virus emerges, a flu pandemic can occur because the human population has little to no immunity against it. The World Health Organization (WHO) is responsible for designating when a disease outbreak has reached a certain pandemic level (WHO, 2009a). Yearly influenza outbreaks do not spread as readily because the population already has some immunity.

The main strategy in reducing the effects of a pandemic influenza is through mass immunization. Mass immunization campaigns have the objective of immunizing large populations over a short period of time and often require the use of locations outside normal health care settings (World Health Organization, 2015).

Studying the management of previous infectious disease outbreaks can lead to better planning and preparedness for future pandemics. Both the Severe Acute Respiratory Syndrome (SARS) in 2003 and the H1N1 flu virus in 2009 have been studied and compared. SARS is particularly important in Canada because, after China and Hong Kong, Toronto was the region most intensely hit by SARS. More than one hundred health care workers were particularly affected, and three died (Health Canada, 2003, p. 20). The H1N1 flu virus reached the level of a global pandemic in June 2009 (WHO, 2009a), and it affected more young and healthy people than regular flu (WHO, 2009b). Many First Nations, Inuit, and Métis communities, pregnant women, and individuals with an underlying medical condition were found to be at an increased risk of severe illness from H1N1 infection (Public Health Agency of Canada [PHAC], 2010). A WHO review of the 2009 H1N1 pandemic (Fineberg, 2014) identified strengths of recently implemented procedures, as well as a number of deficiencies. Community health nursing can use these findings, such as difficulties in decision making under conditions of uncertainty, and challenges in communication among experts, policy makers, and the public, in planning and training.

The issues that were identified after SARS continued to plague nurses working on the front lines during H1N1. Box 14.3 lists the continuing issues from both outbreaks. Most of the issues undermine the ability of public and community health nurses working directly with the public to appropriately perform their work. This not only creates physical and moral stress for the nurses, but also reduces the trust the community has in the government provision of health services. The nurses in the immunization clinics realize that they are the "personal face of the pandemic" because of their personal and professional connections (Hodge, 2014, p. 7).

Two concepts in emergency management can assist community health nurses in dealing with decision making and communication and other issues during a pandemic: surge capacity and continuity of operations plans. **Surge capacity** is the ability to obtain adequate staff and supplies and equipment, and maintain structures and systems, to provide sufficient care to meet the immediate needs of an influx of patients following a large-scale incident or disaster (Adams, 2009). **Continuity of Operations Plans** (COOPs) identify and rank critical services, identify and plan for possible disruption, and allow programs to continue their most important operations.

## Disaster Response

In disaster response, community health nurses are involved in team activities with other sectors, including the police, firefighters, health care personnel, and others as required during and following a disaster. Disasters that have no forewarning, such as terrorist attacks, and other man-made disasters, such as train, plane, or massive vehicle crashes, are particularly difficult to respond to. Natural disasters involving the weather, earthquakes, and viruses provide varying degrees of warning. Response has two approximate phases: the rescue phase and the care phase.

### Rescue Phase

The initial response is to rescue people and stabilize unsafe structures. If there are massive casualties, the next requirement is to triage injured people so that those most injured receive priority treatment. **Triage** is a method for classifying victims according to the severity of their injuries, based on the likelihood of their survival and on the physicians available. Triage takes place in three stages (Pan American Health Organization, 2012):

The team assigned to work on preparedness for pandemic influenza is briefed by the advisor, who helped in the planning, organization, delivery, and evaluation of the 2009 H1N1 mass immunization clinics. She gives them several internal documents and directs them to websites to help them become oriented to flu clinics and mass immunization clinics. She also arranges for each of them to attend different flu clinics. After reviewing the documents and websites, the team decides to look for elements of teamwork, engage community members, and follow a process during the observation of the clinics. They revise the clinic observation checklist provided in Chapter 13 so they can collect consistent information.

The observations in the four locations are quite consistent and show the nurses working as a team and functioning smoothly. In two situations, obviously new public health nurses were learning how to greet people and give the injections by working alongside an experienced nurse. A process was used to guide people to an immunization table and then to the wait area. Each nurse also followed a process with each person that included asking adults about children and older family members, and providing health education on hand washing and safe coughing.

The team's observations contrast sharply with the information they have on mass immunization clinics during H1N1. Although the actual process involved in giving the injection is the same, the student team members realize from their readings that the context surrounding the process would be much more chaotic. In a pandemic, there would be far more people anxiously seeking vaccinations being greeted by an insufficient number of prepared nurses, lack of staffing for critical services, hastily arranged locations, unavailable supplies, and inexperienced support staff to organize people, supplies, and security. The team knows that they can not deal with all of these issues and meet with their advisor to decide what area to consider. She recommends that they deal with surge capacity related to nursing staff. She explains that continuity of operations needs to be addressed but requires negotiation among several department managers.

The advisor does not specify the number of people needed for the surge capacity, but proposes that they brainstorm with staff and others in the community to identify initiatives that could be developed later. The team decides to follow the process for key informant interviews and develop the following five open-ended questions:

1. Do you have experience working in an immunization clinic? If yes: What would be the most difficult part of preparing more nurses for work in mass immunization clinics? If no: What would help to prepare you for work in an immunization clinic?
2. How or where could sufficient nursing and other health care staff be recruited?
3. How could unprepared staff be trained?
4. How could teamwork and support be built into the training and clinic functioning?
5. What other suggestions do you have for preparing people for mass immunization clinics?

The students spend four weeks meeting with from one to three public health nurses whenever they are available. They meet with their faculty instructor to identify who to consult in their nursing program about forming a partnership during an influenza pandemic. They also search the Internet to find relevant resources. Their report includes suggestions such as who to contact at their nursing program about a potential partnership. The team found that their contact was willing to discuss public health access to the nurse training manikins and, in turn, receive clinical placement opportunities related to infection control. The team also suggests recruiting nurses by contacting local nursing organizations to organize a phone or email fan-out system.

The question about teamwork promoted a lot of discussion and seemed very important to everyone. Several ideas were proposed, including support for the idea from the literature about pairing new and experienced nurses. The advisor feels that the suggestions are very worthwhile and that some will certainly end up in the organization's pandemic plan.

**Discussion Topics and Questions**
5. Why was it useful for the team to observe at the regular immunization clinics?
6. How did the team include process in the investigation?
7. What nursing standards and competencies would apply in working on preparation for a pandemic?

1. On-site triage is carried out where victims are found, to distinguish those who need immediate medical care (rapid transport to the victim assembly area) from those who can wait.
2. Medical triage is carried out by medical personnel upon admission to the victim assembly area, and determines what level of care is needed.
3. Evacuation triage classifies victims according to their priority for transfer to a hospital prepared to receive them.

The personnel involved in triage usually have specific training or expertise in determining priorities at each stage. However, depending on the situation, community health nurses, without specific training, may be involved in triage functions using easy-to-follow guides.

Shortly after the disaster, people start reacting in different ways. These reactions, as listed in Box 14.4, can occur in victims, observers, emergency workers, and community members, in the disaster area and in emergency shelters.

Community health nurses have a crucial role at this time to identify symptoms or illnesses that differ from normal reactions (ACHNE, 2008), and identify and help people showing signs of distress. Unusual symptoms that might be the result of a biological or chemical substance require immediate action to alert authorities and to send the people for specialist care.

People showing signs of distress need to know that it is a normal reaction to a disaster. However, the distress may be heightened for some people because the disaster triggers previous traumatic experiences. If the person is part of the response effort, removing them from the immediate environment and giving them time to process their reactions can usually assist them in recovering and returning to their duties. Community members also need to be removed to a quiet place where they can work through the reason for their reactions and possibly talk out their feelings with a receptive person. In both situations, people need to know that this reaction may return at unexpected times.

BOX 14.4
**Feelings and Reactions to Violent Events**

Reactions to stressful events such as a disaster or terrorist attack can affect people in the following ways:

- Physically, including headaches, back pain, stomach aches, diarrhea, problems with sleeping, tightness in neck and shoulders, low energy or general tiredness, loss of appetite or tendency to eat more comforting foods or use more alcohol, drugs, and tobacco.
- Emotionally, including feeling sad, angry, guilty, helpless, numb, confused, discouraged, worried, anxious, and fearful about a reoccurrence. Emotions can come and go like being on a rollercoaster; they may disappear, then return suddenly.
- Thinking, including difficulty in concentrating, thinking about the events, and remembering day-to-day things. Previous sad or difficult times may surface or come out of nowhere when doing something else.
- Sense of safety, including finding it hard to leave home or loved ones, wanting to overprotect children, or be nervous about travelling by plane.

*Source*: Public Health Agency of Canada, 2011.

## Care Phase

In the care phase, people are less likely to be directly injured as a result of the disaster, but they can become ill from the effects. Disasters such as tornados, floods, ice storms, earthquakes, and bombs destroy homes and public services, such as electrical power, water, and sewage. This damage requires the provision of emergency shelters for at-risk or vulnerable people who no longer have a home or cannot manage without public services. **Emergency shelter** is temporary accommodation organized to provide living quarters, food, and assistance with daily living and health care needs during an emergency. The determination of at-risk populations is not straightforward (Minnesota Department of Health, 2013). Certain factors listed in Box 14.5 can place people who are already dealing with difficulties at increased risk for health concerns.

Community health nurses are involved in identifying people at risk during a disaster and directing them to appropriate care services. The most usual care service for those not needing immediate medical care in a disaster is an emergency shelter. When an emergency is declared and the need for emergency shelter identified, usually a charitable organization, such as the Red Cross or Salvation Army in the US and Canada, works with local emergency organizations to provide emergency services. The disaster relief organizations strive to meet people's basic human needs by providing shelter, food, and health and emotional health service, and assist individuals and families in resuming their normal daily activities independently. They also feed emergency workers.

Community health nurses have important roles in caring for people in emergency shelters, possibly in the management of care services and definitely in providing nursing care. The American Red Cross (Springer & Casey-Lockyer, 2014) conducted research on emergency shelter management during disasters occurring between 2005 and 2013 to identify effective procedures and provide accurate data on shelter clients. The new tested procedures, called "Cot-to-Cot," include registration and daily observation and interviews of all shelter clients (Springer, 2013a, 2013b). The initial shelter intake now makes only two observations and asks just two questions of new shelter residents to help them immediately, if needed, and make them aware that help is available.

Within the first 24 hours, or preferably within 6 to 8 hours, the Red Cross nurses institute the Cot-to-Cot system using CMIST. **CMIST** is an acronym that describes a system to help identify access and the functional needs of people in emergency management related to **communication**, **medical needs** (maintaining health), **independence**, **supervision** (services, support, and self-determination), and **transport** (Minnesota Department of Health, 2013; Springer, 2013b; University of New Hampshire Institute of Disability, 2014). The shelter research (Springer & Casey-Lockyer, 2014) indicates that by the third day, clients are more comfortable with the setting, less anxious about the evacuation, more familiar with and trusting of the shelter staff, and thus more able to share their health, mental health, and ADL (activities of daily living) support needs. By 2013, the Red Cross surveillance system was more robust and identified that chronic disease management, minor acute illness, and behavioral health issues were the most common concerns seen in disaster shelters.

Community health nurses, who in most cases might work once or twice in their

The team assigned to work on contributing to plans to manage emergency shelters is placed with the emergency management officer for the city. They wonder at first how to start, but that uncertainty is quickly dispelled. Peter, their advisor, reviews the presentation by J. Springer (2013a) with them and states that the slides titled "Who are your partners?" and "What can your partners bring?" (slides 33 and 34) have the information he needs for preparing plans for emergency shelters. He explains that he already has a list of city departments that would be involved with emergency shelters, but feels that many nongovernment organizations could be included. The team reviews the information they have and draft a list of questions to use. When they next meet with Peter, they have a list of 12 organizations. Peter provides a couple more. One of the students explains that she has been part of a university committee looking at the use of social media in health care. She suggests that this committee would be a good resource. The others agree.

The team and advisor work out an introductory statement for the team to use when they contact people, questions to start the discussion, and the process they will use. They include a question on how organizations communicate with their staff and clients. They feel that the question is important because they want to know if a communication system using some type of Internet device would be feasible. After some discussion, they decide to add a question on specific people who would be interested in helping to manage emergency shelters, rather than just organizations.

At the end of four weeks, the team has identified potential partners who have expertise and resources in working with people who are homeless, blind, hard of hearing, First Nations/American Native, disabled, and have limited English. They have identified organizations that could provide clothing and toys for children. They have found that at least three-quarters of the employees use the Internet at least weekly. Fewer older adults use mobile phones but many use laptops for email and searching the Internet. The majority of other clients, including most new immigrant groups, use mobile phones. The discussion with the university social media committee is also productive. Peter arranges a meeting for them with the city technology department and will provide them with a summary of the results of the question on communication. The team is amazed at how enthusiastic people are to join the city's emergency management efforts. They prepare their report with the list of organizations, contact names and information, and their responses to the questions.

**Discussion Topics and Questions**

8. What process from earlier chapters was used by the team, and how did it differ from the earlier application?

9. How were the social determinants of health and social justice considered in this scenario?

10. What nursing standards and competencies apply to working in an emergency shelter?

career in an emergency shelter, can use the information from the Red Cross and other resources provided in "Website Resources" to adjust their practice to the shelter situation. The best approach is to pace the amount and type of interaction you have with clients based on their ability to respond. For example, in the first few days of being in a shelter, most clients will feel fragile and have difficulty absorbing a lot of information. Therefore, keep information simple and to the point to help them understand how the shelter is set up and how to situate themselves to become more comfortable. Immediate assistance would consist of the provision of first aid, food, water, and a bed. Later, their health, mental health, and activities of daily living would be addressed. When you have observed that clients are somewhat settled, nursing care can move to determining necessary emotional and spiritual support by using effective communication approaches, such as active listening and the 15-minute family interview (see Chapter 9).

Government websites (DisasterAssistance.gov, 2014; Public Health Agency of Canada, 2011) provide extensive information and resources for families, children, and people with disabilities during disaster recovery. Children in particular need additional support. Encourage parents of children under the age of three to consistently reassure them by saying "I will keep you safe." School-age children and adolescents need honest, factual information (e.g., "I don't know right now, but I will tell you when I do"), someone to listen to their feelings, regular routines such as bedtime storytelling, and an assigned role, such as entertaining younger children. They need to be directed away from extensive TV or online viewing of the disaster and into other activities such as drawing, games, or reading.

An emergency shelter quickly becomes a community. Community health nurses can contribute to the health of the community both by following a process to identify and address immediate needs, and later developing a relationship to explore and address less immediate medical, emotional, and social needs. This nursing approach with shelter clients can help them quickly return home once the community environment is safe.

## Recovery

Recovery has no specific start date following an emergency, but people might start talking about being in "recovery mode" when the physical evidence of the disaster starts being removed and they can think of carrying on with their lives with the memory, and not the burden, of the disaster. Recovery involves repairing physical, social, psychological, and economic damage. Actions include clean up and repair of the public and family environment, healing from physical and psychological injuries, and learning to deal with losses.

In recovery, people and governments are more open to consider ways to prevent or reduce the disaster. At this stage, community health nurses help to identify potential hazards related to damaged structures or contaminated water or food. At the community level, a crucial role is to bring the population health perspective to post-disaster evaluation and reconstruction. The community health nursing role is to be involved in the evaluation of process and outcomes (ACHNE, 2008), especially to indicate how health care and services could have been more effective for vulnerable groups during the disaster. They also identify what aspects of the disaster preparation and response were successful and how to build on those aspects to bridge the gaps. By focusing on improving the health of the community, community health nurses can help move disaster reconstruction and policy beyond recovery.

## Summary

Working on the four components of disaster and emergency management provides students and new practitioners the opportunity to apply the skills and knowledge that they have gained throughout this text. They learn to consider community health concepts, such as the social determinants of health and social justice, in working to provide supports for vulnerable people, teamwork when making and carrying out plans together, engaging organizations to bring them into emergency management planning, and following a process. Discussion questions on the application of the community health and public health nursing standards and competencies help to make the guidelines relevant to their developing community health nursing practice.

## Classroom and Seminar Exercises

1. Discuss how the community health process applies to the components of disaster and emergency management.
2. Explain why vulnerable people are more affected by a disaster.
3. Identify which type of disaster would change the type of health services provided in an emergency shelter.
4. Explain how the harnessing of social media would benefit each component of disaster and emergency management.
5. Review each of the three scenarios in the chapter to identify the particular contribution made by the student team.

## References

Adams, L. (2009). *Exploring the concept of surge capacity.* Retrieved from www.nursingworld. org/MainMenuCategories/ANAMarketplace/ANAPeriodicals/OJIN/TableofContents/ Vol142009/No2May09/Articles-Previous-Topics/Surge-Capacity.html

Aliakbari, F., Hammad, K., Bahrami, M., & Aein, F. (2014, July 2). Ethical and legal challenges associated with disaster nursing. *Nursing Ethics.* doi:10.1177/0969733014534877

American Nurses Association. (2013). *Public health nursing: Scope and standards of practice* (2nd ed.). Silver Springs, MD: American Nurses Association.

Association of Community Health Nursing Educators (ACHNE). (2008). *Disaster preparedness white paper for community/public health nursing educators.* Retrieved from www.achne.org/ files/public/DisasterPreparednessWhitePaper.pdf

Baack, S., & Alfred, D. (2013). Nurses' preparedness and perceived competence in managing disasters. *Journal of Nursing Scholarship, 45*(3). doi:10.1111/jnu.12029

British Columbia Ministry of Health. (2013). *Promote, protect, prevent: Our health begins here: BC's guiding framework for public health* (Goal 7, Public Health Emergency Management). Retrieved from www.health.gov.bc.ca/library/publications/year/2013/BC-guiding- framework-for-public-health.pdf

Chiefs of Ontario. (2011). *Housing crisis at Attawapiskat.* Retrieved from www.chiefs-of- ontario.org/housing-crisis

Community Health Nurses of Canada. (2009, May). *Public health nursing discipline specific competencies Version 1.0.* Retrieved from www.chnc.ca/competencies.cfm

Community Health Nurses of Canada. (2010, March). *Home health nursing competencies Version 1.0.* Retrieved from www.chnc.ca/competencies.cfm

Community Health Nurses of Canada. (2011, March). *Canadian community health nursing: Professional practice model & standards of practice.* Retrieved from www.chnc.ca/nursing- standards-of-practice.cfm

DelValle Institute for Emergency preparedness. (2014). *Social media.* Retrieved from https://delvalle.bphc.org/mod/wiki/view.php?pageid=106

Department of Health and Human Services. (2014). *Flu watch.* Retrieved from www.flu.gov/

DisasterAssistance.gov. (2014). *Disaster assistance and information.* Retrieved from www.disasterassistance.gov/

Emergency Management Ontario. (2009). *EM125 exercise program: An introduction.* Retrieved from www.emergencymanagementontario.ca/stellent/groups/public/@mcscs/@www/@emo/documents/abstract/em125.pdf

Emergency Management Ontario. (2010). *Emergency management doctrine for Ontario.* Retrieved from www.emergencymanagementontario.ca/stellent/groups/public/@mcscs/@www/@emo/documents/abstract/ec081624.pdf

Federal Emergency Management Agency (FEMA). (2011). *A whole community approach to emergency management: Principles, themes, and pathways for action* (FDOC 104-008-1). Retrieved from www.fema.gov/media-library-data/20130726-1813-25045-0649/whole_community_dec2011__2_.pdf

Federal Emergency Management Agency (FEMA). (2013). *National preparedness directorate national training and education.* Retrieved from www.training.fema.gov

Federal Emergency Management Agency (FEMA). (2014a). *Ready: Prepare, plan, stay informed.* Retrieved from www.ready.gov/

Federal Emergency Management Agency (FEMA). (2014b). *National incident management system.* Retrieved from www.fema.gov/national-incident-management-system

Fineberg, H. (2014). Pandemic Preparedness and Response—Lessons from the H1N1 Influenza of 2009. *New England Journal of Medicine, 370,* 1335–1342. DOI: 10.1056/NEJMra1208802

Government of Canada. (2013a). 72 hours. *Get Prepared.* Retrieved from www.getprepared.gc.ca/index-eng.aspx

Government of Canada. (2013b). Emergency measures organizations. *Get Prepared.* Retrieved from www.getprepared.gc.ca/cnt/rsrcs/mrgnc-mgmt-rgnztns-eng.aspx

Health Canada. (2003). *Learning from SARS: Renewal of public health in Canada.* Retrieved from www.phac-aspc.gc.ca/publicat/sars-sras/pdf/sars-e.pdf

Hodge, J. (2014). *Canadian healthcare workers' experiences during pandemic H1N1 influenza: Lessons from Canada's response: A review of the qualitative literature.* Retrieved from https://cdn.metricmarketing.ca/www.nccid.ca/files/Evidence_Reviews/HCW_H1N1_Lessons_E.pdf

Jacobson, H., Soto Mas, F., Hsu, C., Turley, J., Miller, J., & Kim, M. (2010). Self-assessed emergency readiness and training needs of nurses in rural Texas. *Public Health Nursing, 27*(1), 41–48. doi:10.1111/j. 1525-1446.2009.00825.x

Katims, L. (2013, October 2). Virtual operations support teams (VOST) harness social media. *Emergency Management.* Retrieved from www.emergencymgmt.com/disaster/Virtual-Operations-Support-Teams-Social-Media.html

Littleton-Kearney, M., & Slepski, L. (2008). Directions for disaster education in the United States. *Critical Care Nursing Clinics of North America, 20*(1), 103–109, viii. doi:10.1016/j.ccell 2007.10.008

Minnesota Department of Health. (2013). *Who might be considered "at risk" populations during disaster and crisis.* Retrieved from www.health.state.mn.us/oep/responsesystems/atriskshort.html

Pan American Health Organization. (2012). 6.1. Pre-hospital management of massive numbers of victims. *Knowledge Center on Public Health and Disasters.* Retrieved from www.saludydesastres.info/index.php?option=com_content&view=article&id=154:6-1-pre-hospital-management-of-massive-numbers-of-victims&catid=205&Itemid=1056&lang=en

Public Health Agency of Canada. (2010). ARCHIVED - Lessons Learned Review: Public Health Agency of Canada and Health Canada Response to the 2009 H1N1 Pandemic. Retrieved from www.phac-aspc.gc.ca/about_apropos/evaluation/reports-rapports/2010-2011/h1n1/context-contexte-eng.php

Public Health Agency of Canada. (2011). *Taking care of ourselves and our families and our communities.* Retrieved from www.phac-aspc.gc.ca/publicat/oes-bsu-02/pdf/communities_e.pdf

Public Health Emergency. (2009). *HHS retrospective on the 2009 H1N1 influenza pandemic to advance all hazards preparedness.* Retrieved from www.phe.gov/preparedness/mcm/h1n1-retrospective/Pages/default.aspx

Public Health Emergency. (2014). *Stay connected.* Retrieved from www.phe.gov/emergency/connect/Pages/default.aspx#state

Public Safety Canada. (2014a). *Federal policy for emergency management.* Retrieved from www.publicsafety.gc.ca/cnt/rsrcs/pblctns/plc-mrgnc-mngmnt/index-eng.aspx

Public Safety Canada. (2014b). *An emergency management framework for Canada* (2nd ed.). Retrieved from www.publicsafety.gc.ca/cnt/rsrcs/pblctns/mrgnc-mngmnt-frmwrk/index-eng.aspx

Registered Nurses of Ontario. (2005). *Position Statement: Vision for nursing in public health.* Retrieved from http://rnao.ca/policy/position-statements/vision-nursing-public-health

Scheller, A., Peck, M., & Olson, D. (2014). Mobile phone use among Medical Reserve Corps coordinators and volunteers: an exploratory study. *Journal of Emergency Management, 12*(3). doi:10.5055/jem.2014.0176

Springer, J. (2013a). *Cot-to-Cot: Identifying access and functional needs in community disaster shelters—What this means and how it applies to public health nursing practice* (PowerPoint presentation). Retrieved from www.maphn.org/Resources/Documents/Springer%20to%20Post%2007%2011%2013.pdf

Springer, J. (2013b). *Registration, Cot-to-Cot and CMIST: Identifying access and functional needs of clients in disaster shelters* (PowerPoint with Voicethread). Retrieved from https://voicethread.com/myvoice/#thread/4547245/23178366/25117391

Springer, J., & Casey-Lockyer, M. (2014). *Translating practice into policy: Disaster nursing and research in the American Red Cross.* Retrieved from https://stti.confex.com/stti/congrs14/webprogram/Paper61290.html

Stangeland, P. (2010). Disaster nursing: a retrospective review. *Critical Care Nursing Clinics of North America, 22*(4), 421–436. doi:10.1016/j.ccell.2010.09.003

Tahirali, J. (2014, May 17). Evacuations start at Attawapiskat due to flooding threat. *CTVNews.* Retrieved from www.ctvnews.ca/canada/evacuation-starts-at-attawapiskat-first-nation-due-to-flooding-threat-1.1826498

University of New Hampshire Institute of Disability. (2014). *Emergency preparedness.* Retrieved from http://iod.unh.edu/Projects/dph/EmergencyPreparedness/ep-personnel/CMIST.aspx

US Department of Education. (2010). *Action guide for emergency management at institutions of higher education.* Retrieved from http://rems.ed.gov/docs/REMS_ActionGuide.pdf

Veenema, T. (2006). Expanding educational opportunities in disaster response and emergency preparedness for nurses. *Nursing Education Perspectives, 27*(2), 93–99.

Weiner, E., Irwin, M., Trangenstein, P., & Gordon, J. (2005). Emergency preparedness curriculum in nursing schools in the United States. *Nursing Education Perspectives, 26*(6), 334–336.

World Health Organization (WHO). (2002). *Disasters and emergencies training package.* Retrieved from http://apps.who.int/disasters/repo/7656.pdf

World Health Organization (WHO). (2009a). *Current WHO phase of pandemic alert for pandemic (H1N1) 2009.* Retrieved from www.who.int/csr/disease/swineflu/phase/en/

World Health Organization (WHO). (2009b). *World now at the start of 2009 influenza pandemic.* Retrieved from www.who.int/mediacentre/news/statements/2009/h1n1_pandemic_phase6_20090611/en/index.html

World Health Organization (WHO). (2015). *Safety of mass immunization campaigns.* Retrieved from www.who.int/injection_safety/toolbox/en/AM_SafetyCampaigns.pdf

# Website Resources

## Education

American Red Cross, *Disaster Training: Disaster Health and Sheltering for Nursing Students*: www.redcross.org/take-a-class/disaster-training
    This two-part, Web-based course introduces nursing students to the role of health care and functional support needs in Red Cross Disaster Shelters. Part One is self-study, online, and can be completed within 60 to 90 minutes. Part Two, for which US nursing faculty must register, is taught by a Red Cross Disaster Health Services RN in the classroom and is a Web-based table-top exercise that takes approximately 2 hours to complete.

Association of Community Health Nursing Educators (ACHNE), *Disaster Preparedness White Paper for Community/Public Health Nursing Educators*: www.achne.org/files/public/DisasterPreparednessWhitePaper.pdf
    The ACHNE white paper identifies the basic essential curricular components for disaster preparedness, including undergraduate competencies for assessment and planning, implementation of interventions, and evaluation of process and outcomes.

## Influenza

British Columbia Centre for Disease Control, *For Health Professionals*: www.bccdc.ca/imm-vac/ForHealthProfessionals/default.htm
    This website for health care providers provides information and videos related to immunization practice and delivery, including the cold chain and immunization competency.

Centers for Disease Control and Prevention, *Guidelines for Large-Scale Influenza Vaccination Clinic Planning*: www.cdc.gov/flu/professionals/vaccination/vax_clinic.htm
    This web page provides recommendations and guidelines for planning large-scale influenza clinics.

Indiana State Department of Health, *The Local Health Department Guide for Hosting a Mass Vaccination Clinic*: http://in.gov/isdh/files/LHDGuideforHostingaMassVaccinationClinic.pdf
    This document provides detailed steps to hosting mass vaccination clinics, from getting started (including how to recruit schools or alternative sites) to evaluation (including worksheets).

Public Health Agency of Canada (PHAC): www.phac-aspc.gc.ca/index-eng.php
    The home page of the PHAC website provides the latest virus notices and travel information.

Public Health Agency of Canada, Immunization Competencies for Health Professionals: www.phac-aspc.gc.ca/im/ic-ci/index-eng.php
    This website offers resources on all aspects of immunization, including biomedical science practice and contextual issues.

World health Organization, *Vaccine Safety Basics e-Learning Course*: http://vaccine-safety-training.org/
    This online course covers characteristics of vaccines, adverse events following immunization, pharmacovigilance, vaccine safety stakeholders, and communication.

**Preparedness**

Centers for Disease Control and Prevention (CDC), Office of Public Health Preparedness and Response, *Zombie Preparedness*: www.cdc.gov/phpr/zombies.htm

CDC's "Zombie Preparedness" website offers a fun way to learn about emergency preparedness. The site provides links to a Zombie blog; a resource for educators with full lesson plans; a graphic novella, *Preparedness 101: Zombie Pandemic*, that demonstrates the importance of being prepared in an entertaining way for people of all ages; and a social media/online page.

Emergency Management Ontario (EMO), *EM125 Exercise Program: An Introduction*: www.emergencymanagementontario.ca/stellent/groups/public/@mcscs/@www/@emo/documents/abstract/em125.pdf

The EMO emergency exercise program is described in stages. It includes a scenario of an airplane disaster and sample forms.

Federal Emergency Management Agency (FEMA): www.fema.gov/

The FEMA website provides extensive information under such categories as "Plan, Prepare & Mitigate," "Disaster Survivor Assistance," "Response and Recovery," "Topics and Audiences," and others related to survival assistance.

Government of Canada, *Get Prepared: 72 Hours*: www.getprepared.gc.ca/index-eng.aspx

This website provides resources and instructions on preparing a 72-hour toolkit for families and for people with disabilities. The site includes a link to a searchable database to identify disasters by location.

Health Canada, *Emergencies and Disasters*: www.hc-sc.gc.ca/hc-ps/ed-ud/index-eng.php

The Health Canada website describes the government's role in, and provides resources for, different types of disasters.

Lessons Learned Information System (LLIS): www.llis.dhs.gov

The LLIS program of Homeland Security provides a wealth of information and frontline expertise on effective planning, training, and operational practices. The "Core Capabilities" tab includes mass care services, community resilience, and disease outbreak, and the "Mitigation Best Practices" is searchable.

MedlinePlus: *Disaster Preparation and Recovery*: www.nlm.nih.gov/medlineplus/disasterpreparationandrecovery.html

The MedlinePlus website offers an extensive list of links in categories such as specific conditions, related issues, videos and games, and topics of interest to children, women, and seniors.

Public Health Agency of Canada (PHAC), *Canadian Emergency Management Agencies/Organizations*: www.phac-aspc.gc.ca/cepr-cmiu/ophs-bssp/ctchin1-eng.php

This PHAC web page provides descriptions and links to Canadian and US emergency/disaster organizations.

Public Health Emergency (PHE), *Stay Connected*: www.phe.gov/emergency/connect/Pages/default.aspx#state

The PHE web page provides links to state and disaster organizations, and courses related to emergency and disaster management.

Ready: Prepare. Plan. Stay Informed: www.ready.gov/

Ready is a FEMA program developed to assist people in planning for a disaster. The website includes information for kids, parents, and educators.

United Nations Office for Disaster Risk Reduction, *Making Cities Resilient: A Toolkit for Local Governments*: www.unisdr.org/campaign/resilientcities/toolkit

This website provides links to case studies, guides, and references, a link to the "10 Essentials" of disaster risk reduction, and a self-assessment tool.


## Response Services including Emergency Shelters

American Red Cross, *Disaster Relief*: www.redcross.org/what-we-do/disaster-relief

Red Cross disaster relief focuses on meeting people's immediate emergency needs caused by disaster. They provide shelter, food, and health and emotional health services to address basic human needs and assist individuals and families in resuming their normal daily activities independently. The Red Cross also feeds emergency workers such as firefighters and police, handles inquiries from concerned family members outside the disaster area, and provides blood and blood products to disaster victims.

Canadian Red Cross, *Emergency Management Professionals*: www.redcross.ca/what-we-do/emergencies-and-disasters/for-emergency-management-professionals-and-voluntary-sector-organizations/emergency-management-professionals

This website explains the role (similar to that of the American Red Cross) of the Canadian Red Cross during a disaster.

Commonwealth of Massachusetts, *Public Safety: Massachusetts Statewide Mass Care Shelter Coordination Plan*: www.mass.gov/eopss/agencies/mema/massachusetts-mass-care-shelter-coordination-plan.html

Developed in 2014, this plan describes local mass care and shelter options that communities may provide, such as personal care sites (warming or cooling centers), locally initiated over-night shelters, and locally initiated multi-community (or regional) shelters. The coordination plan also introduces the concept of State Initiated Regional Shelters.

Centers for Disease Control and Prevention (CDC). *Emergency Preparedness and Response Training Resources*: http://cdc.gov/coca/trainingresources.asp

This CDC website for Clinician Outreach and Communication Activity (COCA) provides timely, accurate, and credible information to clinicians related to training for emergency preparedness and response and emerging public health threats, and fosters partnerships with national clinician organizations to strengthen information-sharing networks.

DisasterAssistance.gov, *Information*: www.disasterassistance.gov/disaster-information

This site provides links to information on disaster-related topics, such as immediate needs, moving forward, community resources, disabilities or access and functional needs, older Americans, children and families, and fact sheets (youth materials).

Medical Reserve Corps of Greater Kansas City, *MRCKC Training: Videos for Volunteers in Disaster Shelters*: www.mrckc.org/shelter-videos.html

The Medical Reserve Corps website provides effective short videos that demonstrate therapeutic practices in a shelter in five categories: the basics (e.g., initiating a conversation), physical care, medical equipment, psychological care, and miscellaneous (e.g., feeding and assisting people who are deaf or blind).

National Mass Care Strategy: http://nationalmasscarestrategy.org/about/

The National Mass Care Strategy website includes resources and outlines its focus on the delivery of mass care services, including household pets, reunification, shelter, feeding, and training and exercises.

Pan American Health Organization, *Knowledge Center on Public Health and Disasters: Health Response in Emergencies and Disasters*: www.saludydesastres.info/index.php?option=com_content&view=article&id=77&Itemid=1019&lang=en

This website is organized into nine health response topics, including health sector interventions and operations, and mass casualty management.

The Salvation Army (Canada), *Emergency Disaster Services*: www.salvationarmy.ca/about/eds/

This Salvation Army (Canada) web page describes their emergency food trucks, training programs, and other emergency relief services.

The Salvation Army (US), *Disaster Relief Services*: http://disaster.salvationarmyusa.org/aboutus/?ourservices

The Salvation Army (US) website describes their services and provides a link to find more about disaster services in each state.

# Tools and Resources
# to Guide Teamwork
# and the Community Project

This appendix includes the tools and resources needed to guide and document team development and the work on community projects on a daily or weekly basis. Since documentation is required in professional practice and promotes learning, these tools and resources support practice by providing structure, guidance, and accountability.

Appendix A.1 provides a list of the tools and resources and indicates where they are described in the text. Appendix A.2 provides the tools and resources for team development, communication, reflection, and evaluation first described in Chapter 2. Appendix A.3 provides the tools and resources that guide the project: the work plan, timeline, and project report. These guides are introduced in Chapters 3 to 5.

## Appendix A.1:
## Tools and Resources Used in Teamwork and Community Project

Table A.1 provides the number, name, and order for each tool and resource in the Appendix. The table also includes the chapter where each is introduced within the text. Teams, instructors, and supervisors can determine which resource is to be used by everyone and which are optional. We strongly recommend that four resources are used: the team agreement, the weekly report, either the work plan and/or the timeline, and the relevant project report.

**Table A.1**

| Number | Name | Chapter Introduced |
|--------|------|--------------------|
| A.2.1 | Pre-clinical assessment[1] | 2 |
| A.2.2 | Team agreement[2] | 2 |
| A.2.3 | Weekly report[2] | 2 |
| A.2.4 | Meeting agenda[1] | 2 |
| A.2.5 | Reflection[1] | 2 |
| A.2.6 | Self-assessment of functioning on team[1] | 2 |
| A.2.7 | Individual assessment of team functioning[1] | 2 |
| A.3.1 | Work plans[3] | 3, 6 |
| A.3.2 | Timelines[3] | 3, 6 |
| A.3.3 | Project reports[2] | 5, 8 |

Notes:
1. Optional
2. Strongly recommended
3. Strongly recommend using either work plan or timeline

# Appendix A.2.1:
## Pre-clinical Individual Assessment Guide

The Pre-clinical Individual Assessment Guide leads you through questions about your previous team experiences. These questions help you become aware of how you feel about team experiences, and provide ideas on how you could build on what was positive and better address what was negative. Your responses will prepare you to contribute to the discussions on the team agreement. Your clinical instructor may ask for a copy of your assessment to gain some understanding of your previous team experiences. You may also find this initial assessment useful when completing your midclinical and final course evaluations.

Name: _____ Date: _____

1. What group experience have you had? (Examples: course work group, community group, work group, professional group)
2. Overall, how would you describe your previous experience?
   ❑ Mostly positive  ❑ Half & half  ❑ Less than half positive  ❑ Not positive
3. Briefly describe a team experience that was particularly rewarding for you.
4. What do you feel contributed to making this a rewarding experience?
5. Based on your past experience, check all the following characteristics that apply to you:

| # | Personal Characteristic | Yes |
|---|---|---|
| 1 | Arrives on time and is prepared to focus on team task | |
| 2 | Takes turn in fulfilling roles, such as facilitator, recorder, reporter | |
| 3 | Does fair share of teamwork | |
| 4 | Admits uncertainty and asks questions to help clarify the situation | |
| 5 | Teaches others by using personal examples or reviewing concepts or assignments | |
| 6 | Readily uses resources such as preceptor, instructor, and written material to help clarify the situation | |
| 7 | Can be counted on to disclose feelings, opinions, and experiences | |
| 8 | Shows respect for others by limiting length of comments, listening to others, and considering their points of view | |
| 9 | Encourages teammates by recognizing their contributions and building on their ideas | |
| 10 | Explores different viewpoints and approaches that may not be appreciated at first | |
| 11 | Uses logic to challenge the thinking and work methods of the team | |
| 12 | Practices reflective thinking and avoids making hasty conclusions | |
| 13 | Responds well whenever others disagree or express criticism | |
| 14 | Keeps trying even when the task becomes demanding | |
| 15 | Expresses optimism about the team being able to achieve success | |

*Sources*: Adapted from Strom, P., Strom, R., & Moore, E. (1999). Peer and self-evaluation of teamwork skills. *Journal of Adolescence, 22*, 539–553; and Woods, D. (1994). *Problem-based learning: How to gain the most from PBL*. Waterdown, ON: Donald R. Woods.

6. What personality type are you? To determine your personality type, go to www.peterursbender.com/quiz/index.html, complete the free personality quiz, and print and attach the results.
7. What contributions could you bring to the group (e.g., previous team or leadership experience, computer skills, presentation skills, ability in a language other than English, cultural perspective, network contacts, etc.)?
8. What has been the most troubling experience you have had with group work?
9. How could this type of troubling group experience be avoided in the future?
10. What do you tend to do when you are faced with conflict or differences in a group?

| Reaction to Conflict | Most of the Time | Half and Half | A Few Times or Never |
|---|---|---|---|
| Accommodate (do what the other person wants, give in) | ❏ | ❏ | ❏ |
| Withdraw (refuse to participate anymore) | ❏ | ❏ | ❏ |
| Compromise (find a middle ground that at least satisfies most) | ❏ | ❏ | ❏ |
| Collaborate (work together to find something that all believe is important) | ❏ | ❏ | ❏ |
| Force (take over decision making and action, leaving little for others to do but follow) | ❏ | ❏ | ❏ |
| Other: | ❏ | ❏ | ❏ |

*Source*: Woods, D. (1994). *Problem-based learning: How to gain the most from PBL* (Box 5.2, pp. 5–7). Waterdown, ON: Donald R. Woods.

11. What thoughts do you have about the population group that you will be working with?
12. What knowledge and skills related to the culture group would be beneficial to you?
13. What rules or guidelines do you like to have about group work? (e.g., What are your timelines? How do you like to work?)
14. What personal goals would you like to accomplish by the end of the project? Indicate at least two (e.g., learn to plan and work to a schedule; be able to express my views when they are different from those expressed by others).
15. What would you like the group to accomplish by the end of the project? Indicate at least one group goal (e.g., we learn to rely on one another) and one project goal (e.g., the people feel that what is produced is worthwhile).

# Appendix A.2.2:
## Team Agreement Guide

The Team Agreement Guide is essential to starting and keeping your team on track both in working well together and completing the project. The team agreement has four sections: team goals, team process, professional accountability, and professional attitude and behavior. The team agreement has been developed over 10 years with student teams in a variety of situations. The team goals provided in the first section have evolved over the years and are consistent with the focus of the text. In other parts of the agreement, the questions are open-ended so you can make adjustments to meet your course and placement requirements.

The team's responses to questions in the agreement provide a reference point for your team and advisors. We strongly advise that you develop your team agreement within the first two weeks of your clinical, so you have a good understanding of each other and what is needed to complete the project. You will refer to the agreement throughout your community clinical experience, when procedures or items need to be changed following the resolution of conflict, and during midclinical and final evaluations. Your agreement needs to be "at the table" when you celebrate the success of your project and teamwork!

Names: _____

Project Title: _____

## Team Goals

- Develop community health nursing practice by completing a community health nursing project.
- Expand knowledge about community health nursing: Identify opportunities to learn about community health nursing beyond our project and manage our work to allow team members to take advantage of these opportunities.
- Develop skills for working in teams.

## Team Process

1. Team and Individual Development (Roles and Responsibilities):
   a. Who will lead the team and coordinate team activities? Who will keep the minutes of team meetings, other activities, and other team documents, and be responsible for submitting the weekly report? Discuss your expectations for the team leader and recorder (see Chapter 2). Identify roles for the other team members.
   b. How will the team ensure that each team member has an opportunity to take on a leadership role, such as rotating through the positions?
   c. What does each team member bring to the team, based on experience? What would team members like to gain from the team experience? How can the team help members to achieve their individual goals? How can the team build a sense of achievement for each member and the team?
   d. How will the team identify and constructively deal with situations that might potentially cause team members to feel dissatisfaction? For example, sometimes a team member might feel that there is an uneven distribution of the team workload.
2. Work Routines: Consider how your team could organize your time within the clinical hours given in the course outline/guidelines.
   a. What work routine would help the team to keep on track during the clinical days? For example, some teams start the clinical day with a meeting to determine an agenda or "to do" list for the day and meet at the end of it to summarize progress and put together the weekly report.
3. Communication and Reporting:
   a. Determine how team members will keep in touch and meet deadlines for reporting.
   b. When, how (email, fax?), and what information is routinely communicated to the clinical instructor and advisor?
   c. When are team reports (team agreement, timeline, final report) due, and how will the team manage them?
   d. What are the procedures to follow if the team is unable to meet a deadline or has to change a planned activity in the community? For example, consider who must be contacted and by whom.
4. Appreciation: How can the team show ongoing appreciation to the agency and agency contact for providing the opportunity to work with them and their clients, and learn about community health nursing?
5. Other: What other items will encourage good teamwork and avoid problems that team members have encountered in the past?

## Professional Accountability

1. Time and Attendance: What are the clinical expectations for attendance from your program and the clinical site, and the expected procedure in case of illness or nonattendance of a team member?

2. Evaluation:
   a. How will this team agreement and other resources, such as the team work plan and self- and team evaluation forms, be used to monitor team progress and encourage team members to share perceptions?
   b. How frequently (other than at midterm and final evaluation) will the team evaluate the points in the team agreement?

## Professional Attitude and Behavior

1. What does it mean for team members to behave in a professional way toward each other, the instructors, agency contacts, staff, and community members? How will the team monitor itself with regard to professional attitude and behavior?
2. Appearance: How will the team promote a professional image that encourages others to have confidence in the ability of team members to develop trusting and responsible relationships? Consider issues such as establishing rapport with the client population, agency/staff meetings, or in special situations (e.g., a presentation to the board). Consider how the team will manage misconceptions and errors by members in a supportive manner that encourages learning.
3. What is the team's policy around sharing feelings about the team within, or outside of, the team and other partnerships?

Team Members:

Signature                                    Date

_____        _____
_____        _____
_____        _____
_____        _____
_____        _____

Clinical Instructor:

_____

Revisions:
Team Members:

Signature                                    Date

_____        _____
_____        _____
_____        _____
_____        _____
_____        _____

Clinical Instructor:

_____

## Appendix A.2.3:
## Weekly Report

The Weekly Report is essential in maintaining communication among team members and advisors. The report keeps the team advisors updated on what is and is not occurring, and provides them an opportunity to provide feedback that can be implemented on the next clinical day. Preparing the report at the end of each day/week helps the team members keep a running summary in mind of what has been accomplished and what needs to happen next.

The Weekly Report serves as documentation for professional accountability, especially when documentation forms are not provided by the placement organization or educational institution. The Weekly Report is completed by the team at the end of each clinical day or week according to timelines determined by your course requirements and are distributed to team members, advisors, and others as required by the designated team recorder. Item "A" of the report is linked to the project plan (A.3.1) or timeline (A.3.2) to ensure that the team is progressing. Often, a blank weekly report form is used as an agenda for the team's first meeting of the day and becomes the minutes/report of what they accomplished at the end.

Distribution List:

Date Completed and Sent:

Team Members Present:

A. Purpose of Activities This Week [linked to project plan/timeline (see Chapters 3 and 4)]

B. Activities, Decisions, Results, and Timing for the Week:

C. Plans for Next Week, Meetings, and Upcoming Activities:

D. Comments or Questions:

E. Team Evaluation:

## Appendix A.2.4:
## Generic Meeting Agenda

The Generic Meeting Agenda guides the team through a sequence of items addressed at most meetings. It can be combined with the items in the weekly report. When the check-in and wrap-up components are used at each meeting, team members feel more connected and prepared to express their feelings. The agenda is especially useful when a meeting involves a few additional people. When 10 or more people are involved, the time for check-in and wrap-up will need to be shortened.

Date:

Time:

Location:

Participants:

1. Welcome, introduction (at first meeting or meeting with new people), and check-in, where each person has 1 to 2 minutes without interruption to express views about team, thoughts, or feelings
2. Adoption of the agenda (review the agenda items and, as a team, add any missing topic that you feel needs to be discussed; you can also determine approximately how much time you want to spend discussing each activity)
3. Acceptance of minutes from last meeting (add action items that need to be discussed to agenda)
4. Item 1 (number of minutes?) (if you know who is responsible for presenting that item, include their name)
5. Item 2 (number of minutes?)
6. Item 3 (number of minutes?)
7. Set next meeting date
8. Wrap-up (round-robin where each person has 1–2 minutes without interruption to indicate what they liked about the meeting and what they would change for the next meeting)

## Appendix A.2.5:
## Types of Questions to Ask during a Reflection On an Event or Experience

Reflection on an event or experience is a requirement of professional practice. These questions can guide your thinking and be adapted to fit your situation. The categories of questions deal with (1) description of event, (2), identifying feelings and thoughts, (3) evaluation of situation, (4) identifying main features, (5) considering alternative strategies, and (6) action plan. Each category has one or more probes that you can use as appropriate for your situation. You may choose to use these questions on your own to deal with an upsetting event or experience or to complete a reflection as part of your clinical practice requirements.

Name: _____

Date: _____

1. Description of event or experience, including:
   - What happened, including when, where, how, and who was involved.
2. Identify feelings and thoughts, such as:
   - What emotions was I feeling as the event happened?
   - What was I trying to achieve?
   - Why was this event important to me?
   - Why did I act the way I did?
   - What happened to others because of my action?
   - What emotions did the others show?
   - How did I know that they had those emotions?
3. Evaluate the situation, such as:
   - What was good about the experience?
   - What was bad about the experience?
4. Identify main features, such as:
   - What features identify my thoughts and emotions before, during, and after the experience?
   - Did my feelings or beliefs affect what happened before, during, and after the experience?
   - In what type of situation have I previously responded in the same way?
5. Consider alternate strategies for situation, such as:
   - What two other approaches could I have taken in this situation?
   - What are the positive and negative aspects of each alternate approach?

6. Action plan, such as:
   - What approach will I use in this type of situation in the future?
   - How will I prepare for this situation in the future?
   - Do I feel more confident in supporting others and myself in this situation? If not, what else can I do?

*Source*: Adapted from Brokenshire, A. (1998). Towards reflective practice: Learning from experience. *Registered Nurse, 10*, 7–8; Johns, C. (1993). Professional supervision. *Journal of Nursing Management, 1*, 9–18; and Gibbs, G. (1999). The reflective cycle. In *Royal College of Nurses: Realizing clinical effectiveness and clinical governance through clinical supervision* (Practitioner Book 1). Oxford: Radcliffe Medical Press.

## Appendix A.2.6:
## Self-Assessment of Functioning on Team

Your assessment of how you are functioning on the team prepares you to contribute to individual and team evaluations. A valuable use of the scale is to identify the items that you rated lower than others with the responses of your team members and to discuss how those items could be improved for each team member. The scale was developed, was tested, and showed high reliability with several classes of nursing students. You may want to use the scale as part of your personal midterm and final course evaluation.

For each behavior item on the left, circle the number on the right that indicates how often you exhibit the behavior:

| | Rarely | | | | Often |
|---|---|---|---|---|---|
| a. I work to keep the team on track. | 1 | 2 | 3 | 4 | 5 |
| b. I share information I have gathered with the team. | 1 | 2 | 3 | 4 | 5 |
| c. I praise others for the support they provide. | 1 | 2 | 3 | 4 | 5 |
| d. I attempt to change things when I see that others are unhappy. | 1 | 2 | 3 | 4 | 5 |
| e. I do a fair share of the work. | 1 | 2 | 3 | 4 | 5 |
| f. I am enthusiastic. | 1 | 2 | 3 | 4 | 5 |
| g. I find I can help in resolving conflict and disagreements. | 1 | 2 | 3 | 4 | 5 |
| h. I encourage others to share their views in team discussions. | 1 | 2 | 3 | 4 | 5 |

## Appendix A.2.7:
## Individual Assessment of Team Functioning

Your assessment of how your team is functioning prepares you to contribute to team evaluations. A valuable use of the scale is to compare the items that you rated as low with the responses of your team members and to discuss how those items could be improved. The scale was developed, was tested, and showed high reliability with several classes of nursing students. You may want to use the scale as part of your personal midterm and final course evaluation.

For each behavior item on the left, circle the number on the right that indicates how often the team exhibits the behavior:

| | Rarely | | | | Often |
|---|---|---|---|---|---|
| a. We willingly contribute our skills and knowledge. | 1 | 2 | 3 | 4 | 5 |
| b. We are proud to be on our team. | 1 | 2 | 3 | 4 | 5 |
| c. We seek input from a variety of sources, including literature and key informants. | 1 | 2 | 3 | 4 | 5 |
| d. We delegate tasks fairly among team members. | 1 | 2 | 3 | 4 | 5 |
| e. We work at maintaining good communication. | 1 | 2 | 3 | 4 | 5 |
| f. We trust each other to do quality work. | 1 | 2 | 3 | 4 | 5 |
| g. We are committed to being frank with each other. | 1 | 2 | 3 | 4 | 5 |
| h. We strive to be flexible. | 1 | 2 | 3 | 4 | 5 |

## Appendix A.3:
## Tools and Resources for Guiding the Community Project:
## Work Plans, Timelines, and Project Reports

The work plans allow the team to document what they have done and accomplished according to the steps and substeps of the community project. The two work plan forms are provided in Appendix A.3.1. The Assessment Work Plan is found in A.3.1a and the Plan, Take Action, and Evaluate Work Plan is found in A.3.1b. The team moves to the second part of the work plan once they have completed the action statements.

The timeline is a Gantt chart that depicts the timing of steps and substeps and is provided in Appendix A.3.2. There are two types of timelines to meet the needs of different situations. If a team plans a project involving assessment, planning, action, and evaluation, they would use the A.3.2a Project Timeline throughout. If a team is not certain, they can start with the A.3.2b Assessment Timeline. The Project Timeline can be revised for different situations, such as a focus on evaluation.

The project report is a required summary document of the project and is provided in Appendix A.3.3. The final report for a project has two formats: the A.3.3a Assessment Project Report or A.3.3b Project Report. The Assessment Project Report ends with recommendations following an assessment. The Project Report includes assessment, planning, action, and evaluation.

The use of the work plan and timeline will vary according to your course requirements. You may be required to use one or the other or both, or they might be optional. Both the work plan and timeline work well with the weekly report.

# Appendix A.3.1a:
## Assessment Work Plan

| Steps, Substeps, & Activities<br>– number and time period | Timeframe, Results Summary, with Completion Date |
|---|---|
| (Name of project)<br>Revision Date: | |
| ASSESS | |
| 1. Orient to community project | |
|   a. Establish relationships | |
|   b. Define the project, population group, and issue | |
| 2. Assess secondary data | |
|   a. Review sociodemographic data | |
|   b. Review epidemiological data on health status | |
|   c. Review previously conducted community surveys and program statistics | |
|   d. Review national and local policy documents | |
|   e. Review literature and best practice guidelines | |
|   f. Summarize secondary data | |
| 3. Assess physical and social environment | |
|   a. Observe and map physical and social environment | |
|   b. Interview key informants | |
| 4. Assess primary data | |
|   a. Select specific assessment methods | |
|   b. Collect data | |
| 5. Analyze assessment data | |
|   a. Assemble assessment data | |
|   b. Analyze and validate data | |
|   c. Develop action statements | |
|   d. Summarize assessment | |
| 9. Evaluate teamwork | |

## Appendix A.3.1b:
## Plan, Take Action, and Evaluate Work Plan

| (Name of project) Revision Date: | |
|---|---|
| **Steps, Substeps, & Activities** (remove Steps 1–5 if continuing from Assessment Work Plan) | **Timeframe, Results Summary, with Completion Date** |
| **ASSESS** | |
| 1. Orient to community project | |
|    a. Establish relationships | |
|    b. Define the project, population group, and issue | |
| 2. Assess secondary data | |
|    a. Review sociodemographic data | |
|    b. Review epidemiological data on health status | |
|    c. Review previously conducted community surveys and program statistics | |
|    d. Review national and local policy documents | |
|    e. Review literature and best practice guidelines | |
|    f. Summarize secondary data | |
| 3. Assess physical and social environment | |
|    a. Observe and map physical and social environment | |
|    b. Interview key informants | |
| 4. Assess primary data | |
|    a. Select specific assessment methods | |
|    b. Collect data | |
| 5. Analyze assessment data | |
|    a. Assemble assessment data | |
|    b. Analyze and validate data | |
|    c. Develop action statements | |
|    d. Summarize assessment | |

## PLAN

6. Plan action

   a. Select priority

   b. Identify goal

   c. Identify strategy and evidence-based intervention

   d. Develop impact and process objectives

## ACT

7. Take action

   a. Tailor the intervention

   b. Make practical arrangements for the delivery of the intervention

   c. Develop evaluation measures

   d. Implement the tailored intervention and conduct evaluation

## EVALUATE

8. Evaluate results and complete project

   a. Analyze evaluation data

   b. Present the results for validation

   c. Draft and complete project report

   d. Conclude relationship with collaborators

   e. Conclude relationship with team

9. Evaluate teamwork

## Appendix A.3.2a:
## Project Timeline

Project Title:

Date:

| Steps and Substeps in Process (week) | 1 | 2 | 3 | 4 | 5 | 6 | 7 | 8 | 9 | 10 | 11 | 12 |
|---|---|---|---|---|---|---|---|---|---|---|---|---|
| **ASSESS** | | | | | | | | | | | | |
| 1. Orient to community project | | | | | | | | | | | | |
|    a. Establish relationships | | | | | | | | | | | | |
|    b. Define the project, population group, and issue | | | | | | | | | | | | |
| 2. Assess secondary data | | | | | | | | | | | | |
|    a. Review sociodemographic data | | | | | | | | | | | | |
|    b. Review epidemiological data on health status | | | | | | | | | | | | |
|    c. Review previously conducted community surveys and program statistics | | | | | | | | | | | | |
|    d. Review national and local policy documents | | | | | | | | | | | | |
|    e. Review literature and best practice guidelines | | | | | | | | | | | | |
|    f. Summarize secondary data | | | | | | | | | | | | |
| 3. Assess physical and social environment | | | | | | | | | | | | |
|    a. Observe and map physical and social environment | | | | | | | | | | | | |
|    b. Interview key informants | | | | | | | | | | | | |
| 4. Assess primary data | | | | | | | | | | | | |
|    a. Select specific assessment methods | | | | | | | | | | | | |
|    b. Collect data | | | | | | | | | | | | |
| 5. Analyze assessment data | | | | | | | | | | | | |
|    a. Assemble assessment data | | | | | | | | | | | | |
|    b. Analyze and validate data | | | | | | | | | | | | |
|    c. Develop action statements | | | | | | | | | | | | |
|    d. Summarize assessment | | | | | | | | | | | | |

| Steps and Substeps in Process (week) | 1 | 2 | 3 | 4 | 5 | 6 | 7 | 8 | 9 | 10 | 11 | 12 |
|---|---|---|---|---|---|---|---|---|---|---|---|---|
| **PLAN** | | | | | | | | | | | | |
| 6. Plan action | | | | | | | | | | | | |
|   a. Select priority | | | | | | | | | | | | |
|   b. Identify goal | | | | | | | | | | | | |
|   c. Identify strategy and evidence-based intervention | | | | | | | | | | | | |
|   d. Develop impact and process objectives | | | | | | | | | | | | |
| **ACT** | | | | | | | | | | | | |
| 7. Take action | | | | | | | | | | | | |
|   a. Tailor the intervention | | | | | | | | | | | | |
|   b. Make practical arrangements for the delivery of the intervention | | | | | | | | | | | | |
|   c. Develop evaluation measures | | | | | | | | | | | | |
|   d. Implement the tailored intervention and conduct evaluation | | | | | | | | | | | | |
| **EVALUATE** | | | | | | | | | | | | |
| 8. Evaluate results and complete project | | | | | | | | | | | | |
|   a. Analyze evaluation data | | | | | | | | | | | | |
|   b. Present the results for validation | | | | | | | | | | | | |
|   c. Draft and complete project report | | | | | | | | | | | | |
|   d. Conclude relationship with collaborators | | | | | | | | | | | | |
|   e. Conclude relationship with team | | | | | | | | | | | | |
| 9. Evaluate teamwork | | | | | | | | | | | | |

# Appendix A.3.2b:
## Assessment Timeline

| Project Title: | | | | | | | | | | | | | |
|---|---|---|---|---|---|---|---|---|---|---|---|---|---|
| Date: | | | | | | | | | | | | | |
| **Steps and Substeps in Process** (week) | **1** | **2** | **3** | **4** | **5** | **6** | **7** | **8** | **9** | **10** | **11** | **12** |
| **ASSESS** | | | | | | | | | | | | |
| 1. Orient to community project | | | | | | | | | | | | |
| a. Establish relationships | | | | | | | | | | | | |
| b. Define the project, population group, and issue | | | | | | | | | | | | |
| 2. Assess secondary data | | | | | | | | | | | | |
| a. Review sociodemographic data | | | | | | | | | | | | |
| b. Review epidemiological data on health status | | | | | | | | | | | | |
| c. Review previously conducted community surveys and program statistics | | | | | | | | | | | | |
| d. Review national and local policy documents | | | | | | | | | | | | |
| e. Review literature and best practice guidelines | | | | | | | | | | | | |
| f. Summarize secondary data | | | | | | | | | | | | |
| 3. Assess physical and social environment | | | | | | | | | | | | |
| a. Observe and map physical and social environment | | | | | | | | | | | | |
| b. Interview key informants | | | | | | | | | | | | |
| 4. Assess primary data | | | | | | | | | | | | |
| a. Select specific assessment methods | | | | | | | | | | | | |
| b. Collect data | | | | | | | | | | | | |
| 5. Analyze assessment data | | | | | | | | | | | | |
| a. Assemble assessment data | | | | | | | | | | | | |
| b. Analyze and validate data | | | | | | | | | | | | |
| c. Develop action statements | | | | | | | | | | | | |
| d. Summarize assessment | | | | | | | | | | | | |

| Steps and Substeps in Process (week) | 1 | 2 | 3 | 4 | 5 | 6 | 7 | 8 | 9 | 10 | 11 | 12 |
|---|---|---|---|---|---|---|---|---|---|---|---|---|
| **EVALUATE** | | | | | | | | | | | | |
| 8. Evaluate results and complete project | | | | | | | | | | | | |
|    a. Analyze evaluation data | | | | | | | | | | | | |
|    b. Present the results for validation | | | | | | | | | | | | |
|    c. Draft and complete project report | | | | | | | | | | | | |
|    d. Conclude relationship with collaborators | | | | | | | | | | | | |
|    e. Conclude relationship with team | | | | | | | | | | | | |
| 9. Evaluate teamwork | | | | | | | | | | | | |

## Appendix A.3.3a:
## Assessment Project Report

[include FINAL in title when complete]

[Name of educational institution and nursing program]

Community Health Nursing Project in Collaboration with [name of agency]

[Project Title]

[Date of Current Draft]

Students:

Agency Advisor:

Clinical Instructor:

Manager:

Key Health Issues of the Population [obtained from secondary data]:

Community of Interest:

Assessment Methods and Timelines:

Validated Key Results/Findings:

Action Statements:

Limitations:

Sustainability:

Recommendations:

Relevance for Community Health Nursing:

Attachments:

## Appendix A.3.3b:
## Project Report

[include FINAL in title when complete]

[Name of educational institution and nursing program]

Community Health Nursing Project in Collaboration with [name of agency]

[Project Title]

[Date of Current Draft]

Students:

Agency Advisor:

Clinical Instructor:

Manager:

Key health issues of the population:

Community of interest:

Assessment methods:

Priority action statement with supporting evidence:

Project goal:

Strategy and evidence-based intervention:

Impact objectives:

Action:

Key findings:

Limitations:

Sustainability:

Recommendations:

Relevance for community health nursing:

Attachments:

# Answer Key to
# Chapter Discussion Questions

# Chapter 1

1. Positive: Opportunity to work fairly independently and creatively in such places as schools and in the areas of maternal health and community safety, possibly promoting the use of car seats and bicycle helmets, or discouraging drinking and driving, or smoking; working to prevent or reduce illness and injury rather than emphasize treatment; daytime work. Less positive: Some may consider it less exciting and demanding than hospital nursing; in some situations, the pay for community nursing may be less than that in hospitals.

2. Community and public health nursing provides a broader context for thinking about health so that when a nurse is doing a dressing in a hospital, treating an injury in the emergency department, helping an older adult reduce the risk of falls, or working on a committee to improve sidewalks, the nurse is also thinking of what caused the injury or risk and what can be done to prevent further problems for that person and other members of the community.

3. Income and social status are reflected in the poor neighborhood, housing, and play areas. The father's unemployment and the poor social environment are apparent because there is no mention of family and friends to assist the mother and to help the father find work.

4. Healthy fresh food is more expensive and difficult to store than packaged foods that are often high in salt, sugar, and preservatives; lack of transportation to a less expensive food store; no safe area to walk; lack of funds for sports.

5. a. An institution might need to be convinced to take some action to increase student activities in the first year. The action could involve events, posters, and/or the Internet. The community might need to be encouraged to increase or improve walking and biking trails and bridges. The state or provincial health or university/college departments could be encouraged to promote active young adults through media campaigns, funds for innovative ideas, and recreation facilities.

   b. The university/college could invite students to join the design committee; seek their opinions through interviews or surveys; or provide the opportunity to vote on different designs.

6. There could be many reasons for safety concerns: inadequate maintenance of roads, housing, and other infrastructure; lack of services; crime; and so on. The municipal services dealing with roads, sidewalks, and lighting would need to be involved; local health services and neighborhood organizations could represent the community. The police services could play a role in traffic safety and dealing with high crime rates. As well, local businesses would be concerned about poor traffic flow and unsafe streets.

7. Learning to talk to groups of students, teachers, and the principal about the concerns they have; providing feedback to the same people as you proceed; and asking for their assistance in taking action.

8. a. All activities could be within the scope of community health nursing practice, but the mandates of local community health organizations or state/provincial public health organizations may vary.

b. Begin all three by speaking to the organizations providing services and the people to determine what is working, what is not working, and what might be done.

c. Other actions could include improving breast-feeding rates; testing well water; working with emergency measure organizations at all levels; organizing community food boxes, clothing exchanges, and home or community lunches for older adults.

9. a. Assessment could be used to determine the best diabetic health program. In assessment, you need to identify first what criteria or guidelines on diabetic education are available for you to review the two programs. You would then use the criteria/guidelines to collect relevant information on the programs from the websites of the community clinics and from the contact person for each of the diabetic programs. The assessment is completed by analyzing the information you have collected to determine the diabetic education program that best meets the criteria. Evaluation could also be used because it follows a similar process.

b. The full community health nursing process could help guide your volunteer experience at an immunization clinic. During your first day or two in your volunteer experience, you will carry out your volunteer assignment while assessing how the clinic functions from when clients arrive to when they leave. Assessment involves making observations and talking with the nurses and support staff about your observations. After a couple of times at the clinic, you may determine from your assessment data that what you have been doing could be expanded or changed to improve the functioning of the clinic and support for clients. Discuss your assessment findings with your supervisor, and if that person is receptive, you could plan a change in what or how you assist. As you take action and implement your plan, continue to note what works well and what does not. Ask staff and clients for their feedback on what you are doing. Evaluate your contribution regularly and at the end of the experience. Discuss your evaluation findings with your supervisor when possible and especially when your experience is ending.

10. The action at the individual level tends to focus on immediate concerns. Action with the community group has a longer time frame and involves improving the group's capacity to take action on their own. For example, the capacity might be learning to organize a meeting to bring together a self-help group.

## Chapter 2

1. They learned to relax and observe rather than trying to do something. They observed the women interacting with their children, and they heard the women's concerns as expressed by the nurse. They also learned to listen to each other.

2. The decision was important because it indicated that the team recognized the expertise of the mothers on what and how they wanted to learn. The team members decided to collaborate with them rather than selecting priorities on their own.

3.  Organized a trip, party, or event with others; acted as a "buddy" for someone who wanted to change their behavior; actively participated in creative or artistic endeavors.

4. a.  The students conducted an assessment, made a plan, and took action. They put up an interactive poster in the cafeteria, planned a contest, and evaluated the results.

   b.  The students collaborated with workers, managers, the Health and Safety Committee, and the occupational health nurse.

   c.  The students worked as a team and with the Health and Safety Committee to plan their work, make decisions, deal with conflict, and take action.

5. a.  If the advisor is a community or public health nurse: Advantages—students have a nursing role model to follow, more opportunity to work at a community rather than group level, and more assistance in completing some aspects of the project. Disadvantages—students may have less flexibility in determining what is done.

   b.  If the advisor is not a community or public health nurse: Advantages—placements without a nurse often provide more opportunity for learning to work with other professionals and nonprofessional staff and for spending more time with vulnerable community groups. Disadvantages—students do not have a nursing role model to follow.

6.  The report requires the team to summarize progress by listing the activities carried out and encourages forward planning for the coming week. Team members are kept up to date, and the clinical instructor and advisor can use the weekly report to monitor the functioning of teams in dispersed locations. In this way, the weekly report provides a record and enables the team to be accountable to each other and to their clinical instructor and advisor.

7.  By discussing and addressing the differences that lead to the conflict in the storming stage, the team can become more cohesive and productive. Conflict is challenging because people might feel that others threaten their values, and they want to avoid confrontation. They might think, "Well, we only have a few weeks left, so it is not worth bringing up problems." However, when ignored, the tension and feelings can build, leading to poor results and bad feelings among team members.

8.  The mentor learns about training someone else and the trainee is able to ask questions and become more confident in the job. As well, there is less opportunity for a breakdown in communication with the team and others.

## Chapter 3

1.  Hours of work; roles and relationships, e.g., reporting arrangements, names and contact information, where you would be located; organization's orientation manual.

2.  Community participation is one of the five principles of primary health care. Facilitating participation is an essential skill for community nurses as community members are likely to have many skills on which to draw. Engaging

community members in health helps to ensure that health programs will be tailored to community needs.

3. There are unlimited possibilities: organizations that run fitness classes (e.g., YM/WCA); health clubs; organizations working with different client groups (e.g., seniors centers); neighborhood associations; health centers; organizations such as banks that want to make a contribution to the community; service clubs; city planners.

4. Students are expected to shape the community project to meet the expectations of the clinical assignment and their learning needs. If time is limited, they will have to set priorities in consultation with the instructor and advisor. Students must be familiar with health literature; have knowledge of statistics; have experience with reviewing and synthesizing health information; and be able to communicate ideas verbally and through slide presentations.

5. Boundaries may include geographical features such as rivers or forested areas, or the built environment, such as major roads, shopping centers, and industrial complexes. Other factors may be used to describe community, such as socioeconomic status (e.g., "a working-class community"); language; ethnicity; and lifestyle. Communities may also be defined by their history or culture (e.g., "Amish community").

6. Students might focus on resources to support activity, such as the natural environment (green spaces, clean air); built environment (traffic, pollution, speed limits); culture (tradition of families walking together in the evening); and safety (crime rates, street lighting, policing).

7. Example provided in text.

8. Needs assessments usually provide information on physical activity. Urban streets with high traffic can be hazardous for cyclists; streets without sidewalks make it difficult to walk; weather, snow, and ice in the winter make sidewalks treacherous—all are examples of how the physical environment influences activity.

9. The decrease beginning with young adults, and continuing, may be associated with transition from school to work/further education, change in family responsibility, pressures of work. Another reason might be loss of exercise partners. Decrease in older adults, possible health issues and social norms around exercise—exercise programs may be geared to younger age groups and costly. All changes might be due to moving away from a well-resourced community.

10. Changes to the environment to promote active living and access to healthy food: School—install bicycle racks, rent-a-bike; provide healthy choices in cafeteria; Workplace—provide a fitness room, green space outside to run at lunchtime; limit alcohol outlets near schools and workplaces.

1.      They might not know about the classes. They might not have money to pay for transportation, babysitting, or for the classes if there are fees. They might be worried that they will not be able to understand what is being said.

2.      Have you heard about classes for women who are pregnant or have a baby? Do you know anyone who has attended a class? Would you like to learn how to look after yourself and your baby when you are pregnant and after having the baby? Would you be able to attend a class for women who are pregnant or have a baby at [name of place where class could be held]?

3.      An advantage was that they could maintain the contacts established by public health with the two volunteers and city staff working within the building. The challenge was learning to work with people from a different culture who speak a different language. They could use the volunteers, staff, and team members who speak Spanish and Cantonese as role models on how and when to approach the women, and as reviewers for any material they develop.

4.      An advantage was that most of the residents of the building spoke English (making communication easier), though public health had not developed contacts with people living/working within the building. One challenge is that the team does not seem to realize that they are not making decisions together. They need to recognize their problem and seek advice and resources (e.g., teamwork in Chapter 2).

5.      Some features could be a drug store/pharmacy, playground, schools, and an Internet connection. Icons could include a grocery cart for a grocery store or a swing for a playground.

6.      If there are a large number of people from the same cultural group, you would likely notice several stores, restaurants, churches, and newspapers catering to the group. These signs would not be apparent if the cultural group had recently arrived. In the latter situation, you might hear people speaking a different language.

7.      Volunteers in the lobby might indicate certain women that others listen to and the times that the women gather. They can describe situations that have occurred, such as a baby becoming very sick or a depressed mother, and how the situation was addressed or could have been addressed better. The city worker can provide information on supports available through the city and whether the women use them or not.

8.      The measures in the English scenario included (a) everyone agreeing that they dreaded the meeting but want to get things resolved, (b) changing their usual meeting process by going outside for a walk and just expressing their feelings, and (c) negotiating changes in how they work together after most feelings have been expressed. Some of your experiences might involve delaying a meeting until tempers have cooled, one or two people taking over and making decisions while the remaining members are resentful, or just persevering with the project without allowing feelings or emotions to emerge. Usually the most effective way involves team members feeling comfortable enough to express their feelings and hear how others are feeling.

9. The team identified the interest in food and the lack of grocery stores in their mapping and key informant interviews.

10. Advantages: Depending on the responses you receive and on body language, you can adjust the questions and your approach to people after each cycle of progressive inquiry. Challenges: A resource called *Simply Put*, prepared by the Centers for Disease Control (2009), explains that subgroups of minority groups often differ greatly from one another and supposedly appropriate images, concepts, and language may not work. They emphasize the need to test messages with the intended audience.

11. Have one member conduct observations in one location, such as the children's playgroup in the corner. One person could observe an aspect of the interactions in the lobby, such as the number of women talking to women/volunteers/ students, say at 20-minute intervals. These observations could provide useful information but might also make the women uncomfortable unless the observer moves around the room and talks to people while making the observations.

12. The team observed that the Tenant Association members were pleased with information about the use of the playground and seemed embarrassed that the issue of finding an indoor place for meetings had previously been dropped. The chair identified two tenants to work with the team and bring back a report to the next meeting. The team's advisor will soon learn of these positive responses and will be able to follow-up with the Association to work on other collaborations possibly involving maternal-child health, immunizations, or healthy eating.

13. The desired group was already meeting and had time, questions, and procedures that had already been used and tested; their advisor acted in the moderator role; and the team was able to delegate tasks and assist each other in preparation.

14. The question starts things off on a positive note. Participants get a chance to express how they feel about their practice. Some, however, may provide a glib answer, such as "I like to help mothers," without any explanation. You could start with the question "Can you describe how something you did in your practice made you feel rewarded?"

15. Advantages: Progressive inquiry encourages the participants themselves to name issues; and questionnaires allow for the systematic collection of responses from more people in the building. The questionnaire provided experience for the team in developing questions and in testing it for public health, and gave them the opportunity to reach out to more women in the building. Disadvantages: It is sometimes difficult to switch from one method to another, and preparation of a questionnaire will reduce the time available to interact with the community group and to complete the action and evaluation.

16. To deal with this ethical issue, you need to explain that you do not have the names of the women and could not identify them because their participation is confidential. You could offer suggestions on how she might ask for women to work with her.

1. Progressive inquiry questions allow the items identified in the two earlier methods to be explored in more depth.
2. The data from the questionnaire increases the number of women involved, and the different approach provides some measure of validation through the triangulation of data.
3. More than half the women participating in the progressive inquiry in the lobby had mentioned this concern. The team wanted to check it out during validation.
4. In the item for "other" food questions, four people indicated that they wanted to know when to start giving food with a spoon. This item is important because it arose as a separate concern of four people without any prompts from the questionnaire items.
5. The analysis could be more difficult if the information comes from different groups, such as a community group and a provider group, since you may not be certain if they interpreted the questions in the same way. Combining data from qualitative methods, such as progressive inquiry and focus groups, with a quantitative method, such as a closed-ended questionnaire, is difficult because the types of data do not usually fit together well and there could be a loss of some of the qualitative information.
6. To maintain confidentiality and anonymity, participants' names are not included in any of the methods and sociodemographic questions are written in broad terms so no particular person can be identified. During the analysis and reporting, information from different sources are combined, which helps to maintain anonymity. Confidentiality and anonymity are important in maintaining both the trust of the community and ethical practice.
7. The team tried out their ideas with the collaborators first. They then asked the women to stand beside the item they supported, which was a clearer response than putting up their hand or filling out a survey.
8. Many of the women were just beginning to learn English. The team wanted to be sure that they were understanding what was being said. By observing the women's body language, they would see from nods and smiles that the women were following the presentation. If the women were frowning or restless, the presenters would need to slow down their delivery and possibly involve interpreters.
9. Lack of money is usually not a feasible concern to address in a short-term project. Longer term projects may include some policy and advocacy aspects, such as increasing welfare payments, or programs such as food baskets or community gardens.
10. Lack of knowledge suggests that providing information will resolve the concern, whereas the evidence suggests broader determinants. As well, the women might feel they are being called stupid or ignorant. The statement on needing appropriate resources or information places the responsibility for the action on the health care provider.

11. The team will find it easier to document the assessment when it is fresh in their minds rather than waiting until the end of the project. They will learn to follow their work plan/timelines and to condense and communicate their achievements in the report (for accountability), and they will have completed a section of the final report by the end of the project.

12. This information helps the collaborators judge the quality of the evidence. People need to know who and how many were involved to determine if the results are relevant.

## Chapter 6

1. You would likely want to learn as much as you can from the community advisor and arrange to spend time at the shelters to get to know the staff and residents.

2. Benefits: Splitting the project into sequential phases allows more people to be involved and continue the project; in regular practice, a change of circumstances often means that you will be required to carry on with work initiated by others; the time and resources spent in the original work will not be wasted and the community will not be disappointed. Challenges: You will need to quickly become acquainted with what has already happened so that others won't feel they are repeating everything; in your review of reports and interacting with the community, you may feel that the action statements do not reflect the present situation; you may have to win the support of the community and collaborators.

3. There was less support for improving the quality of the food, and it was not as life-threatening as shelter from the cold at that time.

4. The priority setting identified the homeless residents as a disadvantaged group lacking shelter from the cold that threatened their health status. The Coalition also recognized the capacity building demonstrated by the homeless residents in helping each other. The homeless residents are not involved in priority setting but will be included in planning and action, thereby providing an opportunity to build on the capacity of the homeless residents.

5. The priority action statement identifies a strength, which can be reinforced. A possible goal would be: "The homeless residents maintain or strengthen their mutual support system."

6. The related-to clause summarizes the assessment data, which informs the need for action. It identifies a lack/deficit that might be corrected, or a strength to be maintained or reinforced. Being consistent with the assessment is important in making the action relevant and therefore sustainable.

7. It might be easier to keep the team on track by asking questions. On the other hand, it might be more effective to work from the description of each objective in Table 6.5 if the questions restrict your thinking.

8. The environmental objective is to have staff and a group of residents in both shelters spread the word about the drop-ins. The staff and residents' knowledge and talking to other residents about the drop-ins changes the social environment to encourage the change in behavior.

# Chapter 7

1. They oriented themselves to the team and project; conducted an Internet search to obtain best practice data and local work-related data; mapped the location by conducting an exploration of the store; used the Health and Safety Committee as key informants; and used progressive inquiry with two shifts of stockers.

2. The project had the support of the Health and Safety Committee and the store manager; the Committee provided statistics supporting the need to reduce back injuries; a Committee member was assigned to work with them; the stockers were interested in learning about reducing back injuries; and promising Internet information on using workshops to reduce back injuries was easily found.

3. The team has chosen a suitable channel for providing information, as described in the Program Cycle. It has sought existing resources, and is consulting with advisors in the development and adjustment of materials. The planned workshop and demonstration will incorporate the four points from the booklet that draw on adult learning theories, including involving workers, hands-on sessions, and problem-solving discussions.

4. Since they need to speak slower, they will not be able to cover as much material as they would with an English-speaking audience. They will likely need to focus on the most pertinent techniques. Since feedback during the workshop depends on participants asking questions, the team will need to consider other ways to get feedback and to encourage discussion.

5. The rehearsal required the team to prepare their content, hear what it sounded like in front of others, and check the timing of each part, thereby giving them confidence. The first pilot test was an opportunity to identify which parts did not engage the audience and to check the timing. This allowed the team to make corrections and adjustments before the first workshop.

6. Most people find it easier to talk about what they themselves did or didn't do; discussing a change you feel another person should make is much more difficult. If team members do not identify an issue on their own, you might find it easier to offer them different options to improve something you noticed.

7. By promoting the benefits of the workshop, more staff are likely to attend and be ready to learn. This means that advertising and marketing would contribute to a positive social environment and improve the impact of the workshop.

8. An efficient use of time is to meet both at the beginning of the day to plan the day's work and at the end of the day to prepare the report and plan the next session. At the meetings, members should update the work plan and/or the Gantt chart, and prepare and follow an agenda and specified time frame. Notices about changes between meetings can be sent by text messages.

9. The team gains an understanding of the actual work environment and has an opportunity to develop a relationship with the stockers. They will learn the type of lifting that is carried out in the store, how to describe and measure each type, and how to identify problem areas related to the physical environment.

10. The numbers are likely unreliable because they are based on a public show of hands, in this case, thumbs, where participants could mimic each other without understanding which lift is correct. It is still useful to ask for the show of thumbs as general feedback and correct any misperceptions if they occur.

# Chapter 8

1. They might be feeling quite prepared because their plan is in place and they have the support of the Health and Safety Committee. On the other hand, they might be feeling overwhelmed because they still have a lot to do before they finish. Or, some or all members of the team may alternate between both feelings. Any of these responses is normal when there is a deadline approaching.

2. The Health and Safety Committee will know about most aspects of the project and will be prepared to continue the work. The team gains the experience of working with people from different backgrounds and has more people to assist with the project work.

3. Prepare a consistent, confidential code for each stocker to prevent duplications. Measures should be clearly defined with a checklist, training and pretesting in the workplace, and a debriefing following training.

4. The percentage used in an impact objective is usually an educated guess, as mentioned in Chapter 6. Many factors, such as a noisy or hot environment, poor equipment, fatigue, language limitations, or fear of failure on the part of the participants can reduce the results. Alternatively, the results might have been accurate only because a lot of different factors came together at the same time. The discussions around why the results met an expected percentage or not is more useful for guiding the discussion and learning how the community functions than whether the guess was accurate or not.

5. Some features of the workplace supported the workshops (e.g., the Health and Safety Committee, a supportive manager, access to community resources). Safe lifting workshops provide the stockers with information and skill, but aspects of the physical environment, such as spaces too cramped to accommodate safe lifting techniques, still need to be addressed by the manager.

6. The audience for the presentation has in-depth knowledge of the workplace and safety issues and can judge whether the intervention was carried out properly, the findings are supported by evidence, and the recommendations are relevant.

7. The report provides credibility to the work that was done and can be used to substantiate changes. The short length makes it quicker to read, and the format ensures that the important elements of the project are included.

8. The team recognized the project collaborators by thanking by them and having them stand during the presentation. They thanked the people involved in the pilot test by putting up a poster, personally thanked the store manager, and wrote a letter commending Letecia.

# Chapter 9

1. You may have had a family member who received nursing care at home after having surgery or was visited by a public health nurse after having a baby. Or you may know an older relative or friend who needed nursing care to deal with a chronic illness.

2. Positive: The person may appreciate the nurse coming to their home because they have difficulty going out; are more comfortable talking to the nurse in their home; can learn ways to care for themselves that work in their home; and have the opportunity for other family members to learn about their care. Less positive: Some people may not welcome a nurse to their home because they feel that the nurse is checking up on them or they are not comfortable with the condition of their house.

3. The diagram made it easier to discuss relationships and people because it is an objective item. The diagram helped to confirm to Julie that Nancy was really interested in her and her family.

4. Julie would be more likely to feel that her ability to care for the baby was in doubt and being tested.

5. The community health nurse asked to talk to both the son and his mother. They sat together in the mother's bedroom. She heard the son's concern about not wanting charity and later provides a couple of different options to give them choices.

6. The most relevant home health nursing competencies (Community Health Nurses of Canada, 2010), under Elements of Home Health Nursing, are "assessment, monitoring and clinical decision making" (p. 11) and "access and equity" (p. 13); and under Foundations of Home Health Nursing, "illness prevention and health protection" (p. 14). The item under Quality and Professional Responsibility would be "professional responsibility" (p. 15). The most relevant public health nursing standards (American Nurses Association, 2013), are Standard 1: Assessment; Standard 3: Outcomes Identification; Standard 7: Ethics; and Standard 11: Communication.

7. The community health nurse used the family as client and family as system approaches in her interactions. She used a circular question to explore the wife's feelings related to her husband.

8. Most home health nurses have limited time to make phone calls, conduct Internet searches, or consult with colleagues.

9. The home health organization could provide an updated list of community resources on their website or support another organization that does. The provision of mobile Internet devices would allow home health nurses to use the Internet to find needed information. The organization needs to make a point of encouraging new nurses to ask questions when they are not sure where to find community resources.

# Chapter 10

1.  A rural area often has higher rates of smoking, obesity, and related diseases such as diabetes, stroke, heart disease, and cancer than similar people in urban areas.

2.  When people talk about what is happening in their area, attend meetings about community issues, attend community events, and talk about "my" or "our" area/town/community, it is a good indication that they feel they belong to a community.

3.  Students were included as collaborators as soon as the team started collecting data. They assisted in collecting data from other students, teachers, and parents. They assisted in making decisions in summarizing data, where to post the data, and identifying leaders and "octopuses."

4.  They involved adolescent students in making decisions that could improve the school culture. They recognized the possible stress experienced by the transfer students and ensured that their responses were obtained.

5.  The team determined the questions and approaches together, went out to their separate locations to use the questions, and compared the responses together before determining new questions. The process is called progressive inquiry (See Chapter 4).

6.  Bev wanted the group to join the country kitchen. She did not say that; she asked for their views and then sat back to allow them to discuss their options freely. When the discussion was winding down, she summarized the different viewpoints, as she heard them, and provided an opportunity for the group to find their own benefits.

7.  They likely saw the benefit for the volunteers of contributing to the community while they learned about healthy eating and for the older adults of enjoying a healthy meal with others without feeling that it was a handout, and, overall, the opportunity the country kitchen provided the county residents to improve life in the county.

8.  They had the opportunity to learn about what occurred before they arrived, the expected long-term outcome, and had time to orient themselves to the community. During their orientation to the community, training of volunteers, and conducting one session of the community kitchen, they were able to gain some understanding of the role of the community health nurse in community capacity building. From their observations and interactions with the community members, the team could appreciate how they could get to know the community better, how the community wanted to be involved, and have some idea of what it might be like being a community health nurse in that community.

## Chapter 11

1.  Health issues: Increasing access to affordable active forms of transportation and exercise resources (sidewalks and bicycle facilities); increasing physical activity (sidewalks, bicycle facilities, crossings, athletic field). Evidence of capacity-building intent: Participation of community members in assessments (walking audits and picture taking) and stakeholder education; development of partnerships between tribal authority, local government, and schools to address broader health and safety concerns.

2.  Skilled communication, good administrator, personable, with knowledge of population. Potential leaders: Person with health and social services background; member of population of interest; possibly someone well known who might draw attention to the group.

3.  Think broadly; for example, community health and social services; transportation; city planners (wheelchair accessibility); business (potential employers).

4.  Use broad questions to open up the discussion. For example, "What experience do you have with this population/issue? I'd like to hear your ideas on how we might get members of X community to participate in our activities. How available are you for meetings and other program activities?"

5.  Advantages for you: Learning opportunity, exposure to wider community organization around exercise, possible job opportunities in the future. Advantages for organization: Possible funding support, opportunity to share experience and influence community action, making connections with other community groups.

6.  First impressions are important, and a failure to make introductions risks discouraging the new members who are likely to bring a needed perspective to the coalition. Reducing the time for budget discussions, however, might alienate members. A compromise solution might be to give brief introductions and arrange to meet with the new members after the meeting.

7.  Negotiate the meeting schedule, possibly the same day/time each month; send out minutes promptly along with a meeting reminder; welcome/recognize attendees; run meeting to time.

8.  Increase the knowledge and skills of members and, if the workshops involve elements of team building and collaboration, can benefit relationships, both of which increase the sustainability of the coalition (CDC, 2012).

9.  Collaborate with coalition partners such as the city planning department, schools, recreation groups, and community associations to encourage community groups to participate in a competition by planting trees to provide shade in play areas and public pools. Add messages about sunscreen protection to handouts and posters illustrating physical activity guidelines with warm weather activities.

# Chapter 12

1. There should not be any restriction for mothers wishing to breast-feed in a public place. (See, in the US: National Conference of State Legislatures, *Breastfeeding State Laws* at www.ncsl.org/research/health/breastfeeding-state-laws.aspx; and in Canada: Infact Canada, *Breastfeeding: It's Your Right* at www.infactcanada.ca/breastfeeding_rights.htm.) Public places with resources for mother and baby, such as a quiet and safe space, some privacy, seating, and facilities for changing diapers, provide a supportive environment. Infact Canada notes that fear of offending others discourages some women from breast-feeding in public.

2. Organizations providing care in the home usually have policies on safe practices for home visits. Health providers and nursing students may be required to maintain immunizations to protect themselves and clients; however, these are usually framed as recommendations.
   Policies on hours of work have potential for health impact, for example, regulations limiting the number of hours worked each day.

3. Community nurses can educate community partners by raising awareness of emerging/best practices on the benefits of supporting breast-feeding in the workplace. Professional organizations can support the objective through member education.

4. Training might be provided in different ways, for example, in-service education; coaching; access to e-learning resources. The 10 steps also require policies and procedures that enable implementation, for example, scheduling time to support breast-feeding mothers.

5. Acknowledge the right of women to decide. Discuss how nurses can best help women to make an informed decision.

6. Ranking will be influenced by personal choice. When weighing the arguments, consider the ease/difficulty of creating positive change in the five areas mentioned. Also consider which women are likely to benefit most from the changes.

7. When reading the article, consider whether both driving and restraining forces are addressed. If only one is addressed, consider what the opposing point of view would be. For example, if the argument focuses on personal rights, an opposing perspective might be what is best for society.

# Chapter 13

1. Evaluation should focus on the program delivered rather than the "program as planned." You can only evaluate the impact of activities delivered on the outcomes being measured. This does not preclude that other factors may have influenced the outcome, given the natural setting of community programs.

2. Advantages: Increases "buy in"; more likelihood of evaluating what is important to the community and taking action on the results. Disadvantages: There may not be support for evaluating theoretically or conceptually. Butterfoss and Francisco (2004) advise that it is important not to go for "easy wins" that do not advance the science.

3. Administer the social network diagram described in Chapter 9 before and after delivery of the program. Compare social network patterns to identify changes, both positive and negative.
   Or, conduct short qualitative interviews (four or five questions) to explore the topic. This might produce more valuable information that could be built on as the program evolves.

4. Program resource requirements, based on the following activities: Preparation and distribution of newspaper articles, leaflet, and a resource package on TB and healthy lifestyles for teachers; public health nurse to screen and refer based on the number of ESL classes; long-term case management, probably a few cases; public health nurse collaboration—time for meetings and planning community support.

5. Access might be impeded by physical barriers, e.g., distance from public transport, inadequate parking, or socio-environmental factors, e.g., language barriers, lack of health coverage, intolerance. Busy clinics, staff shortages, stormy weather, are all factors that compound difficulties and affect data collection. To simplify the task, it might be best to narrow the focus of the observations to one type of barrier and follow randomly selected clients to provide comparative information. Devise a systematic process to select clients, e.g., every fifth person with Nurse A to avoid bias such as choosing someone who looks "friendly."

6. The variety of activities, together with provision of food, might increase participation and encourage mothers to return and maintain the immunization schedule. Other factors, such as staff attitudes, friendliness of clientele, and efficiency of service, might be more influential.

7. Short-term outcomes: Acceptance of the program (e.g., participation rates); satisfaction ratings; increased use of alternative ways to celebrate; fewer ill effects from alcohol and fewer public disturbances; reduced alcohol-related injuries. Long-term outcomes: Reduced use of alcohol by high school students, increase in graduation rates, and reduction of alcohol consumption by high school graduates.

# Chapter 14

1. Examples include H1N1, SARS, measles, pertussis, meningitis.
2. Nurses would use their knowledge to identify people who are isolated or vulnerable in some way, such as those who are disabled, dependent on oxygen, or require medications. Their knowledge and skills in working in the home would be used to determine and provide appropriate care for individuals and families in their homes. If shelters are required, they would use their knowledge in preparing the shelter and their knowledge and skills to care for and support shelter residents physically, mentally, and emotionally.
3. The concepts include a commitment to principles of equity and social justice for vulnerable people, building sustainable relationships and partnerships, and marshaling resources through planning.
4. In Canada, the relevant health nursing standards would be Standard 1: Health Promotion and Standard 2: Prevention and Health Protection. Health promotion is substantiated by the terms "comprehensive assessment of assets and needs" and "variety of information sources including community wisdom"; Prevention and Health Protection, by the terms "identifying potential risks to health including contributing to emergency and/or disaster planning" and "engages in collaborative ... partnerships to address health risks ... recognizing that some individuals and groups are disproportionately affected" (Community Health Nurses of Canada, 2011, pp. 10–13). The applicable competencies are: 4–Partnerships, Collaboration and Advocacy and 5–Diversity and Inclusiveness (Community Health Nurses of Canada, 2009). In the US, appropriate public health standards would be Standard 1: Assessment; Standard 11: Communication; Standard 13: Collaboration; and Standard 15: Resource Utilization (American Nurses Association, 2013).
5. Observation at the clinics helped to orient the students to the layout and functioning of immunization clinics. In this situation, the students came to realize that the regular immunization clinics could be considered the preferred practice and deviations from that would be the risks to quality care that needed to be addressed in a pandemic.
6. The team checked for the use of processes in the immunization clinics and used the key informant process in collecting information from public health staff.
7. In Canada, Standard 7: Professional Responsibility and Accountability in the Canadian Community Health Nursing Standards covers most of the work of the team, since the standard includes appropriate terms such as "assesses and identifies risk management issues," "seeks help with problem-solving," "identifies and acts on factors which affect practice autonomy and delivery of quality care," and "appreciates and develops teamwork skills" (Community Health Nurses of Canada, 2011, pp. 22–23). Standard 2: Professional Relationships is also appropriate because it includes relevant items, such as "builds a network of relationships and partnerships" and "involves ... group ... as active partner ... to identify relevant needs, perspectives and expectations" (Community Health Nurses of Canada, 2011, p. 16). The most relevant Canadian public health nursing competencies are 2–Assessment and Evaluation

and 4–Partnerships, Collaboration and Advocacy (Community Health Nurses of Canada, 2009). In the US, appropriate choices from the public health nursing standards would be Standard 1: Assessment; Standard 10: Quality of Practice; and Standard 13: Collaboration (American Nurses Association, 2013).

8. The team used the key informant interview process defined in Chapter 4. They included many more key informants than is usual in a short-term group project.

9. The team sought out organizations that served and understood the needs of people who likely had low incomes and lower education levels, who spoke different languages and understood different cultures, and who had limited social and physical supports to ensure that their needs would be considered in planning services for emergency shelters.

10. In Canada, the relevant competencies are 4–Partnerships, Collaboration and Advocacy, because their work included items 4.1, 4.2, 4.4, and 4.5 dealing with advocacy for social change, team building, healthy public policies, and involving the community; and 5–Diversity and inclusiveness, because the work includes the three items in the competency: "recognize the determinants of health," "address population diversity," and "apply culturally-relevant and appropriate approaches" (Community Health Nurses of Canada, 2009, p. 7). Appropriate standards would be Standard 4: Professional Relationships and Standard 6: Access and Equity (Community Health Nurses of Canada, 2011). For the US, appropriate standards are Standard 5A: Coordination of Care; Standard 11: Communication; and Standard 13: Collaboration (American Nurses Association, 2013).

# Copyright Acknowledgements

# Index

Page references ending in *b* refer to boxes
Page references ending in *dq* refer to discussion questions
Page references ending in *f* refer to figures
Page references ending in *q* refer to chapter questions
Page references ending in *t* refer to tables
Page references ending in *s* refer to scenarios

care of sick and dying in the home, 260–263
  burden on families, 263
  statistical data, 261, 263
  types of service provided, 260
case finding in home health care, 262
  example of, rural and urban older adults, 277s
  during emergency, 262
  *See also* referral visits
case manager or care coordinator, 277
census data, 78–79
  *See also* community health assessment
circular questions, 271, 277*dq*7
  *See also* Calgary Family Assessment and
    Intervention Models
clinical experience, 173, 175
  source of evidence for practice 173, 175
CMIST (Communications, Medical needs, Independence,
  Supervision, and Transport), 406
coalition, 312–315
  benefits to organizations, 317*t*
  community capacity, (building) and, 313, 314
  community health nurse role and, 309–310, 318*dq*3,
    320, 322, 323*dq*5–7, 332–3*q*1–2, 333*dq*8
  ecological models of health promotion and, 313, 315
  evidence of health status change and, 316
  intersectoral collaboration and, 313
  leadership, 311*dq*2, 317–318, 318*dq*4, 321, 332*q*2
  project assessment, adapted for coalition, 312*t*
coalition formation, 316–333
  advance preparation, 316–318, 332*q*2
  action planning and implementation, 323–330,
    333*dq*9
  community analysis and PRECEDE-PROCEED,
    324–329, 326–329*b*, 327*t*, 328–329*f*
  developing organizational structures, 320–322,
    333*dq*8
  evaluation, 330–331, 332*b*, 333*q*3
  relationships, 319–322
  *See also* PRECEDE-PROCEED model of health
    promotion planning and evaluation
coalition sustainability, 321, 331
Cochrane databases, 175
cold chain, 376s
collaboration, 14–17
  benefits of: development of relevant resources; project
    sustainability, 203, 230*dq*2
  with community group, 53, 202
  family contracts or agreements, 280, 280*f*
  fundamental beliefs guiding community health
    nursing practice, 14, 17
  home care and, 277–281, 279*f*
  interprofessional, interdisciplinary, x, 11, 19, 40,
    318*dq*3, 319*t*, 322
  monitoring, 213
  within project team, 40, 53
  *See also* intersectoral collaboration
collaborative learning, 40, 53
collaborative partnerships, 291
collaborators, 149
  concluding relationship, 246–247
  decision making role in community health nursing
    project, 149
  potential to influence agency policy and program
    goals, 11
  *See also* community participation
commendations, 274
  *See also* Calgary Family Assessment and Intervention
    Models

Commission on Social Determinants of Health (CSDH),
  6, 9
communication types, 205*t*
  *See also* teamwork
communication channel, 204
  choosing, 204–206
  types, 205*t*
community
  defined by geography, common interests and
    social ties, 76
  as social setting or client, 75–77, 352
community-based intervention, 326*b*
community boundaries, 78–79
community capacity, 291, 313, 93*q*1–2
  community health, 8
  goal of community work or means to an end, 77
  measurable dimensions, 313–314
  potential to participate in health planning, 75–76
  *See also* capacity building; social capital
community capacity building and organization strategy
  *See* capacity building; health promotion strategies
community health, 291
  *See also* community capacity
community health assessment
  components, 77
    health status, patterns and variations, 79–82, 81*t*,
      82*t*, 89*dq*9, 89*t*
    health surveys and program statistics, 82–83
    policy documents and guidelines, 84–88, 327*t*
    sociodemographic profile, 78–79, 78*b*
    sources of routinely collected data, 81–82, 83*t*,
      87*dq*8
  conceptual framework guiding assessment, 76–77, 86
  determinants of health and, 80–83, 87*t*, 87*dq*7–8, 88*b*
  documentation and, 88–90
  process, iterative, collaborative, 74–75
  purpose, 74–76, 93
  required knowledge and skills for public health
    practitioner, 25
  sociodemographic profile, examples, 260–261,
    261–263, 296–7, 300–301, 304
  *See also* community health assessment methods;
    determinants of health; know your community;
    present and preferred health situation; primary
    and secondary data; theories, models, and
    conceptual frameworks (selected)
community health assessment methods, 100–130, 199*dq*1
  collecting data, 130
  community mapping, 104–106
  focus groups 123–125
  guided observation, 119–122
  key informant interviews, 107–113
  progressive inquiry, 116–119, 117*dq*10
  questionnaires, 125–129
  required skill for community health nurses, 159
  selecting methods, 129–130, 131*t*
  *See also* analysis of assessment data; community health
    assessment
community health nursing process, 16, 20–23, 23*b*,
  24*dq*9, 35
  community planning models, 20–22
  cyclical process in community program example, 23
  four phases, 3, 16, 404*dq*6
  individual nursing process and, 20–22, 24*dq*10, 27*q*2
community health nursing project, 35
  accountability framework, 53
  collaborative approach, 53, 56s

marketing, 210–211
components: product, price, place, promotion, 210
recruitment and, 211*b*, 212*dq7*, 220*q3*
marketing strategies, 185–186
"marshal resources," 18
*See also* accessibility to resources for health
(mass) health communication strategies, 171*b*
influenza campaign and, 376*s*
one-way communication, 204–205
policy change and, 351–358
social media use in disasters, 397, 407*s*, 409*q4*
types, 205*t*
*See also* health promotion strategies
mass immunization campaigns/clinics, 402, 404*s*
message, 206
checking for cultural appropriateness and plain
language, 201, 203, 207
flu shot, example, 206
message concepts, 206
message content, 207–208
Métis, 326, 402
*See also* Aboriginal people or communities
models and theories. *See* theories, models and conceptual
frameworks
morale, of teams, 43, 45, 47, 51, 61*t*, 90, 93, 158, 218
morbidity data, 73
mortality data, 73


*National Action Plan to Improve Health Literacy*, 201
needs of community or population as a whole, 15–16, 25,
69, 93, 351
approaches to address, 77, 82–83
focus of community assessment, 16, 58
*See also* community health assessment; population
health; "targeting with universalism"
nursing ethics, 19–20
*See also* ethical practice of community health nurses


objectives, 177–186
four questions to use in preparation of, 182
guidelines for preparing, 177, 182–186
SMART criteria and measurement 177, 182–183, 183*b*
types: impact, process, outcome 177–182, 180*f*
*See also* environmental objectives; impact objectives;
program evaluation
observational method, 382–383, 385*dq5*
*See also* guided observation
*Ottawa Charter for Health Promotion*, 163


pandemic, 402–403
continuing issues from SARS and H1N1, 403*b*
mass immunization in, 402
role of World Health Organization in, 402
public participation. *See* community participation
periods of community project teamwork, 55–61
finishing up, 60
getting organized, 55–58
getting things done, 59–60
pilot test, 208, 210
benefits, 209*dq5*
debriefing session, 209*s*
example, for back injury workshop, 209*s*
plain language, 226–227
*See also* health literacy
planning. *See* community health nursing process

planning for action, 165–182, 199*dq2*
health goal, 168–170
health promotion strategies, 170–172, 171*b*
impact objectives, 177–181
intervention, evidence–based, 165, 173–177
priority, 166–168
process objectives, 181–182
*See also* program logic model; program evaluation
policy, 341
example of municipal alcohol policy, 364–365
example of organizational breast feeding policy, 349*b1*
framework for health care, 16, 340
health agency policy assessment, 349*b*
measures to improve health, 345
parts of, 357–359
social justice assessment and, 10
*See also* health policy and healthy public policy
policy change
community health nursing role and, 341, 342*s*, 344*t*,
348*dq3*, 359
decision makers and, 355–356, 360*q1*
evaluation of health status change and, 357
force field analysis and, 353, 354*s*, 354*dq6-7*, 360*q4*
work plan example, 343*t*
policy change process, 342*s*, 347–359, 350*t*
develop action plan, 352–359
evaluate, 359, 366
identify problem, 350–351, 349*b*
implement action plan, 359
policy documents, 84–85, 87*s*
comparison of health agency policies, example, 349*b*
evaluation criteria for, 349*b*
municipal alcohol policy, example, 364–365, 360*q5*
organizational policy, breast feeding, example, 349*b*
population health framework, 85
reflect shift to population health approach, 84–85
source of local and national health goals and priorities,
85, 86
population, levels of intervention, 164*f*
community coalition, 163*s*, 310*s*
community, rural, northern, remote, 300–304,
302–303*s*
disaster and emergency preparation, for, 393*s*, 399*s*,
406*b*, 407*s*
family, 258–282
group, 165*b*, 179–180, 181*t*, 214, 215*t*
multiple, 164*f*, 170,
neighborhood, low income housing, 101*s*, 143*s*
region, 163*s*, 342*s*
sector and system, 206*b*
*See also* disaster and emergency preparation
population groups, by age and gender
adolescents and youth, 295–300, 310*s*, 326–329*b*
adult and older adult women, 206*b*, 342*s*
adults, 163*s*, 198–199*s*, 230*s*, 258*s*, 368*s*
mothers/parents of young children, 101*s*, 143*s*,
179–180, 181*t*, 261–262, 342*s*
older adults, 70*s*, 165*s*, 277*s*, 279*b*, 280*b*, 282–283*s*,
368*s*
school aged children, 15*b*, 177*b*, 280, 280*b*, 310*s*,
326–329*b*
population health, 10, 15, 17, 426
*Adelaide Statement on Health in All Policies* and, 84–85
low–intensity, community wide, and intensive
interventions, with sub–groups, 315
national and international framework and action
guidelines, 85
*See also* Population Health Promotion Model
(the Cube)

source of community health data, 82
public health programs
    mass immunization campaign, 368s, 393s, 404s
    relationship of programs and projects, 37–38
public participation. See community participation

qualitative data, 116
quantitative data, 116
questionnaires, 125–129
    combining with other assessment methods, 143dq2
    distributing questionnaires, 126–127
    ethical review and approval by organization, 123, 125
    example questionnaire with readability at grade 3, 128
    informed consent and, 126, 128s
    preparation and conduct of, 126, 147dq4
    pros and cons of method, 128dq15
    See also analysis of data; community assessment
        methods

readability, 127, 135q2
    questionnaires and, 127
    example questionnaire with Grade 3 readability, 128
    See also health literacy
recommendations, 231
    assessment report and, 155, 155t, 195
    policy change and, 244–245
    presentation and, 236
    project report and, 243–244
recovery phase in emergency management, 408
    role of community health nurses in, 408
recruitment. See marketing
referral, 260, 276
referred visit, 260, 262, 276
reflective process, 16, 50
    in self-assessment, 50, 354s
related-to clause, 152–153, 154dq10, 159q4
    determinants of health and, 153
reliability and validity, of data, 144
    of data sources, 83
resilience, 396
response phase in emergency management, 403–408
    care phase in, 405–408
    emergency shelter management and provision of care
        in, 405–408
    factors that put populations at risk during disasters,
        406b
    feelings and reactions to violent events, 405b
    rescue phase in, 403–405
    role of community health nurses in, 403–408
risk, 394
risk-based, emergency management, 394
rural, northern, remote communities, 300–304
    community health nursing practice in, 304
    food security in, 302–303s

school, school community, 295–300
    assessment in school capacity building, 298–299s
    community health nursing in, 297–300
secondary data. See primary and secondary data
secondary prevention. See levels of prevention
self-assessment, in teamwork, 50
self-selected groups, 43
    See also team
sense of accomplishment, 61–62

sense of community, 291
    associated with academic achievement and health in
        schools, 300
    components: membership, influence, integration and
        fulfillment, shared emotional connection, 292
service delivery outcomes, 374, 377s
service providers, 258
showing appreciation, 246
    contribution to project sustainability and community
        health, 246
    during presentation, 236
    methods of, 246b, 247dq8
skill development activities, 156, 172, 317
    teamwork, 50–51
    See also community health nursing process; health
        education strategies; impact objectives; objectives
SMART criteria, 183, 183b
    example of use, awareness of tobacco industry
        advertising, 183
social and environmental determinants of health.
        See determinants of health
social capital, 330
    See also community capacity, collaboration
social inequities, 6
    See also health equity and inequity
social justice, 10
    framework to support action on social determinants,
        10
    See also health equity and inequity
social media, 397
    in disasters, 397, 397b, 409q4
    in marketing, 208, 211b
social support, 211b
    incentive to recruit participants, 211b
sources of power: position, resources, expertise, personal
        qualities, 356
    See also policy change
stakeholders, 149
    involvement in team decision making, 149
standards and competencies. See community and public
        health nursing standards and competencies
strength and concern, 143
    See also analysis of assessment data; concern and
        strength; issue for action
surge capacity, 402
sustainability, of community health nursing relationships,
    17
    benefit of community participation, 12
    collaborative approaches and, 12, 17, 22
    community presentation as opportunity for, 239
    See also coalition sustainability

tailored intervention, 210–214
    community feedback, in, 206–210, 209dq5–6
    delivery arrangements, 210–212
    development of mammogram message, example, 206b
    Health Communication Program Cycle and, 203–210,
        220q4
    promotion of daily exercise in social media, example,
        208
    recruitment of audience for, 210–212
    training others to take over, 172, 211–212, 217s
    See also intervention; taking action